AF741467

PAIN AND TREATMENT

Edited by **Gabor B. Racz and Carl E. Noe**

Pain and Treatment
http://dx.doi.org/10.5772/57078
Edited by Gabor B. Racz and Carl E. Noe

Contributors

Sang Chul Lee, Young Jae Kim, Fuzhou Wang, Richard Rokyta, Jitka Fricova, Nidal Amin Jaradat, Igor Vasilievich Ukrainets, Elena Mospanova, Larisa Savchenkova, Victor Kuz'min, Anatoliy V. Lyahovsky, Olga V. Gorokhova, Lidiya A. Petrushova, Borja Mugabure Bujedo, Silvia Gonzalez Santos, Amaia Uria Azpiazu, Anxo Rubin Noriega, David Garcia Salazar, Manuel AZCONA ANDUEZA, Linda Le-Wendling, Julia Deloach, Allison Haller, Barys Ihnatsenka, Carl E. Noe, Gabor B Racz, Rajesh Munglani

Published by InTech

Janeza Trdine 9, 51000 Rijeka, Croatia

Copyright © 2015 InTech

Individual chapters are under their authors' copyright and distributed under the Creative Commons Attribution 3.0 license, which allows users to download, copy and build upon published chapters provided that the authors and publisher are properly credited, which ensures maximum dissemination and a wider impact of the authors' work. Any republication, referencing or personal use of the individual chapters or any of their contents must explicitly identify the original source.

Permission for commercial use of the book as a whole, such as (but not limited to) reprint rights, republication, distribution, sales, translation, and reproduction in any and all forms of media, must always be obtained from InTech.

Notice

Statements and opinions expressed in the chapters are these of the individual contributors and not necessarily those of the editors or publisher. No responsibility is accepted for the accuracy of information contained in the published chapters. The publisher assumes no responsibility for any damage or injury to persons or property arising out of the use of any materials, instructions, methods or ideas contained in the book.

Publishing Process Manager Iva Lipovic

Technical Editor InTech DTP team

Cover InTech Design team

First published February, 2015

Printed in Croatia

Additional hard copies can be obtained from orders@intechopen.com

Pain and Treatment, Edited by Gabor B. Racz and Carl E. Noe

p. cm.

ISBN 978-953-51-1629-5

We are IntechOpen, the world's leading publisher of Open Access books

Built by scientists, for scientists

4,000+
Open access books available

116,000+
International authors and editors

120M+
Downloads

151
Countries delivered to

Our authors are among the
Top 1%
most cited scientists

12.2%
Contributors from top 500 universities

CLARIVATE ANALYTICS BOOK CITATION INDEX INDEXED

WEB OF SCIENCE™

Selection of our books indexed in the Book Citation Index
in Web of Science™ Core Collection (BKCI)

Interested in publishing with us?
Contact book.department@intechopen.com

Numbers displayed above are based on latest data collected.
For more information visit www.intechopen.com

For EU product safety concerns:
IN TECH d.o.o., Prolaz Marije Krucifikse Kozulić 3, 51000 Rijeka, Croatia,
info@intechopen.com or visit our website at intechopen.com.

Meet the editors

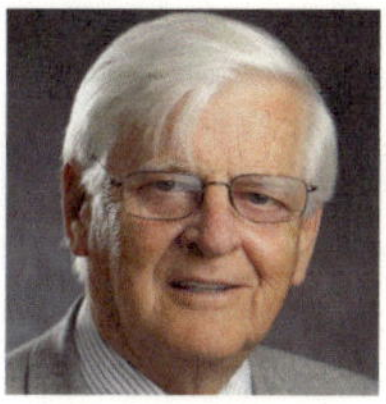

Dr. Gabor B. Racz is a Grover Murray professor and Chairman Emeritus of the Department of Anesthesiology at Texas Tech University Health Science Center in Lubbock Texas, USA. He is a founder of the International Pain Institute at Texas Tech, the World Institute of Pain, and the Texas Pain Society. He is an international leader in the field of pain. He has developed interventional pain management and multiple procedures including the lysis of adhesions that at times are called the Racz Procedure. Has received numerous prizes and awards.

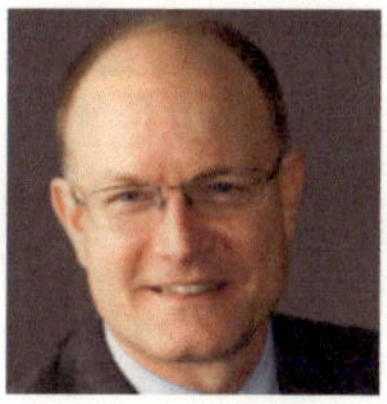

Carl E. Noe, M.D., is a Professor of Anesthesiology and Pain Management at the University of Texas Southwestern Medical Center in Dallas, Texas. He serves as the Director of the Eugene McDermott Center for Pain Management, Pain Division Director and Pain Fellowship Director. He is certified by the American Board of Medical Specialists in Anesthesiology, Critical Care Medicine and Pain Medicine.

Contents

Preface

This second volume of *Pain Management - Current Issues and Opinions,* namely *Pain and Treatment,* is a continuation of the first edition. Authors from multiple regions of the world have contributed chapters based on their experience and expertise. The topics range from the basic chemical science of potential new analgesic compounds to a new chapter on medicolegal issues in clinical pain management. The chapter on Epidural Lysis of Adhesions contains important new information from randomized controlled trials and safety considerations for the procedure. A comprehensive chapter on opioids addresses the evolution of thinking about opioid therapy for chronic pain.

The rapidity of publishing on-line with free downloading access allows readers worldwide to access the latest information about pain from different cultures with the goals of improving patient care and knowledge worldwide. The editors look forward to responses to the book from the global community in a spirit of a united team against the negative consequences of pain. We want to reach many people, and the evidence is clearly seen through the widespread interest in 115,243 downloads of all of the book chapters. There are 196 countries in the world and 159 of them have become aware of the usefulness of the information collected in the first edition of this book. Interested physicians and other readers found the collective hard work of contributors valuable. We are looking forward to an even greater impact from this new edition.

Our warmest wishes,

Professor Gabor B. Racz, MD, ABIPP, FIPP
Texas Tech University Health Sciences Center, Lubbock, Texas, USA

Professor Carl E. Noe, MD, FIPP
University of Texas Southwestern Medical Center, Dallas, Texas, USA

Chapter 1

Medico-legal Aspects of Pain Medicine

Gabor Racz, Carl Noe and Rajesh Munglani

Additional information is available at the end of the chapter

http://dx.doi.org/10.5772/58754

1. Introduction

Deviation from an acceptable standard of care is one of the central issues in a lawyer's mind in any malpractice lawsuit. However, the trigger for a lawsuit is the occurrence of a complication. That is, intense scrutiny of a doctor' practice usually only occurs once harm has occurred to a patient.

Thus avoiding complications is the maxim to follow. Understanding the situations in which complications leading to law suits may arise is most important.

Not all complications will lead to law suits depending on how they are handled and, for example non negligent complications and side-effects may be successfully defended if appropriately consented.

The trend towards more accreditation may reduce rare but serious complications. Many Boards (in the USA) and Faculty of Pain Medicine (in the UK) amongst others and international organizations such as World Institute of Pain (WIP) have introduced standards of training in an attempt to reduce complications rates.

If you are sued, remember no one is going to care more about the result than you do. Pick the best lawyer and experts to defend you.

2. Principles that may help avoid lawsuits

2.1. Physician attitude towards patients

There is evidence that avoiding distressed or angry patients are associated with better outcomes and fewer complaints and lower rates of litigation [1]. Always be respectful and

INTECH
open science | open minds

© 2015 The Author(s). Licensee InTech. This chapter is distributed under the terms of the Creative Commons Attribution License (http://creativecommons.org/licenses/by/3.0), which permits unrestricted use, distribution, and reproduction in any medium, provided the original work is properly cited.

pleasant with patients and communicate with them, this leads to lower rates of complaints and litigation. Patients are treated in private but you practice in public, in front of a jury of your peers [2-5].

2.2. Minimizing errors during conduct of interventional procedures

Steps to promote safety for interventional pain procedures include the "time out" where activity stops and the team of the patient, nurses and physicians verify the patient's identity, the diagnosis, the procedure, the side of the procedure (right or left), a valid consent form, allergies and other critical information before proceeding with the procedure. Labeling syringes and marking the site of the procedure is also helpful. Numerous deaths have occurred from erroneous labeling and administering the wrong drug.

Performing the correct procedure for a specific pain problem is more important than performing an alternative procedure first because it may be less expensive.

The practice of performing series of procedures and the use of algorithms of multiple procedures is non-specific and needs to be refined to be not only more cost effective but to reduce risk.

The use of physician extenders is a risk factor for medical-legal disputes in pain management. Physician standards of care are the standard that patients expect and the evolving practice of pain management does not lend itself well for delegation of decision making for opioid prescribing and procedure selection [6].

Monitoring the patient, having venous access and having equipment for anaphylactic reactions and other emergencies is advisable for procedures other than simple peripheral injections.

2.3. The increasing use of anticoagulation

Anticoagulation has become very common in the United States, as has daily aspirin therapy. The management of these medications before and after pain management procedures is problematic since existing data does not answer all questions. Discontinuing aspirin has been associated with stroke and myocardial infarction; however, new platelet function tests are markedly abnormal with one 325 mg tablet per day. Patients with mechanical valves or recent coronary stints or pulmonary emboli are not good candidates for discontinuing anticoagulation. Coordination with the anticoagulant managing physicians is important when these patients need procedures.

Discontinuing platelet inhibitors has more advocates than opponents but the risk of bleeding versus infarction is a subject that is well suited for a discussion with the patient's other physicians and with the patient.

3. Medical malpractice

Medical legal issues may arise in the form of a lawsuit, brought by a patient or their representative or from a hostile action from a licensing agency, a hospital privilege committee, a medical society, an insurance company or government health plan, a certifying board or other government agency or non-government party.

3.1. Four conditions constitute a malpractice claim

1. A duty must exit between a physician and the patient. In other words, a doctor –patient relationship must exist.
2. the duty must have been compromised by negligence.
3. the patient must have suffered damages.
4. the alleged negligence must be proven to have caused the damages.

3.1.1. Related to the above concepts is the burden of proof test

In order to bring a successful claim against you, the patient, or other person bringing the claim, has to prove on the balance of probabilities:

Breach of duty – that the treatment was such that no reasonable practitioner would have delivered that care

3.1.2. Causation and negligence

Causation – that the breach of duty or negligence caused or contributed to the injury, loss or damage suffered, and that the patient would not have suffered that injury without the breach Causation, or proof that damages resulted from negligence and were not coincidental, has a threshold of being more likely that not, other wise know as the 50.1% test

Both these tests have to be established to prove negligence [7].

Negligence, or a breech of duty, is a deviation from the standard of care. Standard care is the care provided by a reasonable and prudent physician of the same specialty and under the same circumstances, otherwise known as the Bolam test [8].

3.2. Effects of medical malpractice of healthcare delivery

Physicians claim that medical malpractice liability increases healthcare costs and limit access to care for which there is now increasing evidence [9]. There is some evidence that practicing "defensive medicine" probably worsen outcomes.for patients [10].

Advocates of the medical malpractice system argue that malpractice insurance premiums are a result of poor insurance company management. The Harvard Medical Practice Study in 1990 reposted that only a small fraction of patients with negligent injuries sued and that more suits were in order rather than less.

3.3. Tort and it's reform

A tort is a civil wrong that causes injury, exclusive of a breach of contract. Medical malpractice is a tort resulting from negligence, which is defined as conduct that falls below the standard established by law for the protection of others against unreasonable risk of harm. An intentional tort may arise when informed consent is not obtained.

Tort reform initiatives have proposed several ways to reduce the costs of malpractice awards. [11, 12]

Caps on noneconomic damages limit the amount of money that can be awarded for pain and suffering. Some jurisdictions have limits of $250,000. Economic damages cover medical expenses, lost wages and costs of re-education and/or rehabilitation.

Caps on punitive damages limit the amount of money awarded for conduct that is beyond negligence and includes fraud or evil. Advocates for caps have argued that evidence must be "clear and convincing" rather than "a preponderance" before punitive damages are awarded [13]. It has been argued that a portion of punitive damages go to a fund for a public purpose rather than to the plaintiff.

Abolishing joint and several liability would prevent each defendant from being liable for 100% of the damages. The principle of joint a several liability serves to assign liability equally to all defendants rather than allow defendants to divide responsibility based on their portion of conduct.

The collateral source rule allows plaintiffs to be compensated twice for the same injury. Abolishing this rule would result in an offset of damages based on other resources such as insurance payments and disability payments [14].

Contingency fee limits would require attorneys to be paid based on the amount of work they perform rather than a percentage of the awarded damages but in other jurisdictions such as the UK there are imperatives which state the costs in a case must be proportionate [15]

Statues of limitations require malpractice lawsuits to be filed within a time period from the injury. In the UK this is generally accepted to be 3 years in most circumstances [16]. If an injury is not discovered immediately or of the injured person is a child, the limitation is frequently expanded to allow a suit to be brought. A newborn baby is obviously unable to file a lawsuit but can when adulthood is reached. In the UK the statute of limitation only starts when the child reaches 18 [17] Medical records tend to degrade after years and memory is of limited help. These factors disadvantage the defense of a physician though the advent of electronic records may prove helpful in this respect.

4. The American society of anesthesiologists closed claims study

The ASA closed claim study has resulted in a number of reports regarding pain management and related liability. The number of claims against anesthesiologists for pain management doubled between 1985 and 1989. It doubled again between 1990 and 1994 [18]. Claims for postoperative pain management increased from 6% during the 1980's to 8% in 2000 [19].Claims from chronic pain management increased from 7% between 1985-1994 to 12% between 1995-2004. [20]

In a large report, the number of claims increased since the 1980's before pain management began to grow as a specialty. Deaths from epidural injections were associated with epidural injection of local anesthetic and opioid. Nerve damage and pneumothorax were reported to be most common causes of claims. Intra-thecal pump mishaps were also associated with deaths. [21]

44% of medication errors have been related to incorrect dosing, 30% are related to wrong drug administration, 10% are related to contraindicated drugs and 8% are related to incorrect timing of administration. [22]

Most medication claims are associated with medication misuse and both patient and physician conduct contribute to a high proportion of deaths.

Medication management claims were associated with men with back pain who were prescribed long acting opioids and also taking other psychoactive medications and had signs of medication misuse. [23]

Blocks accounted for 84% of claims during the 1990s. [24]

50% of nerve injury claims involved spinal cord injury. Pneumothorax from trigger point injections has been a common claim. [25]

Spinal cord injuries have been reported to be associated with cervical procedures in women under general anesthesia. [26]

22% of chronic pain claims are related to cervical procedures and the injuries are commonly permanent and disabling.

Brain damage and death were associated with epidural steroid injection only when used with local anesthetic or opioid [21].

Ultrasound guided nerve blocks have been associated with fewer claims [27].

Other factors have been reported as a part of the closed claim study.

Agreement among experts in malpractice cases has been shown to correlate poorly. (k 0.37] [28]

However, publishing and publicizing examples of questionable expert testimony has been discouraged for legal reasons. [29]

Malpractice insurance rates vary widely from $15,000 to $64,000 per year depending on the states' legal system and award amounts over time [30].

The recommended amount of malpractice insurance coverage varies but 1-3 million dollars per claim and 3-6 million dollars in aggregate have been proposed [31].

The closed claims study data is limited statistically because it reports the numerator but not a denominator, so trending is difficult to evaluate. However, it clearly serves a good purpose in identifying potential problems.

The closed claims study does not include information from non-anesthesiologists and pain management has become a multi-specialty field with a variety of specialists performing procedures oftentimes with little training.

In the State of Georgia, one malpractice insurance carrier no longer offers coverage for physiatrists who perform trigger point injections because of the high rate of pneumothorax. The use of a 25 or 30 gauge needle and fanning injections is associated with pneumothorax. Fanning injections with a small gauge needle tends to produce multiple punctures along the same track rather than injecting in multiple directions as intended with the fanning motion. The reason is that the small gauge needle lacks the stiffness necessary to overcome the "grip" of the muscle and has a "woodpecker effect" producing multiple punctures of the pleura. Using 22 gauge needles for trigger point injections or avoiding fanning, we have not seen this problem.

5. Some complications and their mechanisms

25 plus years of serving as an expert in 350-400 cases (GBR) as well taking into account the UK perspective (RM) has revealed some patterns of complications and likely mechanisms. Many cases settle and no record of the complication is made and valuable information is lost. The following section represents some of that information.

With increasing emphasis on treatment of pain, there has been recognition of recurring patterns of complications. Therefore once understanding reaches a broad base of practicing clinicians, a reduction of these serious but rare complications should be possible.

5.1. Pneumothroax

Pneumothorax is a complication for trigger point injections. Frequently the needle used was 25 G or smaller. These needles bend easily and when "fanning" injections are made, the needle tract is uncontrollable. A "woodpecker" effect can result with multiple holes in the pleura and a pneumothorax requiring a chest tube is a common trigger for a lawsuit. Medicare will no longer pay for treatment of a pneumothorax from a central line placement and similar reimbursement patterns may be forthcoming for pain related complications.

5.2. Injections near the cranium

This same mechanism can occur with other injections. For example, injecting a painful scalp scar after craniectomy for acoustic neuroma has resulted in local anesthetic being injected intracranially.

5.3. Cervical sympathethetic injections

Cervical nerve root injection occurs after cervical sympathetic (stellate ganglion) block using the classic technique. Needles directed to Chassignac's tubercle are directed to the vertebral artery and cervical nerve root. Local anesthetic injection may result in immediate seizures or paralysis but delayed complications may result from subdural blocks after patients have been discharged. Patients should be monitored for longer periods of time in an environment with full resuscitative personnel and equipment. A lesson learned from this is that the needle tip migrates into a nerve or artery where injection occurs. The new Bella D needle (Epimed, International) has a sealed tip and a side port for directional injection, and may reduce this occurrence.

5.4. Spinal transformainal injections and the erroneous concept of a "safe" area for injection

Deaths after transforaminal injections have occurred and the notion of a "safe" avascular area in the posterior foramen has been shown to be false. Local anesthetic injection or arterial injury can result in catastrophic spinal cord injury and/ or death. Huntoon has demonstrated arterial supply in each posterior cervical neuroforamina which effectively discredits the concept of a safe area [32]. The increasing number of cases of catastrophic neurological injury in the lumbar region following otherwise supposedly correct injection appropriate have also undermined the concept of this "safe" area and an alternative site; Kambins triangle has been alternatively proposed [33] [34].

Unfortunately catastrophic has occurred following injection of saline, contrast and steroid and is not prevented by digital subtraction angiography [35] The onset of neurological signs may be delayed and may be associated with the lack any obvious untoward effects at the time of a test dose of local anesthetic which was used to confirm epidural placement. The authors suggested Utilizing blunt needles or larger bevel needles in place of sharp, cutting needles may minimize the chances of this event occurring. Subdural injections may also be associated causes vasospasm and infarction.

5.5. The debate over sharp versus blunt needles

Sharp needles by their very design minimize the feedback produced as bodily structures are penetrated. This means there will be minimal awareness of vascular, neural and spinal cord structure with needle advancement. Such injections seem to be associated with more lawsuits. The dural can be more easily punctured and local anesthetic and corticosteroid preparations can be injected.

Despite the fact no randomized controlled data exist for sharp needle injection safety, serious concerns have been raised. Sharp needle movement after initial placement seems to be a factor as well. In response The Bella D needle has been designed in an attempt to reduce punctures and migration associated with small movements. The tip is blunt and a side port is located proximal to the tip. Blunt needles have been shown to be less likely to puncture nerves and arteries in animal studies [36]. Interscalene block complications have also been associated with sharp needles. Intra-cord injections, quadriplegia, Brown-Sequard and brachial plexopathy have been reported. The true incidence of major complications is unknown. Sweet reported one death and several hematomas in a series of 7000 foramen ovale procedures. This may be a similar complication rate for pain procedures

The RX-2 coude (Epimed International) epidural needle has a second stylet, which is blunt to convert the needle tip from sharp to blunt to reduce the incidence of a dural or venous laceration when rotating the needle in the epidural space. The second stylet is placed once the epidural space is reached but before any rotation. The blunt tip stylet projects 1mm beyond the tip of the needle and acts as a guard to the sharp edge of the needle.

The RX-2 coude needle is gaining wider acceptance for epidural needle and catheter placements as well as spinal cord stimulation electrode placements.

A lesson learned is that every case of spinal cord injury and death until has been associated with the use of sharp needles by direct trauma or the mechanism of arterial penetration and comprise of the arterial supply. Experimental studies suggest that blunt needles have not been associated with arterial wall penetration [36].

The available clinical information and animal data supporting the use of blunt needles only applies to blunt needles and cannot be extrapolated to pencil point tip needles. Pencil point tip needles are designed to penetrate the dura and have not been studied with regard to puncturing arteries and nerves.

The pencil tip needles have not been studied regarding perforation into nerves or arteries. The blunt needles have been shown not to perforate from 18 gauge to 25 gauge.

The disastrous vascular and neurological complication seen with stellate ganglion procedure should theoretically be avoidable using the Bella D needle. Most of these complications seem to be related to the classic C 6 approach to Chassaignac's tubercle. The teaching to make bony contact and then pull back 1mm is an inexact process and the needle tip and injection can be placed in an artery or nerve. Cases of immediate or delayed total spinal block, brain or spinal cord infarction have occurred. Using the Bella D needle placed at the lateral body of C7 may reduce the incidence of these complications.

Whilst some of the evidence does suggest blunt needles may be safer, the first cases of spinal cord injury the use of blunt needles are now being reported to be associated with vascular spread [37]

The curved, blunt RF (Racz-Finch) needle is being used increasingly in an attempt to avoid intraneural, intracord and intra-arterial placement especially with the use of particulate corticosteroids. Thus far, no cases involving these needles have surfaced.

The curved blunt needle must be used with an introducer but once it is placed, it can be used as a percutaneous navigation devise (PND) and directed around other structures to the target area.

This same concept is behind the Rx 2 coude and the 14-gauge spinal cord stimulation electrode epidural needle, which can be used to steer the electrode safer and in less time.

5.6. Particulate steroids

Patients with acute and chronic pain have received steroids in neuraxial blockade for many years. There has been recent controversy about their efficacy but also about the possibility of neurological complications associated with the use of particulate steroids such as methylprednisolone, triamcinolone and betamethasone. In contrast dexamethasone is a non-particulate steroid with less platelet aggregating properties [38].

Scanlon et al reported that in the USA between 1998 and 2003, the number of cervical and thoracic TF ESI almost doubled. They noted at the time of writing 27 cases of brain and spinal cord infarction following TF ESI and their survey revealed a further additional 78 cases following a survey of 1400 or so physicians despite a response rate of approximately only 21%. In no case was the use of non-particulate steroid dexamethasone associated with adverse neurological outcomes. Depomedrone, a particulate steroid was 7 times more likely to have been used in cases where there was evidence of brain and spinal cord infarction than either triamcinalone or betamethasone. No cases were reported with dexamthasone. However it could be argued this simply reflected a frequency of use rather than a propensity to cause problems.

In particular it was hypothesized inadvertent intra-arterial injections of particulate steroids is thought to lead to spinal cord ischaemia by blocking of small arterioles and secondary catastrophic neurological and other complications and indeed studies showed that methyl prednisolone and triamcinolone were more likely to aggregate than dexamethsone or betamethasone, sometimes up to 100um in diameter on microscopic slides which have the theoretical ability to block small arteries [39]. [40] [41] [42].

Use of contrast and aspiration is no guarantee that vascular uptake has not or will not take place. The overall incidence of intravascular uptake during lumbar spinal injection procedures as determined by contrast enhanced fluoroscopic observation is 8.5%. Preinjection aspiration failed to produce a flashback of blood in 74% of cases that proved to be intravascular upon injection of contrast dye [43] Despite this evidence, a survey in 2012 suggested a significant proportion of UK pain consultants continued to use particulate steroids for cervical injections and even greater proportion for lumbar root injections [44]. A clinical negligence barrister in the UK has commented the current position of UK pain consultants who continue to use particulate steroids is uncertain in terms of breach of duty if they haven't offered patients the probably safer option of non particulate steroids even if they continue not to accept the evidence as regards of particulate steroids. [45].

5.7. Unreliability of the ligamentum flavuum as a loss of resistance sign

Anatomical studies have shown the inconsistent presence of the ligamentum flavuum. Ligamentum flavum resistance is an unreliable sign in the cervical spine and the first resistance appreciated may be the dura or cord. [46] This means that intracord injection may easily occur with interlaminar epidural steroid injections with Tuohy spinal needles using "loss of resistance" techniques as the latter is an unreliable sign in these circumstances.

5.8. Spinal haematomas and peri venous counter spread

Subdural, subarachnoid or intra-cord needle placements followed by injections of contrast, local anesthetic or corticosteroid can produce spinal cord injury, paralysis and death.

The cervical venous plexus is predominantly lateral and ventral as opposed to the thoracic, which is predominantly posterior. Epidural hematomas are usually upper thoracic and lateral recess stenosis compounds the problem.

Lawsuits are rare when an epidural hematoma is diagnosed early and surgical decompression is carried out expeditiously [47]. A second opinion consult should be obtained if the first surgeon wishes to delay surgical treatment of an acute epidural hematoma though conservative management has been described [48]

Peri-venous counter spread (PVCS) has been reported and occurs when epidural injection leads to pressure building on one side which forces flow to the opposite side [49]. If fluid is unable to escape the spinal canal, pressure can compress the cord and produce quadriplegia. When recognized, the patient should flex and rotate the neck. Then causes the pars of the facet joints to slide over one another and enlarge the neural foramina. This provides an escape route for injected material and pressure release.

This procedure has become a standard of practice and is described in multiple publications. It should be used to spread cervical injectate and allow lateral run-off.

When pressure builds up, the patient will complain of ipsilateral pain possibly spreading bilaterally. Neck and arm pain precede chest pain and spinal cord ischemia. Numbness, weakness and paralysis can be prevented by repetitive exercises.

PVCS has been described as a mechanism for acute compression, which may be relieved by repetitive chin to shoulder flexion exercises. These movements increase the size of the cervical canal, allowing spread of injectate and pressure reduction. Thoracic catheter placement and advancement to the cervical level in the lateral epidural space may reduce the risk of compartmental injection by opening lateral run off. The practice of avoiding the lateral epidural space may predispose patients to loculation and syrinx formation.

We recommend caution or avoidance of epidural injections in patients with a syrinx, arnold chiari malformations and arachnoiditis. Paralysis and other severe neurological complications have been seen. [50, 51]. The only effective treatment for injecting the wrong contrast is irrigation of cerebrospinal fluid with saline. Injections in patients with arachnoiditis is hazardous because dissection can occur into the subdural space and loculation can occur leading to circulatory compromise to the spinal cord.

5.9. Sub-occipital injections

Sub-occipital injections have been associated with the "locked in phenomenon", brain stem infarction and death. Injectate can tract retrograde along the occipital nerve and dissect into the CNS.

Sub-occipital decompression has not been associated with the "lock in" phenomenon. 10 cases of complications with intraneural injection have occurred but not with the use of the Stealth (Epimed, International) 20-gauge 2" needle aimed just below and slightly posterior to C1. The "locked in" phenomenon, while rare, is an example of the importance of recognizing an emergency and being able to respond with resuscitative measures.

5.10. Arachnoiditis

It is still not clear what causes arachnoiditis, though epidural injection of modern drugs are unlikely to be associated with such a complication. In contrast intrathecal injection of steroids has been associated with histological changes in animal studies and also probably humans [52] [53]. Studies of epidural steroids and contrast suggest greater changes with the injection of contrast media. [54]. Therefore contrast injection should be limited to agents, which are safe for intrathecal use.

The cause of a recent report of urological problems and severe dense foot drop following a few days post blind caudal injections for contralateral radicular pain is uncertain but infection has been postulated for the arachnoiditis seen on imaging [55]. Recently, a 30 million dollar lawsuit was brought after a patient developed arachnoiditis after multiple wet taps during attempted spinal cord stimulator electrode placement. The allegation was that an epidural blood patch caused the arachnoiditis. The medical records weighed 97 pounds and the trial lasted 2 weeks but the defense prevailed. Nevertheless, it is not uncommon for the Tuohy type needle to enter the subdural space without the physician recognizing it. Cerbrospinal fluid may not appear during the procedure.

5.11. Radiofrequency of the medial branches

In principal radiofrequency of the medial branch seems to be an inherently safe procedure [56]. It is however important to warn patients about post operative soreness and inconsequential long term numbness due to lesioning of the lateral branch [57]. Such procedures may have poorer prognoses in those patients who appear to catastrophize and alternative treatment offered, certainly initially [58], though subsequently such procedures can be beneficial to the overall pain and psychological state [51, 59].

Radiofrequency procedure complications and medicolegal cases include instances where sharp needles enter nerves or arteries and where injection created pressure, which is transmitted to a distant structure. Additionally, thermocoagulation of unintended structures, such as the vagus nerve during a C2-3 facet denervation, can occur. Permanent losses of voice and hoarseness have been complications. The vagus nerve courses slightly anterior and lateral to the target [60]. For this reason, performing bilateral upper cervical facet denervations at the same sitting is not advisable. Patients should be brought back for the second side. In addition, weakness of cervical muscles can occur resulting in a permanent inability to raise the head. [61]

5.12. Complications of opioid therapy

The prescription of a strong opioids is a significant therapeutic which can be associated with poor outcomes including overdose and death. It is important that the rational for such a prescription is fully documented with informed consent [62].

Opioid rotation in the presence of benzodiazepines is associated with respiratory arrest. Outpatient spinal opioid trials are as well. Many patients receive psychiatric care in secrecy to avoid insurance premium increases. These patients may not disclose their complete medication list and may be taking centrally acting drugs without the knowledge of the pain physician. Urine drug testing may help to some degree but many drugs are not routinely tested. Opioid rotation, at least at high does, should not be done in one stroke [63] [64]. One opioid can be reduced while another one titrated.

Some centers now recommend benzodiazepine tapering before optimization/ rotation of opioid therapy especially in the elderly.

Methadone, while inexpensive, is falling out of favor due to deaths associated with its use for chronic pain [65]. Spinal opioid trials are best done as an inpatient [66] [67].

Many patients take herbal products and the pharmacologic effects of these products are unknown but should be documented as there is growing evidence that they may interact with more standard pharmaceutical agents.

6. Informed consent

Written informed consent should be obtained before any procedure to document education of the patient regarding risks of the procedure and to fulfill the legal requirement and avoid a charge of battery.

In Texas, new laws require specific language for informed consent for three types of pain procedures.

6.1. Neuroaxial procedures (injections into or around spine)

Failure to reduce pain or worsening of pain

Nerve damage including paralysis (inability to move)

Epidural hematoma (bleeding in or around spinal canal)

Infection

Seizure

Persistent leak of spinal fluid, which may require surgery

Breathing and/or heart problems including cardiac arrest (heart stops beating)

http://dx.doi.org/10.5772/58754

6.2. Peripheral and visceral nerve blocks and/or ablation

Failure to reduce pain or worsen pain

Bleeding

Nerve damage including paralysis (inability to move)

Infection

Damage to nearby organ or structure seizure

6.3. Implantation of pain control devices

Failure to reduce pain or worsening of pain

Nerve damage including paralysis (inability to move)

Epidural hematoma (bleeding in or around spinal cord)

Infection

Persistent leak of spinal fluid which may require surgery

6.4. Brief comments as regards serving as an expert witness

Before serving as an expert witness, one must feel comfortable holding themselves out as experts. Many fine physicians are not experts and the expert must have a curriculum vitae and enough experience to qualify as an expert in a court of law. Experts must limit their expert opinion to their area of expertise. Being an expert in one area does not qualify one to be an expert in a related by different area. Medical societies may expel members for testifying against other members if the testimony is unprofessional.

Second, before committing to serve as an expert, the records should be reviewed. No conflict of interest should exist between the expert and either party to a lawsuit. For example, one should avoid defending or testifying against a business partner or a business competitor. Testifying against another physician is a difficult task, as is, defending a doctor who has had a serious complication. Each side will have compelling arguments and the expert must be completely comfortable with the testimony they will give. While physicians are given considerable leeway to testify, the expert's reputation is at stake as much as the defendant's. The expert should make certain that the attorney, who calls them to testify, is aware of what the expert is willing to say and what the expert is not willing to say before any trial is scheduled. Experts must be willing to make themselves available once they have committed to a case. Court schedules change and delays are inevitable. Fees for serving as an expert should be in a similar range with what the physician would generate during the same time in practice, plus any expenses for travel, etc.

The medical legal aspects of pain management are unlikely to become less complex with time. Physicians need to increase their activity in specialty societies and political action committees in order to avoid the consequences of remaining silent.

7. Summary

This chapter has been but a brief introduction to how to reduce complications and by taking on board some of the messages in the chapter we hope you will not find a two or three period of your life being dominated by litigation with your professional and personal integrity being scrutinized in a harsh way.

Primum non nocere, or first do no harm is the maxim to follow. An awareness of the likely scenarios for complications, recognizing both patient, disease and technique related factors associated with such adverse outcomes and avoiding them can achieve a great deal in continuing to both enjoy ones clinical practice and get a good night's sleep.

We as the authors, intend to expand this chapter significantly in future years based on our experience of having to deal with many such cases in the medicolegal setting. We wish you well and invite you to share any cases with us that you might wish us to consider including in future years, to inform and educate us all.

A summary of some potential complications of injection and other therapies and how to avoid them

PROCEDURE	COMPLICATION	MECHANISM	POTENTIAL SOLUTION
Thoracic and cervical trigger point injection	Pneumothorax	25-30 g needle Fanning technique	22 g Avoid fanning
Transforaminal	Spinal cord or vertebral artery injection	Sharp needle intravascular or intraneral penetration	Use a blunt needle use
Single shot epidural steroid injection	Subdural injection	Dural laceration from sharp touhy or spinal needle	Use of blunt needle e.g RX 2 coude
Epidural needle palcement	Intracord injection	Initial loss of resistance is deep to epidural space due to inconsistant ligamentum flavum at cervical levels	Entry level at t 2 Catheter placement to cervical level :use contrast
Occipital block-	total spinal from injection in foramen magnum, intra-arterial injection and local anesthetic toxicity, occipital nerve injury, hematoma		Use of 20 gauge stealth needle and suboccipital decompression technique. Use of contrast and avoid large volumes

PROCEDURE	COMPLICATION	MECHANISM	POTENTIAL SOLUTION
Cervical transforaminal steroid injections	total spinal, vertebral artery injury, cerebellar hemorrhage, spinal cord infarct	Use of sharp needle	Use of blunt coude needle Avoid particulate steroid
Cervical interlaminar steroid injections	spinal cord injury, epidural hematoma, epidural abscess, loculation of injectate	Use of sharp needle	Use of blunt needle Rx 2 coude epidural needle
Cervical sympathetic block	total spinal, pneumothorax, horner's syndrome, recurrent laryngeal nerve block, brachial plexus block, intravascular injection and seizure, pneumochylothorax	Classic technique	Use of C7 lateral body technique blunt needle with Bella D needle
Atlanto occipital block	ataxia	Central local anesthetic effect	Minimize local anesthetic volume
Cervical 3 facet denervation	Hoarseness	Vagus nerve injury	Avoid bilateral procedure
Bilateral cervical injections	Respiratory arrest	Bilateral phrenic nerve blockade	Avoid bilateral procedure
Cervical facet injection	total spinal, spinal cord injury	Medial needle placement	Frequent use of Anterior posterior flouroscopic localization
Intercostal block	pneumothorax	Plural puncture with sharp needle	Use of flouroscopy and fixation of needle at skin puncture site
Lumbar sympathetic block	retroperitoneal hematoma, lymphatic injury	Vascular structure puncture	Use of blunt coude needle
Lumbar transforaminal injection	paraplegia	Segmental Arterial injection	Use of blunt coude and avoid deep foraminal placement Avoid particulate steroid
Lumbar sympathetic block Hypogastric plexus block	impotence, bladder dysfunction	Autonomic block	Avoid bilateral procedure

Author details

Gabor Racz[1], Carl Noe[2] and Rajesh Munglani[3]

1 Texas Tech University Health Science Center, Lubbock Texas, USA

2 University of Texas Southwestern Medical Center, Dallas Texas, USA

3 West Suffolk Hospital Cambridge University Hospitals Trust, Bury St Edmunds, UK

References

[1] NICE. CG88 Low back pain: Early management of persistent non-specific low back pain. NICE Clinical Guidelines: NICE; 2009.

[2] Rudol G, Rambani R, Saleem MS, Okafor B. Psychological Distress Screen as Predictor of Outcome of Epidural Injection in Chronic Lower Back Pain. Bone & Joint Journal Orthopaedic Proceedings Supplement. 2013;95(Supp 20):17-.

[3] Domino J, McGovern C, Chang KW, Carlozzi NE, Yang LJ. Lack of physician-patient communication as a key factor associated with malpractice litigation in neonatal brachial plexus palsy. J Neurosurg Pediatr. 2014;13(2):238-42.

[4] Hamasaki T, Takehara T, Hagihara A. Physicians' communication skills with patients and legal liability in decided medical malpractice litigation cases in Japan. BMC Fam Pract. 2008;9:43.

[5] Improving Communication, Cutting Risk: MPS New Zealand; 2012 [cited 20 1]. 10-1]. Available from: http://www.medicalprotection.org/newzealand/casebook-january-2012/improving-communication-cutting-risk.

[6] Jackson JZ. HW, ATC, Hahn, CK. Physician Assistants ; Liability and Regulatory Issues 2012. Available from: http://www.mdmc-law.com/tasks/sites/mdmc/assets/Image/MDAdvisor_FALL_12_ONLINE_FINALrev.pdf.

[7] MPS. Clinical negligence claims-what to expect. 2013.

[8] Bolam v Friern Hospital Management Committee. Wikipedia2014.

[9] Manner P, A. Practicing defensive medicine-Not good for patients or physicians. AAOS Now. 2007;Jan/Feb.

[10] DeKay ML, Asch DA. Is the defensive use of diagnostic tests good for patients, or bad? Med Decis Making. 1998;18(1):19-28.

[11] Cohen H. Medical Malpractice Liability Reform: Legal Issues and Fifty-State Survey of Caps on Punitive Damages and Noneconomic Damages. Received through the CRS Web: The Library of Congress, 2005 Contract No.: Order Code RL31692.

[12] Office CB. Medical Malpractice Tort Limits and Health Care Spending. Background Paper: The Congress of the United States; 2006.

[13] Shearer P. Punitive Damage Awards, Caps and Standards. 2007 Contract No.: 2003-R-0743.

[14] Association ATR. Collateral Source Rule Reform.

[15] Lord Neuberger of Abbotsbury MotR. Proportionate Costs. Fifteenth Lecture in the Implementation Programme; The Law Society2012.

[16] Limitation Act 1980. Wikipedia.

[17] Limitation Periods in the UK. Wikipedia.

[18] Kalauokalani D. Malpractice Claims for Nonoperative Pain Managment: A Growing Pain for Anesthesiologists? ASA Newsletter. 1999;63(6):16-8.

[19] Bird M. Acute Pain Management: A New Area of Liability for Anesthesiologist. ASA Newsletter. 2007;71(8).

[20] Liau D. Trends in Chronic Pain Management Malpractice Claims.. ASA Newsletter. 2007;71(8).

[21] Fitzgibbon DR, Posner KL, Domino KB, Caplan RA, Lee LA, Cheney FW, et al. Chronic pain management: American Society of Anesthesiologists Closed Claims Project. Anesthesiology. 2004;100(1):98-105.

[22] Sandnes D, Stephens L, Posner K, KB D. Liability Associated with Medication Errors in Anesthesia: Closed Claims Analysis. Anesthesiology. 2008;109(A770).

[23] Fitzgibbon DR, Rathmell JP, Michna E, Stephens LS, Posner KL, Domino KB. Malpractice claims associated with medication management for chronic pain. Anesthesiology. 2010;112(4):948-56.

[24] Fitzgibbon D. Liability Arising From Anesthesiology-Based Pain Management in the Nonoperative Setting. ASA Newsletter. 2001;65(6):12-5.

[25] Domino K, Fitzgibbon D. Clinical lessons in chronic pain management from the Closed Claims Project. ASA Newsletter. 2004;68(2):25-7.

[26] Rathmell JP, Michna E, Fitzgibbon DR, Stephens LS, Posner KL, Domino KB. Injury and liability associated with cervical procedures for chronic pain. Anesthesiology. 2011;114(4):918-26.

[27] Lee L, Posner K, Kent C, Domino K. Complications Associated With Peripheral Nerve Blocks: Lessons From the ASA Closed Claims Project. Int Anesthesiol Clin. 2011;49(3):56-67.

[28] Posner KL, Caplan RA, Cheney FW. Variation in expert opinion in medical malpractice review. Anesthesiology. 1996;85(5):1049-54.

[29] Caplan R, Posner R. The expert witness: Insights from the Closed Claims Project.. ASA Newsletter. 1997;61(6):9-10.

[30] Domino K. Availability and Cost of Professional Liability Insurance.. ASA Newsletter. 2004;68(6):5-6.

[31] Cheney F. How Much Professional Liability Coverage Is Enough? Lessons From the ASA Closed Claims Project.. ASA Newsletter. 1999;63(6):19,21.

[32] Huntoon MA, Martin DP. Paralysis after transforaminal epidural injection and previous spinal surgery. Reg Anesth Pain Med. 2004;29(5):494-5.

[33] Alturi S, Glaser SE, Shah RV, Sudarshan G. Needle position analysis in cases of paralysis from transforaminal epidurals: consider alternative approaches to traditional technique. Pain Physician. 2013;16(4):321-34.

[34] Glaser SE, Shah RV. Root cause analysis of paraplegia following transforaminal epidural steroid injections: the 'unsafe' triangle. Pain Physician. 2010;13(3):237-44.

[35] Chang Chien GC, Candido KD, Knezevic NN. Digital subtraction angiography does not reliably prevent paraplegia associated with lumbar transforaminal epidural steroid injection. Pain Physician. 2012;15(6):515-23.

[36] Heavner JE, Racz GB, Jenigiri B, Lehman T, Day MR. Sharp versus blunt needle: a comparative study of penetration of internal structures and bleeding in dogs. Pain Pract. 2003;3(3):226-31.

[37] Ilkhchoui Y, Koshkin E. A blunt needle (Epimed(®)) does not eliminate the risk of vascular penetration during transforaminal epidural injection. Surg Neurol Int. 2013;4(Suppl 5):S404-6.

[38] Scanlon GC, Moeller-Bertram T, Romanowsky SM, Wallace MS. Cervical transforaminal epidural steroid injections: more dangerous than we think? Spine (Phila Pa 1976). 2007;32(11):1249-56.

[39] Tiso RL, Cutler T, Catania JA, Whalen K. Adverse central nervous system sequelae after selective transforaminal block: the role of corticosteroids. Spine J. 2004;4(4): 468-74.

[40] Baker R, Dreyfuss P, Mercer S, Bogduk N. Cervical transforaminal injection of corticosteroids into a radicular artery: a possible mechanism for spinal cord injury. Pain. 2003;103(1-2):211-5.

[41] Derby R, Lee SH, Date ES, Lee JH, Lee CH. Size and aggregation of corticosteroids used for epidural injections. Pain Med. 2008;9(2):227-34.

[42] Lyders EM, Morris PP. A case of spinal cord infarction following lumbar transforaminal epidural steroid injection: MR imaging and angiographic findings. AJNR Am J Neuroradiol. 2009;30(9):1691-3.

[43] Sullivan WJ, Willick SE, Chira-Adisai W, Zuhosky J, Tyburski M, Dreyfuss P, et al. Incidence of intravascular uptake in lumbar spinal injection procedures. Spine (Phila Pa 1976). 2000;25(4):481-6.

[44] Tharakan L, Gupta S, Munglani R. Survey of current UK practice in use of fluoroscopy, contrast material and steroids in neuraxial injections Pain News. 2012:3.

[45] Nash A. Use of particulate steroids in neuraxial injections: a common but negligent practice? Pain News. 2012:2.

[46] Lirk P, Kolbitsch C, Putz G, Colvin J, Colvin HP, Lorenz I, et al. Cervical and high thoracic ligamentum flavum frequently fails to fuse in the midline. Anesthesiology. 2003;99(6):1387-90.

[47] Chien GC, McCormick Z, Araujo M, Candido KD. The Potential Contributing Effect of Ketorolac and Fluoxetine to a Spinal Epidural Hematoma following a Cervical Interlaminar Epidural Steroid Injection: A Case Report and Narrative Review. Pain Physician. 2014;17(3):E385-95.

[48] Makris A, Gkliatis E, Diakomi M, Karmaniolou I, Mela A. Delayed spinal epidural hematoma following spinal anesthesia, far from needle puncture site. Spinal Cord. 2014.

[49] Smith HS, Racz GB, Heavner JE. Peri-venous counter spread-be prepared. Pain Physician. 2010;13(1):1-6.

[50] Chiapparini L, Sghirlanzoni A, Pareyson D, Savoiardo M. Imaging and outcome in severe complications of lumbar epidural anaesthesia: report of 16 cases. Neuroradiology. 2000;42(8):564-71.

[51] Smith AD, Jull G, Schneider G, Frizzell B, Hooper RA, Sterling M. Cervical radiofrequency neurotomy reduces central hyperexcitability and improves neck movement in individuals with chronic whiplash. Pain Med. 2014;15(1):128-41.

[52] Lima RM, Navarro LH, Carness JM, Barros GA, Marques ME, Solanki D, et al. Clinical and histological effects of the intrathecal administration of methylprednisolone in dogs. Pain Physician. 2010;13(5):493-501.

[53] Latham JM, Fraser RD, Moore RJ, Blumbergs PC, Bogduk N. The pathologic effects of intrathecal betamethasone. Spine (Phila Pa 1976). 1997;22(14):1558-62.

[54] Kitsou MC, Kostopanagiotou G, Kalimeris K, Vlachodimitropoulos D, Soultanis K, Batistaki C, et al. Histopathological alterations after single epidural injection of ropi-

vacaine, methylprednizolone acetate, or contrast material in swine. Cardiovasc Intervent Radiol. 2011;34(6):1288-95.

[55] Nanjayan SK, Swamy GN, Yallappa S, Bommireddy R. Arachnoiditis following caudal epidural injections for the lumbo-sacral radicular pain. Asian Spine J. 2013;7(4): 355-8.

[56] Cheng J, Abdi S. COMPLICATIONS OF JOINT, TENDON, AND MUSCLE INJECTIONS. Tech Reg Anesth Pain Manag. 2007;11(3):141-7.

[57] Kornick C, Kramarich SS, Lamer TJ, Todd Sitzman B. Complications of lumbar facet radiofrequency denervation. Spine (Phila Pa 1976). 2004;29(12):1352-4.

[58] Smith AD, Jull G, Schneider G, Frizzell B, Hooper RA, Sterling M. A comparison of physical and psychological features of responders and non-responders to cervical facet blocks in chronic whiplash. BMC Musculoskelet Disord. 2013;14:313.

[59] Smith AD, Jull G, Schneider G, Frizzell B, Hooper RA, Dunne-Proctor R, et al. Cervical radiofrequency neurotomy reduces psychological features in individuals with chronic whiplash symptoms. Pain Physician. 2014;17(3):265-74.

[60] Chinosornvatana N, Woo P, Sivak M, Sung C-K. Iatrogenic Unilateral Vocal Fold Paralysis after Radiofrequency Lesioning for Cervical Facet Joint Denervation. The Laryngoscope. 2009;119(Supplement S1):S29.

[61] Stoker GE, Buchowski JM, Kelly MP. Dropped head syndrome after multilevel cervical radiofrequency ablation: a case report. J Spinal Disord Tech. 2013;26(8):444-8.

[62] Munglani R. Numbers needed to heal, numbers needed to harm, numbers needed to kill: reflections on opioid therapy and the primary duty of medicine. Pain News. 2013;11(1):5.

[63] Fine PG, Portenoy RK, Rotation AHEPoERaGfO. Establishing "best practices" for opioid rotation: conclusions of an expert panel. J Pain Symptom Manage. 2009;38(3): 418-25.

[64] Centre MGDNP. Practice Toolkit. Canadian Guideline for Safe and Effective Use of Opioids for Chronic Non-Cancer Pain. Michael G. DeGroote National Pain Centre: Michael G. DeGroote National Pain Centre.

[65] Prevention CfDCa. Prescription Painkiller Overdoses: Methadone 2014. Available from: http://www.cdc.gov/features/vitalsigns/methadoneoverdoses/.

[66] Rathmell JP, Miller MJ. Death after initiation of intrathecal drug therapy for chronic pain: assessing risk and designing prevention. Anesthesiology. 2009;111(4):706-8.

[67] Coffey RJ, Owens ML, Broste SK, Dubois MY, Ferrante FM, Schultz DM, et al. Mortality associated with implantation and management of intrathecal opioid drug infusion systems to treat noncancer pain. Anesthesiology. 2009;111(4):881-91.

Chapter 2

4-Hydroxyquinolin-2-ones and their Close Structural Analogues as a New Source of Highly Effective Pain-Killers

Igor V. Ukrainets, Olga V. Gorokhova,
Nidal Amin Jaradat, Lidiya A. Petrushova,
Elena V. Mospanova, Larisa V. Savchenkova,
Victor E. Kuz'min and Anatoliy V. Lyahovsky

Additional information is available at the end of the chapter

http://dx.doi.org/10.5772/57402

1. Introduction

Despite the most unflattering epithets and fear, pain was and still remains the normal response of any living organism on strong physical, chemical or mechanical stimuli. It has the most important protection function in nature – at just the right time pain immediately signals about appearance of exogenic or endogenic destructive effects on a certain organ [1-6], and it is simply necessary for the organism's survival as a biological unit. Unfortunately, it presents not only by disagreeable sensation. Being rather complex psychophysiological phenomenon pain (especially strong and continued) is often accompanied by very powerful emotional stresses [7-9], which can rapidly exhaust the body's adaptation resources and cause the serious disorders of its vital functions. Obviously it is for this reason that International Association for the Study of Pain considers pain as a global factor causing problems in modern society not only of medical, but also of socio-economic character [10-13].

Pains of various origin and pain syndromes occur so often as it is difficult to find a person among the world population that does not know this feeling. Hence it is not surprising that pain-killers are among the most popular and often used drugs. The drug arsenal of this pharmacological group that is available in modern medicine is exceedingly wide [14]. However, even under such conditions the appropriate pain relief is not always successful. The cause of it can be side effects and, as a consequence, numerous contraindications and restric-

INTECH
open science | open minds

© 2015 The Author(s). Licensee InTech. This chapter is distributed under the terms of the Creative Commons Attribution License (http://creativecommons.org/licenses/by/3.0), which permits unrestricted use, distribution, and reproduction in any medium, provided the original work is properly cited.

tions in using drugs [15]. That is why the vital task of pharmaceutical and medical chemistry is the search of new, highly effective and, most notably, safe pain-killers.

Quinoline as a basic structure of such investigations is of special interest. The precondition of it is the natural origin, practically unlimitted synthetic potential and, of course, the analgetic action, which is inherent to many of its derivatives. For example, quinine (**1**, Figure 1) – the main alkaloid of cinchona tree bark – does not only inhibit malaria parasites actively, but reveals nonspecific analgesic properties. It potentiates the action of narcotic and nonnarcotic analgesics, thanks to which it has been widely used in the composition of finished drug combinations for headache. Lysergic acid diethylamide (**2**, more known under abbreviation LSD) created semisynthetically as a vigorous psychodelic is currently prohibited to therapeutic use by the laws in most countries. Nevertheless, in spite of its illegal status, researchers continue to be interested in LSD because of its unique medicinal properties. In particular, it has been found that as an analgesic this substance acts more effectively and sustained than opiates in low doses that do not cause any psychologic effects. And as for inhibition of cluster headaches – a rare syndrome causing particularly intensive pain, it has no equal at all for the present [16].

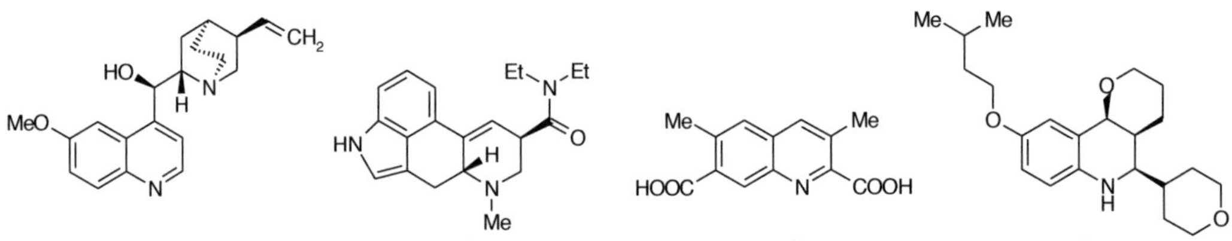

Figure 1. Natural (**1**), semisynthetic (**2**) and synthetic (**3** and **4**) quinoline analgesics

Natural resources are limited and not always reproducible. Besides, isolation of biologically active substances from the plant or animal raw material, their subsequent purification and standardization is, as a rule, difficult and time-consuming. That is why it is quite natural that the search of new analgesics of the quinoline Internet resources reveals a lot of publications concerning the given topics [17-23]. Thus, promising substances are created based on various derivatives both quinoline (**3**) itself and its hydrogenized analogs (**4**).

2. Synthesis and analgesic activity of 1-allyl-4-hydroxy-6,7-dimethoxy-2-oxo-1,2-dihydroquinoline-3-carboxylic acid *N*-R-amides

Until recently 4-hydroxyquinolin-2-ones have not even mentioned as analgesics in scientific literature. Only some years ago the situation turned over when based on preliminary virtual screening we obtained hydrochlorides of [(alkylamino)alkyl]amides of 1-allyl-4-hydroxy-6,7-dimethoxy-2-oxo-1,2-dihydroquinoline-3-carboxylic acid as potential opioid receptor antagonists [24]. Further pharmacological research has confirmed the presence of "calculated" biological properties of the compounds synthesized. At the same time it has been noted that some substances do not block the pain-killing action of narcotic analgesics, but vice versa, prolong it greatly. It is this obsevation that has become the first step for conducting extensive studies in purposeful research of substances with a new type of the pharmacological effect on a living organism for this class of compounds, i.e. potential pain-killers, in the range of 4-hydroxyquinolin-2-ones derivatives.

The beginning of this big and complex work was the synthesis of 1-allyl-4-hydroxy-6,7-dimethoxy-2-oxo-1,2-dihydroquinoline-3-carboxylic acid alkyl-, hydroxyalkyl-, *cyclo*-alkyl-, arylalkyl- and hetarylalkylamides (**6**, Figure 2) carried out by the reaction of methyl 1-allyl-4-hydroxy-6,7-dimethoxy-2-oxo-1,2-dihydroquinoline-3-carboxylate (**5**) with the corresponding primary amines in boiling methanol [25, 26].

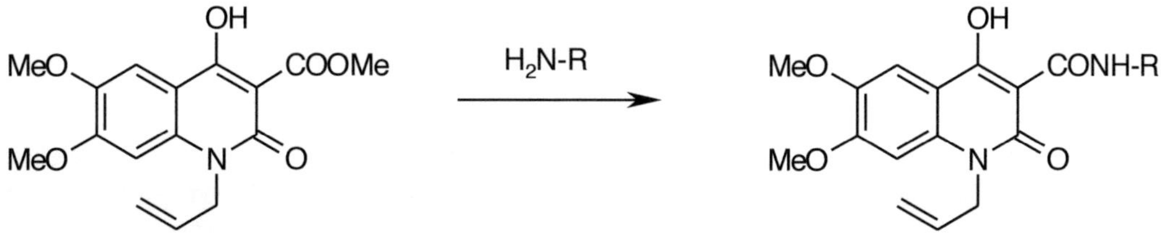

5 **6**

Figure 2. Synthesis of 1-allyl-6,7-dimethoxy-4-hydroxy-2-oxo-1,2-dihydroquinoline-3-carboxamides (**6**)

The screening test of analgesic properties of 1-*N*-allylsubstituted amides **6** convinced us in correctness of the chosen direction – each and all compounds revealed the analgesic effect to a greater or lesser degree in oral introduction to white rats in the dose of 0.00005 Mol/kg (on the average it is approximately 20 mg/kg) [25, 26]. While carrying out the biological experiments the animals were treated in accordance with the European Convention for Protection of Vertebrate Animals used for Experimental and Other Scientific Purposes. Of 50 samples studied with the general formula **6** approximately half of them do not yield Diclofenac in activity, and three of them (**6**, R = -$(CH_2)_2OH$, -$CH_2C_6H_4$-Cl-4 or furfuryl) even exceed one of the most powerful nonnarcotic analgesics Ketorolac. In the experiments of the given series the standard model of rectal mucosa irritation by electric current was used. Therefore, the central component influencing on the nociceptive system is present in the mechanism of the analgesic action of amides **6**. One regularity that can be interesting for future research has come to our attention. It is clearly traceable in all groups of compounds with the same aromatic ring in the arylalkylamide fragment, e.g., benzyl- → 2-phenylethyl- → 3-phenylpropylamide; 4-chlorobenzyl- → 2-(4-chlorophenyl)ethylamide, etc. It appeared that the farther the aromatic substituent from the amide nitrogen atom is, the less are the analgesic properties of the corresponding 1-allyl-4-hydroxy-6,7-dimethoxy-2-oxo-1,2-dihydroquinoline-3-carboxylic acid arylalkylamides.

3. Chemical modification of 1-allyl-4-hydroxy-6,7-dimethoxy-2-oxo-1,2-dihydroquinoline-3-carboxamides

After revealing a new biological activity in compounds of any chemical class usually the complex of works directed to improvement of their pharmacological and(or) pharmaceutical properties follows. This methodology being generally recognized and traditional for medical chemistry consists in gradual introduction of various structural modifications into a basic molecule allowing to have changes in its characteristics in the right direction. We tried to implement such approach in practice in our further research; by its result the theoretically important regularities of the "structure – activity" relationship at least can be determined. And if one is fortunate (the element of chance is always present in such works), it is realistic to reveal the promising lead compounds with a practical significance concerning the solution of the problem dealt with.

3.1. Halocyclization in 2-bromomethyl-7,8-dimethoxy-5-oxo-1,2-dihydro-5*H*-oxazolo[3,2-*a*]quinoline-4-carboxamides

The ability of 1-*N*-allylsubstituted 4-hydroxyquinolin-2-ones to cyclize readily in oxazoloquinolines [27] while interacting with the molecular bromine in acetic acid was used by us for transformation of amides **6** described above into their tricyclic derivatives **7** (Figure 3). This interesting reaction occurs instantly and quantitatively, but its direction is insensitive to the structure of substituents and it always primarily occurs as bromocyclization [28, 29]. Nevertheless it should be remembered that carrying out such reactions requires the strict observance of the equimolar ratio of reagents. It is clear that the lack of bromine will lead to partial transformation of allyl derivatives **6** into oxazoloquinolines **7**. However, the excess of bromine is also inadmissible since in this case formation of complexes of di(2-bromomethyl-5-hydroxy-7,8-dimethoxy-4-R-carbamoyl-1,2-dihydrooxazolo[3,2-*a*]quinolinium) ditribromides with bromine [25] or (if there is structural background for it) bromination of the molecule's amide fragment are possible [26].

According to the data of the biological research transfer from bicyclic 1-allyl-4-hydroxy-6,7-dimethoxy-2-oxo-1,2-dihydroquinoline-3-carboxamides **6** to their tricyclic oxazoloquinoline derivatives **7** as such does not have a significant effect on analgesic properties and, therefore, it is not likely to be considered practical. Nevertheless, rather high reactivity of 2-bromomethyl oxazol fragment of these compounds in relation to various nucleophiles allows conducting more profound transformation into 2-aminomethyl- (**8**) or 2-methylene- (**9**) oxazoloquinolines that have not studied yet pharmacologically and even into 1-acetonyl derivatives (**10**) [27]. Taking into account immensely wide synthetic possibilities the probability of success in future studies concerning these directions remains at the very high level.

3.2. 1-*N*-Allyl group removal

The next variant of the chemical modification of 1-allyl-4-hydroxy-6,7-dimethoxy-2-oxo-1,2-dihydroquinoline-3-carboxamides (**6**) was obvious and simple removal of 1-*N*-allyl

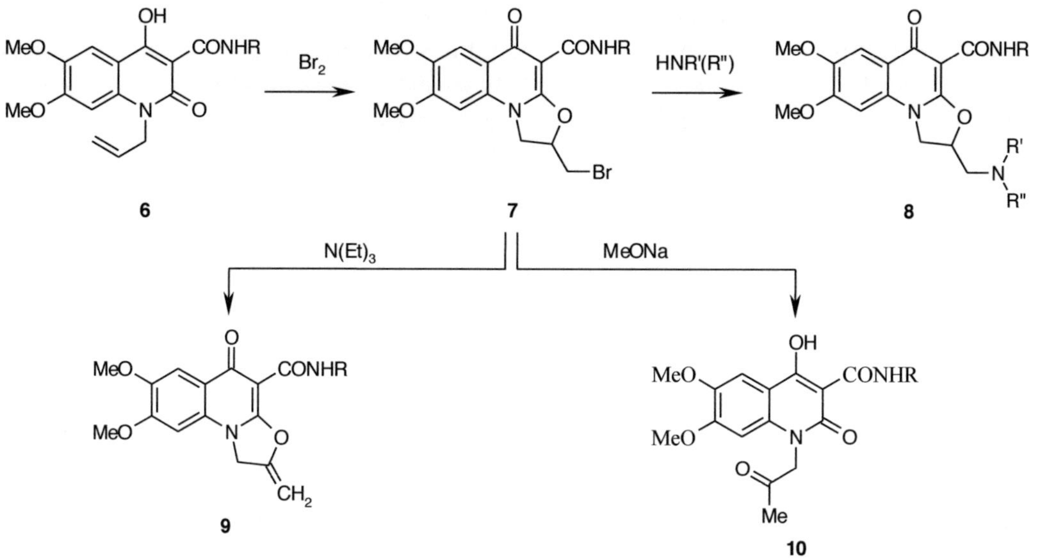

Figure 3. Synthesis and chemical transformations of 2-bromomethyloxazolo[3,2-*a*]quinoline-4-carboxamides (**7**)

substituent from the basic molecule. More specifically, obtaining of the target products only externally looks like removal of 1-*N*-allyl fragment. In reality the first stage of alkylation for initial methyl 4,5-dimethoxyanthranilate is simply excluded from the synthetic scheme of amides **6** obtaining [30].

Lower esters of 4-hydroxy-2-oxo-1,2-dihydroquinoline-3-carboxylic acids have a high reactivity [31-34]; due to it their transformation into various *N*-R-amides usually causes no complications. That is why problems arosen in amidation of dimethoxy substituted ester **11** by primary alkylamines appeared to be unexpected to a great extent. For example, after the synthesis in boiling DMF used because of the low solubility of ester **11** in other organic solvents, along with target alkylamides **12** formation of a noticeable amount of 4-hydroxy-6,7-dimethoxy-1*H*-quinoline-2-one was observed (**13**). The cause of appearance of this admixture proved to be water present in the reaction mixture; its effect could be eliminated by amidation at the temperature of about 80 °C. As a result a great number of target alkyl-, hydroxyalkyl-, *cyclo*-alkyl- and arylalkylamides of 4-hydroxy-6,7-dimethoxy-2-oxo-1,2-dihydroquinoline-3-carboxylic acid (**12**, Figure 4) have been obtained with high yields and purity [35, 36]. Anilides and hetarylamides **12** do not form in these conditions. The more rigid conditions are necessary for their synthesis such as the temperature of approximately 120 °C and quite little amount of DMF (1-2 ml per 0.01 mol) [37, 38]. It is of interest that in a greater volume of the solvent amidation of alkyl 4-hydroxy-2-oxo-1,2-dihydroquinoline-3-carboxylates by anilines and hetarylamines takes place incredibly slow.

The analgesic activity of seventy 4-hydroxy-6,7-dimethoxy-2-oxo-1,2-dihydroquinoline-3-carboxamides in empty position 1 with the general formula **12** has been studied in white mice. In the experiments the classical model of "acetic acid induced writhing" [39] allowing to estimate the peripheral component of the pain relieving effect of the tested samples has been used. We immediately note that simplification of the structure of the objects under research initiated by us did not affect their biology cardinally – in this set of experiments there were no examples of complete or substantial loss of analgesic properties.

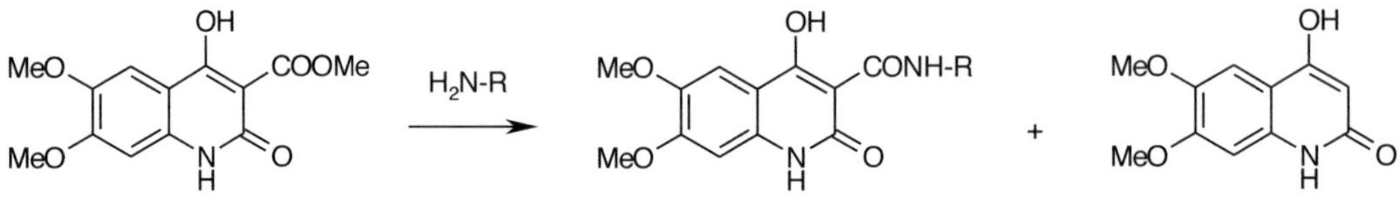

11 12 13

Figure 4. Synthesis of 4-hydroxy-6,7-dimethoxy-2-oxo-1,2-dihydroquinoline-3-carboxamides (**12**)

Most alkylamides **12** demonstrate a moderate and statistically significant ($p \leq 0.05$) analgesic effect comparable with Piroxicam at the same dose (20 mg/kg, orally) [35]. Hydroxyl or alkoxyl groups at the terminal carbon atom of amide fragments only decrease the activity. And transfer from alkylamides with the normal structure to their cyclic analogs is not so unambiguous. For example, in the case of propyl derivatives the transformation mentioned is accompanied with almost complete loss of analgesic properties. However, with prolongation of alkyl chains the effect changes to the opposite one – *cyclo*-pentyl - and *cyclo*-hexylamides **12** are more active than their acyclic analogs. Of all the group of alkyl-, hydroxyalkyl- and *cyclo*-alkylamides only propylamide (**12**, R = Pr) is worthy. It has demonstrated the better results on the "acetic acid induced writhing" model than Piroxicam, and even than more effective drugs Nabumetone and Diclofenac.

Arylalkylamides **12** are of much greater interest. Many of them do not yield, and some of them even exceed generally accepted analgesics used in tests by their analgesic action in much lower doses [36]. Thus, the structural biological regularity found while studying 1-*N*-allylsubstituted amides **6** has been confirmed once more, namely, with introduction of the aryl ring into the alkylamide fragment the activity increases, but with its moving from the nitrogen amide atom it gradually decreases.

Involvement of new classes of compounds, in particular anilides (**12**, R = Ph or substituted Ar) [38], in the range of the objects under research has supplemented this regularity with one more observation that is important for future investigations – the total absence of any methylene bridge between nitrogen amide atom and aryl substituent reflects negatively on analgesic properties.

In the group of hetarylamides only pyridine derivatives (**12**, R = Py or 2-Py-Me) [37] synthesized as structurally related carbonyl analogs of Piroxicam have been studied. The biological testing of these compounds has shown that the majority of them are approximately equal to Piroxicam by the level of their analgesic activity. In the range of isomeric unsubstituted pyridylamides a distinct dependence of their analgesic action on the position of the nitrogen atom in the pyridine fragment: $3 < 4 < 2$ is observed. In the next group of isomers – monomethyl substituted pyridyl-2 amides – there are somewhat different regularities: although C-methylation of the pyridine ring promotes intensification of analgesic properties, however, in general, the effect appears to be insignificant and, furthermore, with low sensitivity to the methyl group position.

Hetarylalkylamides of 4-hydroxy-6,7-dimethoxy-2-oxo-1,2-dihydroquinoline-3-carboxylic acid (**12**, R = picolyl-2, 3 or 4; furfuryl or tetrahydrofurfuryl) should be particularly mentioned. The bioisosteric replacements methodology [40-43] used in medical chemistry fruitfully and for a long period of time was the theoretical background for the synthesis of these compounds. In classic case implementation of this approach is replacement of an atom or a group of atoms with another ones having approximately the same size, shape and similar electronic configuration [44]. It is expected that after such modification a substance will possess the biological effect, which is close to the initial structure, and, probably, the more expressed one [45]. Based on these particular considerations we substituted the phenyl ring in the most active compound studied – *N*-benzyl-4-hydroxy-6,7-dimethoxy-2-oxo-1,2-dihydroquinoline-3-carboxamide (**12**, R = CH_2Ph) – by pyridinic or furan nuclei being isosteric to it. According to the results of pharmacological studies transfer to tetrahydrofuran and especially furan derivatives has been recognized as unsuccessful as it led to the marked loss of the analgesic activity. But Ph → Py replacement appeared to be really bioisosteric. Moreover, in this case the strength of the effect is determined by the position of a heteroatom in the pyridinic cycle: 4-Py ≤ Ph = 2-Py < 3-Py. A significant enhancement of analgesic properties of *N*-(3-pyridylmethyl)-4-hydroxy-6,7-dimethoxy-2-oxo-1,2-dihydroquinoline-3-carboxamide (**12**, R = CH_2Py-3) was a solid argument for choosing it as a lead compound at the given stage of our research.

3.3. Modification of the benzene moiety of quinolone ring

The next fragment of our research is devoted to making modifications into benzene and (or) other moieties of the quinolone ring only exclusively by the lead compound (Figure 5).

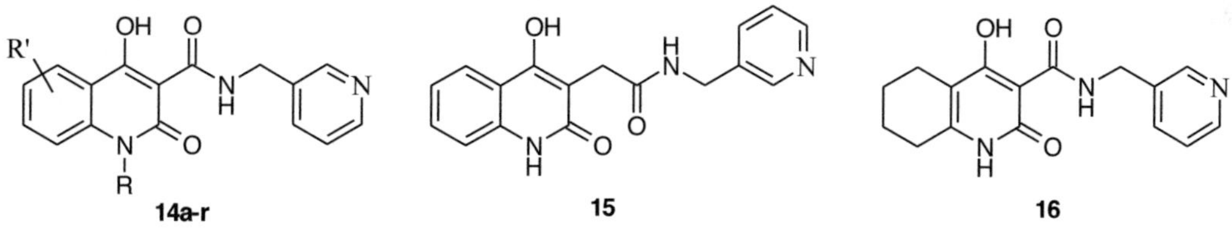

14a-r **15** **16**

Figure 5. Structural analogs of the lead compound modified in benzene and other moieties of the quinolone ring

Pharmacological testing of this group of substances (Table 1) has demonstrated that on the model of "acetic acid induced writhing" with oral administration in the dose of 20 mg/kg they all are highly active analgesics, which do not yield or exceed the known drugs taken in the doses that correspond to their ED_{50} [46]. Therefore, there is every reason to believe that generally substituents in the quinolone ring affect weakly the analgesic properties of 4-hydroxy-2-oxo-1,2-dihydroquinoline-3-carboxamides. Nevertheless, *N*-(3-pyridylmethyl)-4-hydroxy-6,7-dimethoxy-2-oxo-1,2-dihydroquinoline-3-carboxamide has still retained its leading positions. In particular, it has been found that removal of one methoxy group from its molecule (amides **14a,b**), as well as 1-*N*-ethylation (amide **14j**) result in some decline of analgesic properties. Halogens in the benzene moiety of the molecule (amides **14c-i**) cause the similar effect; therefore, their presence should be also admitted as undesirable. The exception is only 6-bromine derivative **14g** appeared to be even somewhat more active than the lead compound. But in the whole, increase of the activity is quite negligible (see Table 1). In addition, in this case it is necessary to consider the possible increase of toxicity due to the presence of a halogen atom in the molecule.

Compound	R	R'	Analgesic activity (decrease in the amount of "acetic acid writhing", %)	Compound	R	R'	Analgesic activity (decrease in the amount of "acetic acid writhing", %)
14a	H	6-OMe	64.3	**14k**	H	H	70.6
14b	H	7-OMe	60.2	**14l**	Me	H	61.4
14c	H	6-F	51.2	**14m**	Et	H	50.2
14d	H	6,7-F_2	48.6	**14n**	All	H	75.9
14e	H	6-Cl	54.6	**14o**	Pr	H	74.3
14f	H	7-Cl	67.9	**14p**	Bu	H	63.1
14g	H	6-Br	78.3	**14q**	*i*-Bu	H	59.0
14h	H	6,8-Br_2	54.2	**14r**	Am	H	57.8
14i	H	6-I	69.7	**15**	–	–	45.0
14j	Et	6,7-$(OMe)_2$	63.4	**16**	–	–	80.7
Lead compound (20 mg/kg)			75.3	**Metamizole sodium** (55 mg/kg)			35.1
Piroxicam (20 mg/kg)			34.5	**Diclofenac** (5 mg/kg)			51.6
Piroxicam (92 mg/kg)			50.0	**Nabumetone** (50 mg/kg)			50.7

Table 1. The analgesic properties of picolyl-3-amides **14-16** on the the "acetic acid induced writhing" model ($p \leq 0.05$)

Cheap and more available synthetically picolyl-3-amides without substituents in the benzene moiety of the molecule (**14**, R' = H), especially 1-*N*-allyl (**14n**) and 1-*N*-propyl (**14o**) derivatives, demonstrated excellent indices. However, separation of 3-carboxamide and quinolone fragments by the methylene bridge, i.e. transfer to *N*-(3-pyridylmethyl)-2-(4-hydroxy-2-oxo-1,2-dihydro-3-quinolinyl)acetamide (**15**), influences on the analgesic activity negatively. According to the results of the primary screening it should be recognised that the most successful chemical modification of the lead compound is removal of both methoxy groups with the simultaneous reduction of the benzene moiety of the quinolone ring – *N*-(3-pyridylmethyl)-4-hydroxy-2-oxo-1,2,5,6,7,8-hexahydroquinoline-3-carboxamide (**16**) appeared to be the most powerful analgesic of the given group. Unfortunately, after thorough analysis of all the pros and cons we had to refuse the further study of some highly reactive compounds for various reasons. Amides **14k-r**, for instance, were published earlier as objects for searching antituberculous drugs [47]. Therefore, their proper patent protection as analgesics is already impossible in principle. In case of hexahydroderivative **16** we faced another problems that were more serious.

3.4. Polymorphism of *N*-(3-pyridylmethyl)-4-hydroxy-2-oxo-1,2,5,6,7,8-hexahydroquinoline-3-carboxamide

A high analgesic activity of *N*-(3-pyridylmethyl)-4-hydroxy-2-oxo-1,2,5,6,7,8-hexahydroquinoline-3-carboxamide (**16**) found during the primary pharmacological screening caused, of course, an intense interest in it as a potentially new lead compound. However, the second sample of amide **16** sent to the biological laboratory unexpectedly demonstrated the result approximately two times lower than the first one. And they both were the products of the same synthesis! Multiple repeated experiment under the similar conditions for both samples simultaneously confirmed finally the significant differences in their analgesic properties. At first there were even doubts that we dealt namely with amide **16** in both cases. But NMR spectroscopy and combined gas chromatography mass-spectrometry assuaged these doubts rapidly and confirmed the absolute identity of the first and second samples.

Amide **16** is insoluble in water and it was introduced orally to the experimental animals as a fine aqueous suspension stabilized by Tween-80. Since the tested substance entered the organism as a solid, then the crystalline structure became one of the most probable factors influencing considerably on its biological properties [48]. The tendency of many substances to form various crystalline modifications (polymorphism) has attracted the attention of scientists for a long time. In particular, drug polymorphism is capable to change their characteristics so cardinally that currently all serious pharmaceutical manufacturers can not ignore this problem. And the government regulatory authorities also pay attention to the issues of obtaining, determination, description, purity and properties of crystalline forms of products used in pharmacy. As a result – today registration of a new drug in many countries of the world has become impossible without such information. It should, however, be recognised that although polymorphism has turned into an individual science, but it still remains an unsolved phenomenon of nature to a large extent. Until the present researchers only state the fact of formation of one or another polymorphic modifications of a substance. For the present one fails to predict theoretically or calculate this process and, particularly, predetermine conditions providing formation only the necessary polymorph.

Taking into account the given data we consider expedient to conduct the study of the phase composition of highly and lower active samples of *N*-(3-pyridylmethyl)-4-hydroxy-2-oxo-1,2,5,6,7,8-hexahydroquinoline-3-carboxamide (**16**) by the methods of X-ray powder and single-crystal X-ray structural analysis. Tailing of most peaks on the X-ray powder diffraction patterns complicated their analysis greatly and allowed to state with certainty only the fact that each sample consisted of several phases in various ratios. A thorough microscopic analysis led to similar results, but at the same separate shiny triclinic crystals suitable for conducting the single-crystal X-ray structural research were observed in the total powder mass of the active sample (Figure 6).

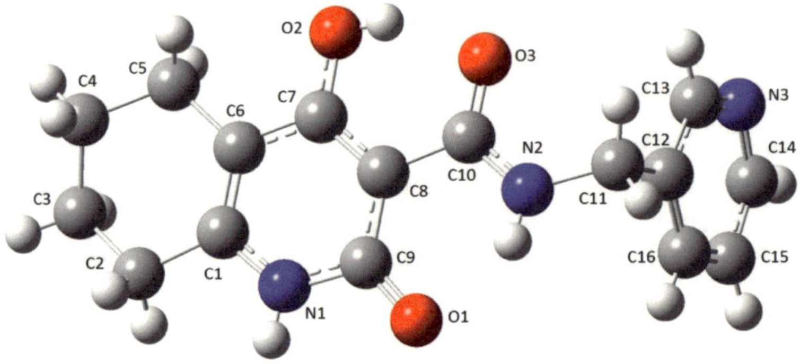

Figure 6. The structure of 1,2,5,6,7,8-hexahydroquinoline-3-carboxamide **16** molecule with numbering of the atoms

In the independent part of the elementary cell of this crystalline phase of amide **16** two molecules – **A** and **B** differing in some geometric parameter were found. The cyclohexone fragment in each of these both molecules is disordered by two *half-chair* conformations – **A1** and **A2**, **B1** and **B2** (folding parameters [49]: $S = 0.69$, $\Theta = 35.4°$, $\Psi = 29.9°$ in **A1**; $S = 0.81$, $\Theta = 34.3°$, $\Psi = 29.7°$ in **A2**; $S = 0.87$, $\Theta = 32.3°$, $\Psi = 25.1°$ in **B1**; $S = 0.57$, $\Theta = 39.4°$, $\Psi = 28.4°$ in **B2**). Deviation of atoms $C_{(3)}$ and $C_{(4)}$ from the mean-square plane of the rest atoms of the cycle is -0.34 and 0.34 Å in **A1**, 0.40 and -0.40 Å in **A2**, 0.50 and -0.35 Å in **B1** and -0.28 and 0.28 Å in **B2**, respectively. The carbamide fragment of the substituent at atom $C_{(8)}$ is in the plane of the quinolone cycle [the torsional angle is $C_{(7)}$–$C_{(8)}$–$C_{(10)}$–$O_{(3)}$ is -0.3(8)° in **A** and -4.3(8)° in **B**]; it is promoted by formation of intramolecular hydrogen bonds: $O_{(2)}$–H…$O_{(3)}$: (H…O 1.77 Å, O–H…O 149° in **A**, H…O 1.75 Å, O–H…O 150° in **B**) and $N_{(2)}$–H…$O_{(1)}$: (H…O 2.02 Å, N–H…O 135° in **A**, H…O 2.00 Å, N–H…O 135° in **B**). Formation of the given hydrogen bonds leads to electron density redistribution in this fragment of the molecule: bonds of $O_{(1)}$–$C_{(9)}$, $O_{(3)}$–$C_{(10)}$ and $C_{(7)}$–$C_{(8)}$ are extended, and bonds of $O_{(2)}$–$C_{(7)}$ and $C_{(8)}$–$C_{(9)}$ are shortened comparing to their mean values. 3-Picolyl substituent is in the antiperiplanar position in relation to $C_{(8)}$–$C_{(10)}$ bond [the torsional angle is $C_{(11)}$–$N_{(2)}$–$C_{(10)}$–$C_{(8)}$ is 173.4(5)° in **A** and 169.6(5)° in **B**], and its aromatic cycle is in *–sc*-conformation in relation to $C_{(10)}$–$N_{(2)}$ bond and noticeably turn to $N_{(2)}$–$C_{(11)}$ bond [torsional angles are $C_{(10)}$–$N_{(2)}$–$C_{(11)}$–$C_{(12)}$ are -83.7(6)° in **A** and -78.2(7)° in **B**; $N_{(2)}$–$C_{(11)}$–$C_{(12)}$–$C_{(16)}$ -68.6(7)° in **A** and -69.7(7)° in **B**]. In the crystal of molecule **A** and **B** owing to several intramolecular hydrogen bonds of C–H…π stacking-dimers **A-A** and **B-B** are formed by the "head-to-tail" type (the distance between π-systems is 3.8 Å).

In the low active sample of amide **16** such crystalline phase has not found and it is probably the cause of decrease of its biological activity. This conclusion is not final, of course, since any polymorphic modification of amide **16** in the pure form has not been obtained and studied (as, for example, it was successful in the case of 6-hydroxy-*N*-(4-methoxyphenyl)-4-oxo-1,2-dihydro-4*H*-pyrrolo[3,2,1-*ij*]quinoline-5-carboxamide [50] passing clinical trials as a new quinolone diuretic). The external factors caused the changes of the phase composition of the second sample are not clear yet. Nevertheless, based on the available data it is definitely arguable that *N*-(3-pyridylmethyl)-4-hydroxy-2-oxo-1,2,5,6,7,8-hexahydroquinoline-3-carboxamide (**16**) highly prone to polymorphism. And what's the main – it is not likely reasonable its further study as a potential pain-killer until at least the conditions, which would allow obtaining polymorphic modifications of this substance that are entirely highly active in regard to pharmacology and, not least importantly, with the guarantee of their stability while storing, are found.

4. Structure, physicochemical and analgesic properties of 4-R-2-oxo-1,2-dihydroquinoline-3-carboxylic acids

Even skimming of the scientific literature devoted to 4-hydroxyquinoline-2-ones reveals an extremely wide spectrum of biological properties that are common to these compounds. At the same time in the range of derivatives of 4-hydroxy-2-oxo-1,2-dihydroquinoline-3-carboxylic acids the overwhelming majority of publications is devoted to *N*-R-amides and products of their further chemical transformations. Esters are investigated much more rarely and the data concerning acids are practically absent at all. Meanwhile, being the basis of many *N*-R-amides possessing a high analgesic activity, 4-hydroxy-2-oxo-1,2-dihydroquinoline-3-carboxylic acids themselves also are of a certain interest as possible pain-killers.

4.1. 4-Hydroxy-2-oxo-1,2-dihydroquinoline-3-carboxylic acids and their close analogues

There are few methods for obtaining 4-hydroxy-2-oxo-1,2-dihydroquinoline-3-carboxylic acids known at present; moreover, all of them are similar and based on transformation of the corresponding esters [51]. It is our opinion that the most successful of them is hydrolysis in the AcOH–HCl–H_2O system, which allows to obtain target products with good yields and purity, as well as to avoid decarboxylation. It is this method that has been used in the synthesis of 4-OH-derivatives **17-19** (Figure 7, Table 2). Acids **20a,b** unsubstituted in position 4, their 4-chloro- (**20c**) and methyl (**20g-j**) derivatives are much more stable to decarboxylation and can be obtained by the common alkaline hydrolysis of lower alkyl esters of the corresponding quinoline-3-carboxylic acids. Only in the case of 4-alkyl- and 4-arylamino derivatives (**20e,f**) another synthetic scheme was used – interaction of alkylamines or anilines with 2-oxo-4-chloro-1,2-dihydroquinoline-3-carboxylic acids [51]

The ionization constants of the compounds synthesized determined by potentiometric titration show that they all are relatively weak acids. At the same time their dissociation constants (p*K*a) by the carboxy group consistently correlate with the influence of substituents present in the quinolone ring (Table 2). Of special note are 4-amino derivatives: 4-amono group (acid **20d**) possessing electron-donor properties decreases acidity of COOH-group so greatly that it

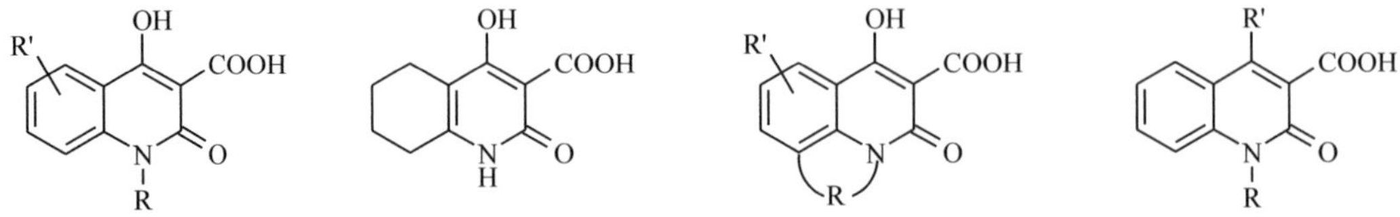

17a-o 18 19a-c 20a-j

Figure 7. 2-Oxo-1,2-dihydroquinoline-3-carboxylic acids

could not be determined by potentiometric titration (the measurement rang is p*K*a ~ 14). The benzyl substituent in 4-amino group (acid **20e**) does not change the situation, and only aryl fragments (for example, 4-chlorophenyl in acid **20f**) promote some enhancement of acid dissociation of carboxyl. By comparison it is notable that many known drugs of nonnarcotic analgesics group (for example, Diclofenac or Ketorolac, Table 2) are so strong acids, from the chemical standpoint, that even being as salts they exert the ulcerogenic action and, therefore, have a lot of contraindications [52].

The study of the analgesic activity of acids **17-20** has been carried out by the method used when testing 1-*N*-allylsubstituted amides **6** described above. Thus, the experimental data obtained testify that in an hour after introduction of the tested compounds the pain threshold increases in all experimental animals by 7.2-77.3% comparing to the initial level (Table 2). In other words, in spite of significant differences in the potency of the effect exerted all acids **17-20** without any exception reveal analgesic properties. Thus, if the first representative of 4-hydroxy derivatives group – acid **17a** – does not yield Diclofenac in its activity, then introduction of N-alkyl, benzyl or phenyl substituents (acids **17b-g**) leads to the marked decrease of the analgesic action. At the same time carbamoylethyl derivative **17h** exceeds all the reference drugs used, including the narcotic analgesic Tramadol, by its analgesic effect.

In most cases modification of the benzene moiety of 4-hydroxy-2-oxo-1,2-dihydroquinoline ring (acids **17i-o, 18, 19**) negatively reflects on biological properties. Nevertheless, highly active compounds have been also found in this range. For example, 6-bromo-4-hydroxy-2-oxo-1,2-dihydroquinoline-3-carboxylic acid (**17l**) appeared to be a more powerful pain-killer than Tramadol. It is interesting that 6-bromo derivative appeared to be also the most active in the case of picolyl-3-amides **14** (see Table 1). However, additional bromine atom in position 8 (acid **17m**) almost completely deprives the molecule of analgesic properties. 4-Hydroxy-2-oxo-1,2,5,6,7,8-hexahydro- and 1-allyl-4-methyl-2-oxo-1,2-dihydroquinoline-3-carboxylic acids (**18** and **20i**, respectively) exceeding nonnarcotic analgesics Diclofenac and Ketorolac by specific activity and yielding Tramadol a little are also worthy.

However, of all 4-R-2-oxo-1,2-dihydroquinoline-3-carboxylic acids **17-20** considered we think 4-benzylamino derivative **20e** attracts the most interest. With its high analgesic activity this compound is surprisingly a very weak acid. That is why unlike Diclofenac and Ketorolac there should not be any serious gastrointestinal disorders with its possible medical application (at least in such pronounced form).

http://dx.doi.org/10.5772/57402

Compound	R	R'	pKa^{COOH}	Analgesic activity (increase of the pain threshold, %)
17a	H	H	7.16	34.1
17b	Me	H	7.49	28.6
17c	Et	H	7.53	13.9
17d	All	H	7.30	14.4
17e	Pr	H	7.61	7.8
17f	Bn	H	7.15	17.2
17g	Ph	H	6.91	17.0
17h	$CH_2CH_2CONH_2$	H	7.06	77.3
17i	H	6-F	6.87	10.4
17j	H	6-Cl	6.76	7.2
17k	H	7-Cl	Insoluble	13.8
17l	H	6-Br	6.69	69.1
17m	H	6,8-Br_2	5.69	8.7
17n	H	6-I	6.63	34.6
17o	H	6,7-$(OMe)_2$	7.68	10.4
18	–	–	8.25	54.9
19a	$(CH_2)_2$	H	7.20	17.1
19b	$(CH_2)_3$	H	7.61	8.7
19c	$(CH_2)_2CH(Me)$	9-F	7.32	15.9
20a	H	H	8.74	30.5
20b	Pr	H	8.99	21.2
20c	Et	Cl	6.29	8.7
20d	H	NH_2	> 14	52.4
20e	H	NH-Bn	> 14	75.4
20f	H	NH-C_6H_4-Cl(4)	10.48	19.6
20g	H	Me	7.15	36.7
20h	Et	Me	7.10	33.4
20i	All	Me	6.95	51.5
20j	Pr	Me	7.17	15.6
	Diclofenac (10 mg/kg)		4.15	34.1
	Ketorolac (10 mg/kg)		3.49	46.4
	Tramadol (25 mg/kg)		-	57.2

Table 2. Acidic and analgesic properties of 2-oxo-1,2-dihydroquinoline-3-carboxylic acids **17-20**

4.2. 4-*N*-R-Substituted 2-oxo-1,2-dihydroquinoline-3-carboxylic acids and functional derivatives thereof

Naturally the combination of characteristics of 4-benzylamino-2-oxo-1,2-dihydroquinoline-3-carboxylic acid (**20e**) that are important for a possible future drug have not gone unnoticed. This compound is of a real interest as an intermediate leading structure in the search of potential pain-killers with improved properties. With the purpose of revealing the structural fragments affecting the most actively manifestation of analgesic properties the synthesis of series of the closest analogs of this compound and their pharmacological screening have been carried out.

The first representative of modified derivatives was 4-benzylaminoquinoline-2-one (**21**, Figure 8) obtained readily by decarboxylation of the parent structure **20e** or by the reaction of 4-chloro-2-oxo-1,2-dihydroquinoline-3-carboxylic acid with benzylamine in high-boiling solvents [53]. As it turned out, removal of the carboxy group from the molecule results in substantial reduction of the analgesic activity – at the same time the ability to increase the pain threshold three times decreases comparing to the initial acid **20e** (see Table 3). Esterification of the carboxy group (ethyl ester **22a**), 1-*N*-ethylation of the quinolone ring (acid **23**), as well as esterification with the simultaneous 1-*N*-alkylation (1-*N*-propylsubstituted ester **22b**) lead to the similar consequences. The result obtained is a convincing proof of the essential role of the carboxy group in exhibiting the biological effect, first of all. Introduction of 1-N-alkyl substituents, as judged by the examples described, is undesirable; though in general their impact is not so definite and it can be the subject of further study in principle.

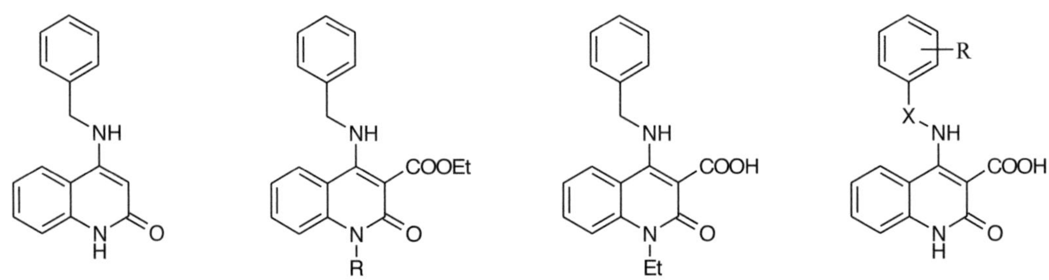

21 **22a,b** **23** **24a-p**

Figure 8. Modified analogs of 4-benzylamino-2-oxo-1,2-dihydroquinoline-3-carboxylic acid (**20e**)

Taking into account the abovementioned facts all our further efforts concerning the chemical modification of 4-benzylamino-2-oxo-1,2-dihydroquinoline-3-carboxylic acid (**20e**) were directed to make changes entirely to the benzyl moiety of its molecule. The synthesis of 4-N-R-substituted quinoline-3-carboxylic acids **24a-p** was carried out according to the scheme of the same type by interaction of the corresponding primary amines with 4-chloro-2-oxo-1,2-dihydroquinoline-3-carboxylic acid in boiling ethanol (i.e. under conditions intentionally excluding the possibility of decarboxylation).

The chemical modification of the benzyl moiety of acid **20e** conducted can be conditionally divided into three separate directions. The first two deal with separately the methylene unit or phenyl ring, respectively, the third involves both groupings simultaneously. The pharmacological testing has demonstrated that removal of the methylene bridge separating the secondary amino group and the aromatic ring (4-N-phenylsubstituted acid **24a**) is equal to decarboxylation described above by its effect on the analgesic properties, i.e. it also results in about three times decrease of the activity (Table 3). The replacement of the methylene unit by ethylene and, especially, propylene chains should be also considered unsuccessful. If with trasfer to 2-phenylethyl derivative **24b** the analgesic effect though twice decreases, but still remains at the level of Diclofenac, then in the case of 3-phenylpropylsubstituted acid **24c** it is practically lost at all.

Methylation of the methylene unit of acid **20e** has brought the unexpected results. As a result of such transformation one asymmetrical carbon atom appears in the molecule, hence, the final product can be racemic mixture **24d** or one of the enantiomers with *S*- or *R*-configuration of the chiral center (**24e** or **24f**, respectively). In the synthesis of these compounds racemic and optically pure 1-phenylethylamines are used; that is why the structure of aminoquinolines **24d-f** obtained on their basis is without any doubt. Depending on the spatial structure of the biological target and a number of other factors optical antipodes can exert both the same pharmacological properties and the properties varying so widely. Thus, preservation of the activity by a racemate usually observed in practice at the same level in the first case and its essential decrease or even its complete loss in the second case are quite logical. In this connection a rather high analgesic activity of racemic 1-phenylethylsubstituted quinoline-3-carboxylic acid **24d** on the background of optically pure enantiomers **24e** and **24f** that are absolutely inert in biological respect appears to be somewhat unexpected. The test substances introduced to the experimental animals as aqueous suspensions are insoluble in water and that is why it is not improbable that the cause of the effect found is in differences of crystalline forms. But the final conclusion on this point can be made only after special additional research.

The second direction of the chemical modification of lead compound **20e** is represented by 4-benzylamino-2-oxo-1,2-dihydroquinoline-3-carboxylic acids **24g-n** containing substituents in the aromatic ring of the benzyl fragment. Unfortunately, in all the examples considered a stable tendency to decrease analgesic properties is observed irrespective to the nature of the substituents introduced and their position in the ring (Table 3).

And finally, the third way of modification of 4-N-benzyl substituent of acid **20e** intending introduction of changes into the methylene unit and the aromatic ring simultaneously is presented only by two compounds – optically active 4-[1-(4-methoxyphenyl)-ethylamino]-2-oxo-1,2-dihydroquinoline-3-carboxylic acids **24o** and **24p**. Here, the influence of the spatial configuration of asymmetric carbon on the strength of the analgesic effect is clearly visible: *S*-enantiomer **24o** is noticeably more active than its *R*-antipode **24p**. It is also interesting to note the fact that the methyl group introduced separately into the methylene unit (acid **24e**) or 4-methoxy introduced into the aromatic ring (acid **24l**) lead to the complete loss of the analgesic properties by basic structure **20e**. However, the effect of the same substituents introduced

Compound	R	X	Analgesic activity (increase of the pain threshold, %)
21	–	–	24.8
22a	H	–	18.0
22b	Pr	–	28.8
23	–	–	7.6
24a	H	none	26.0
24b	H	$(CH_2)_2$	35.2
24c	H	$(CH_2)_3$	7.5
24d	H	(±) CH(Me)	40.1
24e	H	*S*(+) CH(Me)	2.2
24f	H	*R*(–) CH(Me)	2.0
24g	4-F	CH_2	35.0
24h	2-Cl	CH_2	42.7
24i	4-Cl	CH_2	18.1
24j	4-Me	CH_2	20.5
24k	2-OMe	CH_2	5.8
24l	4-OMe	CH_2	11.9
24m	3,4-$(OMe)_2$	CH_2	28.3
24n	3-O-CH_2-O-4	CH_2	32.2
24o	4-OMe	*S*(+) CH(Me)	46.1
24p	4-OMe	*R*(–) CH(Me)	31.6

Table 3. Analgesic properties of 4-amino-2-oxo-1,2-dihydroquinolines **21-24** on the model of rectal mucosa irritation by electric current ($p \leq 0.05$)

simultaneously is not any more categorical. In particular, the activity of acid **24o** remains unchanged at the level of one of the most powerful nonnarcotic analgesics Ketorolac.

Thus, according to the results of the research performed the conclusion can be made that in the structure of 4-benzylamino-2-oxo-1,2-dihydroquinoline-3-carboxylic acids the carboxy group plays a key role in the process of binding with receptors beyond any doubt. The benzyl group is one more important structural fragment providing a large interaction with a biological target. At the same time the role of 1-*N*-alkyl substituents is not so simple and requires more profound study. The significance of the benzene moiety of the quinolone ring, as well as the secondary amino group in position 4 remains completely unclear.

4.3. The crystalline structure of 2-oxo-4-(1-phenylethylamino)-1,2-dihydroquinoline-3-carboxylic acids as the factor that their analgesic activity

When studying biological properties of substances containing asymmetric carbon various situations are possible such as: enantiomers show the same clinical picture [54]; only one isomer stipulates the desirable effect, whereas the second one is low active or inactive at all [55]; enantiomers reveal quite different (sometimes directly opposite) physiological properties [56]; one of the isomers is unambiguously harmful [57]. It is clear that only in the first case drugs prepared on the basis of optically active compounds can be racemic mixtures. In all other situations it is expedient to use one of the enantiomers. However, it should be remembered that actually sometimes even under the most favorable pharmacological indications in favor of one of the optical isomers a drug racemate enters the market after all since obtaining the required optically pure enantiomer presents various difficulties [58].

One more varient of manifestation of biological properties by chiral compounds is theoretically possible, and it can occur in practice (although quite rarely), when a racemate appears to be much more active than enantiomers [59]. Frequently this phenomenon is explained by synergy of effects that are inherent to each of the optical isomers individually (see, for example, a detailed study of the mechanism of the analgesic action of Tramadol [60]). We came up against a similar situation while investigating 2-oxo-4-(1-phenylethylamino)-1,2-dihydroquinoline-3-carboxylic acids **24d-f**. However, there are some differences, which can not be explained only by synergy – racemate **24d** (**R**) appeared to reveal the marked analgesic activity on the background of enantiomers **24e,f** (**E**) being practically inert in the biological respect. We tried to find out the cause of this effect in this section.

Acids **24d-f** are insoluble in water and introduced orally as aqueous suspensions to the experimental animals. That is why previously we made an assumption about possible dependence of the pharmacological action on the crystalline structure of the substances under study, the more especially as there are many examples of interactions of such kind [48].

The X-ray diffraction analysis has demonstrated that optically pure enantiomers *S*- and *R*-configuration **24e,f** obtained independently have the same crystalline structure and, as we might expect for chiral compounds, they are crystallized in the noncentrosymmetric space group $P2_1$ [53]. On the contrary, racemate **24d** crystallizes in the centrosymmetric space group $P2_1/n$.

The comparative analysis of the structure of the racemic and enantiomeric molecules (on the example of an isomer with *R*-configuration of the chiral center) of 2-oxo-4-(1-phenylethylamino)-1,2-dihydroquinoline-3-carboxylic acids has show that it is generally rather similar. In both cases the heterocycle, nitrogen atom $N_{(2)}$, carboxide and carboxy group are in the same plane with accuracy to 0.02 Å (Figure 9), it is conditioned by formation of two strong intramolecular hydrogen bonds: $N_{(2)}$–$H_{(2N)}$...$O_{(2)}$ [H...O 1.81 Å, N–H...O 146° in the enantiomer structure and H...O 1.74 Å, N–H...O 150° in the racemate] and $O_{(3)}$–$H_{(3O)}$...$O_{(1)}$ [H...O 1.43 Å, O–H...O 148° in **E**, H...O 1.59 Å O–H...O 154° in **R**]. As a result of formation of hydrogen bonds a marked electron density redistribution also occurs in the quinolone fragment as evidenced by bond lengthening of $O_{(1)}$–$C_{(9)}$ to 1.273(1) Å in **E** and to 1.268(2) Å in **R**, $O_{(2)}$–$C_{(10)}$, to 1.234(2) Å in **E** and to 1.225(2) Å in **R** comparing to their mean value of 1.210 Å, as well as the bond of $C_{(7)}$–$C_{(8)}$ to 1.410(2) Å in **E** and to 1.418(2) Å in **R** (the mean value is 1.326 Å). At the same time some bonds are shortened on the contrary: $O_{(3)}$–$C_{(10)}$ to 1.316(1) Å in **E** and to 1.327(2) Å in **R** (1.362 Å), $C_{(8)}$–$C_{(9)}$ to 1.420(2) Å in **E** and to 1.433(2) Å in **R** (1.455 Å).

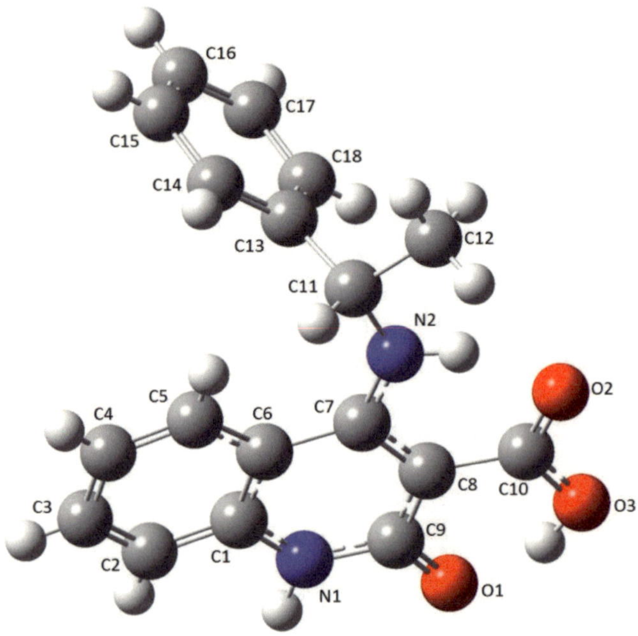

Figure 9. The structure of 2-oxo-4-(1-phenylethylamino)-1,2-dihydroquinoline-3-carboxylic acids **24d-f**

The substituent at the amino group is in *syn*-periplanar conformation in relation to $C_{(6)}$–$C_{(7)}$ bond [the torsional angle is $C_{(11)}$–$N_{(2)}$–$C_{(7)}$–$C_{(6)}$ -19.7(2)° in **E** and -1.6(2)° in **R**] and turn in such way that the methyl group is in *–ac*-orientation in relation to $C_{(7)}$–$N_{(2)}$ bond in the structure **E** and in *ap*-orientation in **R** [the torsional angle is $C_{(7)}$–$N_{(2)}$–$C_{(11)}$–$C_{(12)}$ -143.0(2)° in **E** and 171.3(1)° in **R**]. The phenyl substituent is practically perpendicular to $C_{(7)}$–$N_{(2)}$ bond and somehow turn to $N_{(2)}$–$C_{(11)}$ bond in the enantiomer structure [torsional angles are $C_{(7)}$–$N_{(2)}$–$C_{(11)}$–$C_{(13)}$ 94.6(2)° and $N_{(2)}$–$C_{(11)}$–$C_{(13)}$–$C_{(14)}$ 10.7(2)°]. In the racemate the phenyl substituent is in *–sc*-conformation in relation to $C_{(7)}$–$N_{(2)}$ bond and noticeably turn to $N_{(2)}$–$C_{(11)}$ bond [torsional angles are $C_{(7)}$–$N_{(2)}$–$C_{(11)}$–$C_{(13)}$ -67.3(2)° and $N_{(2)}$–$C_{(11)}$–$C_{(13)}$–$C_{(18)}$ -36.3(2)°]. Such position of the substituent at the amino group leads to appearance of a strong repulsion between it and atoms of the aromatic cycle of the quinolone fragment [shortened contacts are $H_{(5)}$...$C_{(11)}$ 2.46 Å in **E** and 2.44 Å in **R** (the sum of van der Waal radii is 2.87 Å), $H_{(5)}$...$H_{(11)}$ 2.07 Å in **E** and 1.98 Å in **R** (2.34 Å), $H_{(5)}$ ...$C_{(13)}$ 2.42 Å in **E** and 2.57 Å in **R** (2.87 Å), $H_{(11)}$...$C_{(5)}$ 2.65 Å in **E** and 2.75 Å in **R** (2.87 Å), $H_{(5)}$

...$C_{(14)}$ 2.77 Å in **R** (2.87 Å), $C_{(11)}...C_{(5)}$ 3.09 Å in **E** and 3.10 Å in **R** (3.42 Å), $C_{(13)}...C_{(5)}$ 3.30 Å in **E** and 3.22 Å in **R** (3.42 Å)]. As is known [61], the benzene ring is conformationally flexible and under the influence of the environment can be rather deformable. From these considerations we have sugested that the steric strain in the enantiomer structure is partially compensated by disflattening of the aromatic cycle of the quinolone fragment, distortion in some torsional angle, as well as some pyramidalization of nitrogen atom of the amino group [53]. In the racemate structure the steric strain is compensated only by the substituent's deviation at atom $C_{(7)}$ from the quinolone fragment plane [the torsional angle is $C_{(5)}–C_{(6)}–C_{(7)}–N_{(2)}$ -7.6(2)°]. The shortened intramolecular contacts of $H_{(2)}...H_{(1N)}$ 2.23 Å in **E** and 2.29 Å in **R** (2.34 Å), $H_{(12a)}...H_{(2N)}$ 2.24 Å in **E** (2.34 Å), $H_{(12b)}...C_{(18)}$ 2.78 Å in **E** (2.87 Å) and $H_{(14)}...N_{(2)}$ 2.51 Å in **E** (2.67 Å) have been also found in the molecule.

Packing of molecules in crystals of chiral and racemic 2-oxo-4-(1-phenylethylamino)-1,2-dihydroquinoline-3-carboxylic acids is much more different. For example, molecules of pure enantiomers form endless zigzag chains in the crystal along the crystallographic line [0 1 0] owing to intermolecular H-bonding of $N_{(1)}$-$H_{(1N)}...O_{(2)'}$ ($-x$, $0.5+y$, $1-z$) H...O 2.15 Å, N–H...O 148° (Figure 10). In turn, these chains form stacks along the crystallographic line [1 0 0], in which the distance between the aromatic cycle of the bicyclic fragment and π-system of carbonyl and carboxy groups of adjacent molecules is 3.37 Å; it allows to suggest the existence of stacking interaction between them. The intermolecular C–H...π hydrogen bond of $C_{(16)}–H_{(16)}...C_{(9)'}$ (x, y, $1+z$) (H...π 2.84 Å, C–H...π 152°) has been also found in the enantiomer crystal.

In the crystal of racemate the molecules of 2-oxo-4-(1-phenylethylamino)-1,2-dihydroquinoline-3-carboxylic acid form centrosymmetric dimers owing to intermolecular H-bonding of $N_{(1)}$-$H_{(1N)}...O_{(1)'}$ ($1-x$, $1-y$, $-z$) H...O 1.79 Å, N–H...O 175° (Figure 11). The distance between π-systems of adjacent dimers (3.49 Å), as well as degree of their overlapping allow to assume the existence of stacking interaction. Adjacent dimers are bound with each other by weak intermolecular hydrogen bonds of C–H...π: $C_{(12)}–H_{(12b)}...C_{(10)'}$ (x, $1+y$, z) (H...π 2.81 Å, C–H...π 130°) and $C_{(11)}–H_{(11)}...C_{(9)'}$ (x, $1+y$, z) (H...π 2.85 Å, C–H...π 145°).

Thus, the research conducted shows the essential distinctions in the crystalline structure of enantiomeric and racemic 2-oxo-4-(1-phenylethylamino)-1,2-dihydroquinoline-3-carboxylic acids. It is known [48] that it is this factor that often determines the most important pharmacokinetic determinants of the drug biological action such as bioavailability, distribution in tissues, metabolic rate, etc. Therefore, it can serve as a prime cause of differences in analgesic properties of the substances studied. It is evident that specific packing of the racemate molecules in the crystal promotes their easy bioavailability – hence it is its higher activity. The satisfactory evidence of this conclusion is the fact that the mechanical racemate of 2-oxo-4-(1-phenylethylamino)-1,2-dihydroquinoline-3-carboxylic acids obtained by a simple mixing of equimolar amounts of optically pure enantiomers **24e** and **24f** without subsequent crystallization (it is its fundamental difference from the true single-crystal racemate **24d** described above) is no different by the biological properties from the chiral products composing it. In other words, bioavailability of enantiomers of 2-oxo-4-(1-phenylethylamino)-1,2-dihydroquinoline-3-carboxylic acid **24e,f** remains low irrespective of how they are introduced into the organism of an experimental animal – individually or as a simple mechanical mixture.

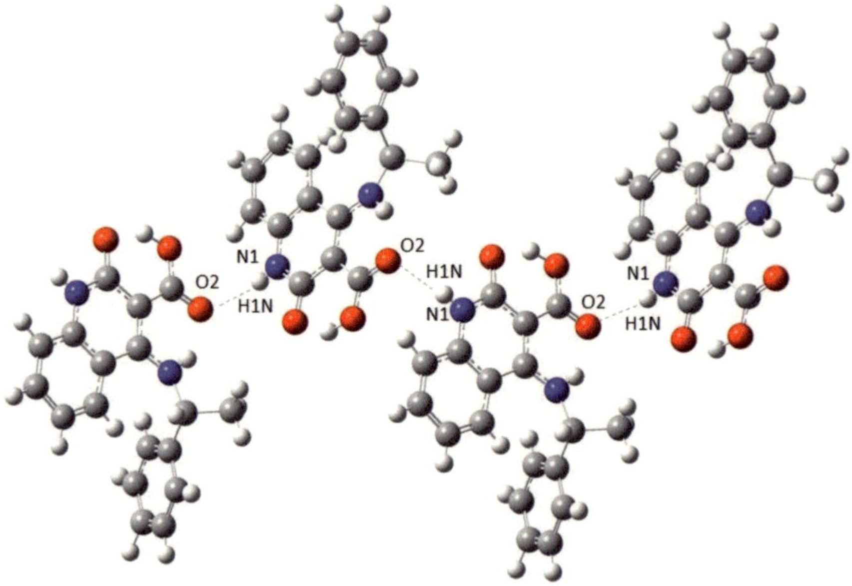

Figure 10. Zigzag chains formed in the crystal by the molecules of enantiomers **24e,f**. The dotted lines indicate the intermolecular hydrogen bonds

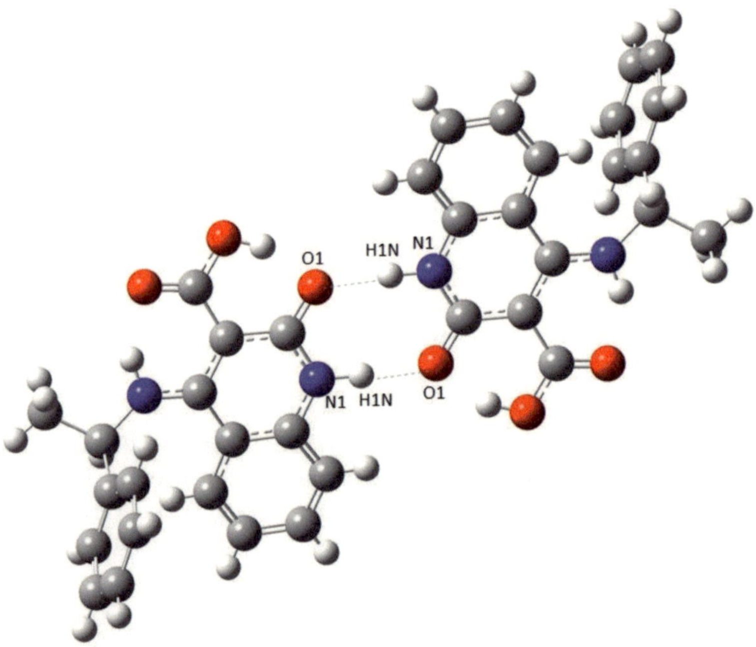

Figure 11. Centrosymmetric dimers formed in the crystal by the molecules of racemate **24d**. The dotted lines indicate the intermolecular hydrogen bonds

Taking this circumstance into account the research of the phase composition revealing the biological activity of a single-crystal racemate is of interest. The X-ray phase analysis [62] performed has demonstrated that the sample is single-phased and fully corresponds to the racemate's structure determined for a single crystal. Impurity lines, including those that could refer to the structure of one of the enantiomers crystallized in group $P2_1$ on the powder diffraction pattern have not been found. Since the parameters of a primitive unit cell of the crystals of enantiomer (**E**) and racemate (**R**) differ markedly, one may state that the X-ray phase analysis was carried out with considerably fine precision.

4.4. 4-(Hetarylmethyl)amino-2-oxo-1,2-dihydroquinoline-3-carboxylic acids

The conception of bioisosteric replacements suggested at the beginning of the last century [44] currently remains one of the most powerful means for creating effective and safe medicines [40-43]. Its application allows not only to optimize biologically active substances already known, but to reveal new structures with the similar or related properties and so to enhance the patent protection of a future drug.

This methodology has proven its value completely while working with 4-hydroxy-6,7-dimethoxy-2-oxo-1,2-dihydroquinoline-3-carboxamides (**12**). That is why we attempted once more to use it in our research – now for modification of 4-benzylamino-2-oxo-1,2-dihydroquinoline-3-carboxylic acid (**20e**), which we made by the classical isosteric replacement of the benzene ring with the heterocycle being similar in many physical and chemical characteristics. As is known [44], they are pyridine, thiophene and in some way furan.

The target 4-(hetarylmethyl)amino-2-oxo-1,2-dihydroquinoline-3-carboxylic acids **25a-f** (Figure 12) have been synthesized by the interaction of the corresponding primary amines with 4-chloro-2-oxo-1,2-dihydroquinoline-3-carboxylic acid [63]. In parallel with hetarylmethyl amino substituted acids **25a-f** cyclohexyl derivative **25g** has been obtained. Of course, this compound cannot be classed to heteroanalogs of acid **20e**, however, the possibility of finding additional information concerning the key functional groups owing to it became a solid ground to its synthesis. By these reasons the reaction of 4-chloro-2-oxo-1,2-dihydroquinoline-3-carboxylic acid with some secondary amines has been studied. Unfortunately, the corresponding quinoline-3-carboxylic acids with tertiary amino groups in position 4 appeared to be extremely unstable substances readily decarboxylized in boiling ethanol immediately after their formation. As a result, we succeded only in isolating 4-N-R,R'-aminoquinolin-2-ones **26** and **27**. Nevertheless, there is a benefit from the experiments carried out. Firstly, they allow to clarify that 4-amino-2-oxo-1,2-dihydroquinoline-3-carboxylic acids are relatively stable only with the presence of even one proton in the amino group. Secondly, the substances obtained are themselves of interest for pharmacological research as a particular type of new structural analogs of the basic molecule. And still, the initially entirely specific task set of this experiment – explain the role of 4-NH-proton in the process of binding of 4-benzylamino-2-oxo-1,2-dihydroquinoline-3-carboxylic acid with a biological target – has not be solved yet.

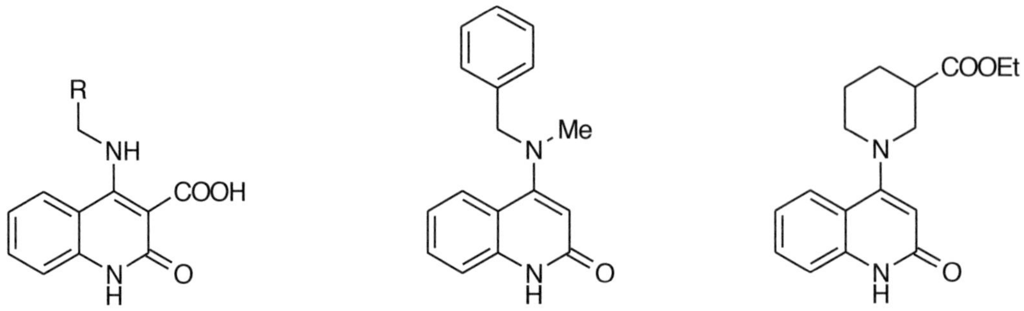

25a-g **26** **27**

Figure 12. Heteroanalogues of 4-benzylamino-2-oxo-1,2-dihydroquinoline-3-carboxylic acid (**20e**)

The analgesic activity of aminoquinolines **25-27** has been studied under conditions being similar to those in testing quinoline-3-carboxamides **12.** Analysis of the data presented in Table 4 shows that our replacement of the aromatic ring of the benzyl fragment in 4-benzylamino-2-oxo-1,2-dihydroquinoline-3-carboxylic acid by isosteric heterocycle is mainly accompanied with some decrease in the analgesic properties. In the case of pyridine derivatives the dependence of the potency of the effect exerted on the position of the nitrogen atom is distinctly visible. Thus, pyridine-3-ylmethylamine substituted acid **25b** does not practically differ from benzyl analog **20e** by its activity, whereas *ortho*-isomer **25a** yields it more than three times.

Benzene has much more similar physical and chemical characteristics with thiophene then with furan [44]. Therefore, it is quite regular that thiophenemethyl derivative **25f,** but not furfuryl analogs **25d,e,** is closer to benzyl prototype **20e** by its biological properties.

Compound	R	Analgesic activity (decrease in the amount of "acetic acid writhing", %)	Compound	R	Analgesic activity (decrease in the amount of "acetic acid writhing", %)
25a	2-Py	21.8	**25f**	Thiophen-2-yl	49.1
25b	3-Py	65.4	**25g**	*cyclo*-C_6H_{11}	46.5
25c	4-Py	34.9	**26**	–	40.3
25d	Furan-2-yl	39.5	**27**	–	16.2
25e	5-Me-furan-2-yl	39.5	**20e**		69.8

Table 4. Analgesic properties of aminoquinolines **25-27** on the model of "acetic acid induced writhing" ($p \leq 0.05$)

Cyclohexylmethylamine substituted acid **25g** deserves individual attention, first of all, because it maintains rather strong influence on the pain reaction in spite of a significant conformation rearrangement of 4-N-fragment subjected to modification as compared to a flat benzyl prototype. This example testifies the possible perspectives of the given direction development involving hydrogenized analogs of other molecular systems, including heterocyclic ones, in the range of the objects studied.

We came to the conclusion of necessity to continue our research after testing 4-N-R,R'-aminoquinoline-2-ones **26** and **27**. The reason for this was a surprisingly high analgesic activity of 4-(benzylmethylamino)-1*H*-quinoline-2-one (**26**). As previously thought [53], removal of the carboxy group from the molecule inevitably resulted in the essential decrease of analgesic properties. However, as it happens, the presence of 3-carboxy group is already not always necessary for 4-aminoquinoline-2- ones with two substituents in 4-amino group.

5. (4-Hydroxy-1-methyl-2-oxo-1,2-dihydroquinolin-3-yl)acetic acid and its esters

Pain and inflammation belong to the most widespread signs accompanying numerous pathological states. To eliminate these manifestations NSAIDs are currently widely used; among them derivatives of aryl- and hetarylacetic acids – Diclofenac, Aceclofenac, Indometacin, Clinoril, Etodolac, etc., occupy an important place [14, 52]. In this regard, involvement of (4-hydroxy-2-oxo-1,2-dihydroquinolin-3-yl)acetic acid and its derivatives in searching new pain-killers conducted by us is logical and regular.

The synthesis of the initial (4-hydroxy-1-methyl-2-oxo-1,2-dihydroquinolin-3-yl)acetic acid (**28**, Figure 13) has been carried out by acylation of methyl *N*-methylanthranilate with β-methoxycarbonylpropionyl chloride with subsequent treatment of the intermediate sodium anilide by methylate in methyl alcohol. The mixture of methyl esters of quinolin-3-yl)acetic and benzoazepine-4-carboxylic acids formed in the course of this reaction is subjected to hydrolysis and recyclization into the same final product – (quinolin-3-yl)acetic acid **28** when treating with the aqueous solution of KOH [64]. Esterification of this compound catalyzed by acids gives alkyl (4-hydroxy-1-methyl-2-oxo-1,2-dihydroquinolin-3-yl)acetates (**29**) with high yields; they are also of interest for pharmacological testing.

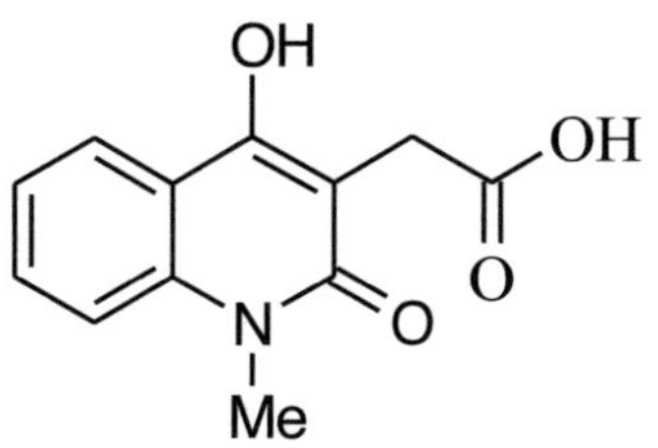

28

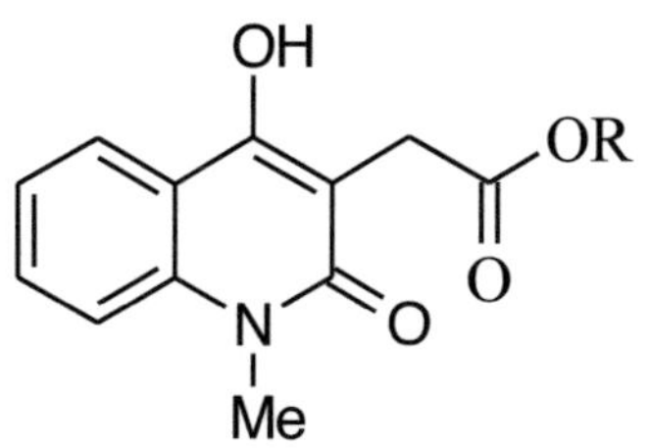

29a-i

Figure 13. (4-Hydroxy-1-methyl-2-oxo-1,2-dihydroquinolin-3-yl)acetic acid and its esters

One of the characteristic criteria of efficiency for anti-inflammatory drugs is the anti-exudative action. In this regard we began testing the biological properties of the compounds synthesized with studying their effect on the exudative phase of acute aseptic inflammation. The research was conducted on the model of carrageenan edema in mice [65]. As a reference drug the classic nonsteroidal anti-inflammatory drug – Diclofenac in the dose of 8 mg/kg (ED_{50}) was used. The results obtained show that the initial quinoline acetic acid **28** in the equimolar dose to Diclofenac can decrease the carrageenan edema size by 23.1% (Table 5). Esterification affects the anti-exudative properties especially successful. Among the compounds synthesized the substances, which do not practically yield Diclofenac in their activity (esters **29b,f,h**) and even exceed it somehow (allyl ester **29c**) have been found. In this range of compounds the interesting dependence has been revealed – transfer from esters with the normal *O*-alkyl chains to derivatives of the *iso*-structure is accompanied almost complete loss of the anti-inflammatory action.

But for the analgesic properties of quinolinylacetic acid **28** and its esters **29** ("acetic acid induced writhing", $p \leq 0.05$, details see Quinoline-3-carboxamides **12**) this structural biological regularity is not already characteristic. Although here most of esters appeared to be much more active than the initial acid.

Compound	R	Anti-inflammatory activity(edema reduction, %)	Analgesic activity (decrease in the amount of "acetic acid writhing", %)
28	–	23.1	28.5
29a	Me	12.7	64.2
29b	Et	45.5	54.4
29c	All	52.5	24.1
29d	Pr	20.4	33.9
29e	*i*-Pr	3.1	39.3
29f	Bu	46.2	50.2
29g	*i*-Bu	27.3	50.2
29h	C_5H_{11}	44.5	35.9
29i	*i*-C_5H_{11}	9.6	22.1
Diclofenac (8 mg/kg)		49.8	–
Diclofenac (5 mg/kg)		–	51.6

Table 5. Anti-inflammatory and analgesic properties of quinolinylacetic acid **28** and its esters **29** ($p < 0.05$)

The X-ray diffraction study of the spatial structure of the most powerful pain-killer from the esters group – methyl quinolinylacetate **29a** – has allowed to determine that the quinolone ring in the molecule of this compound is incompletely planar: the torsional angle $C_{(1)}$–$N_{(1)}$–$C_{(9)}$–$C_{(8)}$ is -5.8(2)° (Figure 14). Hence, a shortened intramolecular contact of $H_{(5)}...O_{(2)}$ 2.40 Å (the sum of van der Waal radii 2.46 Å) appears. The methoxycarbonyl fragment of the substituent at atom $C_{(8)}$ is located orthogonally to the plane of the bicycle and turn a little in relation to $C_{(8)}$–$C_{(10)}$ bond [torsional angles are $C_{(7)}$–$C_{(8)}$–$C_{(10)}$–$C_{(11)}$ 93.9(1)° and $C_{(8)}$–$C_{(10)}$–$C_{(11)}$–$O_{(3)}$ -19.7(2)°]. The methyl group is in *ap*-conformation in relation to $C_{(10)}$–$C_{(11)}$ bond [the torsional angle is $C_{(12)}$–$O_{(4)}$–$C_{(11)}$–$C_{(10)}$ 178.3(1)°].

A rather strong repulsion has been detected between atoms of the methyl group at atom $N_{(1)}$ and adjacent atoms of the carbonyl group $C_{(9)}$–$O_{(1)}$ and hydrogen atom in peri-position of the benzene ring; shortened intramolecular contacts of $H_{(2)}...C_{(13)}$ 2.53 Å (2.87 Å), $H_{(2)}...H_{(13c)}$ 2.27 Å (2.34 Å), $H_{(13c)}...C_{(2)}$ 2.74 Å (2.87 Å) and $H_{(13a)}...O_{(1)}$ 2.24 Å (2.46 Å) testify about it.

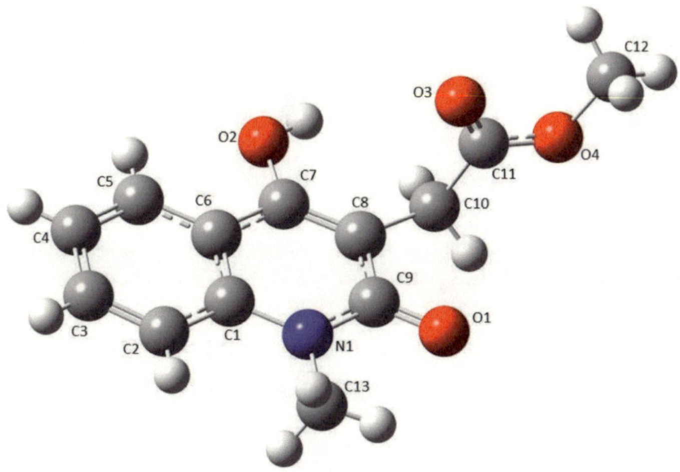

Figure 14. Structure of the methyl quinolinylacetate **29a** molecule with numbering of the atoms

Molecules of methyl quinolinylacetate **29a** form endless zigzag chains in the crystal (Figure 15) along the crystallographic line [0 0 1] owing to intermolecular H-bonding of $O_{(2)}$–H...$O_{(1)'}$ (x, 0.5 - y, 0.5 + z) H...O 1.76 Å, O–H...O 160°. It seems that formation of this hydrogen bond stipulates $C_{(9)}$–$O_{(1)}$ 1.251(1) Å bond lengthening comparing to its mean value 1.210 Å. The system of intermolecular C–H...π hydrogen bonds: $C_{(12)}$–$H_{(12a)}$...$C_{(5)'}$ (x, 0.5 - y, -0.5 + z) H...π 2.78 Å, C–H...π 172°; $C_{(13)}$–$H_{(13a)}$...$C_{(11)'}$ (x, 0.5 - y, -0.5 + z) H...π 2.84 Å, C–H...π 138° and $C_{(13)}$–$H_{(13b)}$...$C_{(5)'}$ (-x, 1 - y, 1 - z) H...π 2.81 Å, C–H...π 148° has also been found in the crystal.

A comparative analysis of X-ray diffraction data of methyl quinolinylacetate **29a** and its ethyl analog **29b** [66] reveals a remarkable resemblance not only the peculiarities of the spatial structure of these compounds, but their crystalline packing as well. In this connection and taking into account the abovementioned examples of a significant influence of the crystalline structure of 4-hydroxyquinolin-2-ones on their biological activity, the related analgesic properties of esters **29a** and **29b** are quite logical. In addition, significant differences in the anti-inflammatory action of these substances are an eloquent evidence of the fact that the crystalline structure is though important, but not the only factor determining the pharmacological properties of a substance.

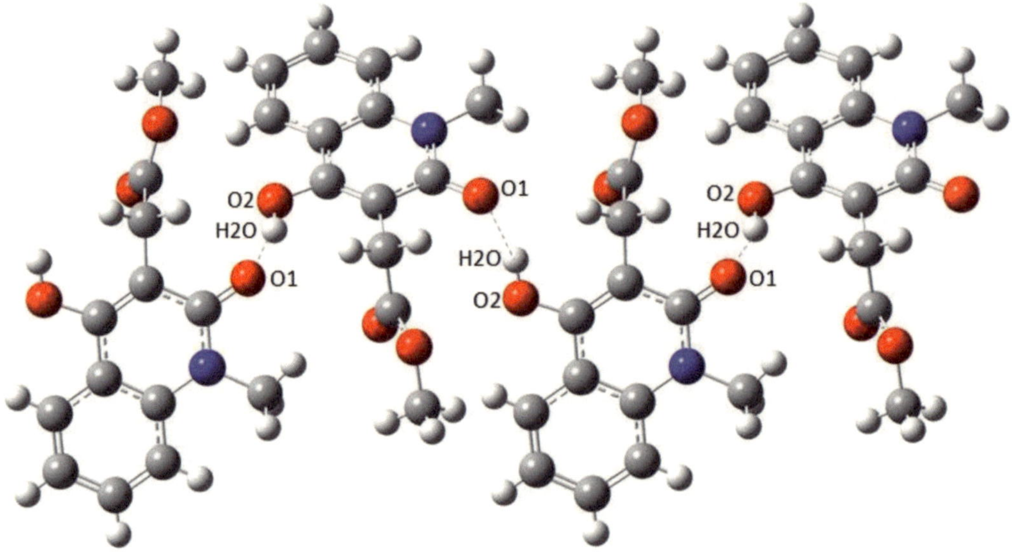

Figure 15. Endless zigzag chains formed in the crystal by molecules of methyl quinolinylacetate **29a**. The dotted lines indicate the intermolecular hydrogen bonds

6. The study of *N*-(3-pyridylmethyl)-4-hydroxy-6,7-dimethoxy-2-oxo-1,2-dihydroquinoline-3-carboxamide as a promising pain-killer

According to the results of the primary pharmacological screening only one compound – *N*-(3-pyridylmethyl)-4-hydroxy-6,7-dimethoxy-2-oxo-1,2-dihydroquinoline-3-carboxamide (**12**, R = CH_2Py-3) has been selected as a lead compound from the large group of 4-hydroxy-6,7-dimethoxy-2-oxo-1,2-dihydroquinoline-3-carboxamides, their closest structural analogs and some derivatives. After oral introduction to white mice in the dose of 20 mg/kg this compound is able to reduce the number of writhings caused by intraperitoneal injection of acetic acid by 75.3 % (see Table 1). Picolyl-3-amide **12** has also demonstrated a high activity – 81.1% ($p < 0.05$) – on the model of "kaolinic writhings" used for research of the peripheral component of the analgesic effect [65].

The effect of the lead compound on the central component of the nociceptive system has been studied *in vivo* on the models involving the central mechanisms of the pain formation: thermal or electric irritation of the murine paw, as well as thermal irritation of the rat's tail and electric stimulation of the rat's tailhead [65]. All experiments have been carried out according to the same scheme: *1* – determination of the initial level of algesthesia in all animals induced by the appropriate nociceptive irritator; *2* – oral introduction of picolyl-3-amide **12** to the experimental animals in the dose of 20 mg/kg and the solvent to the control group of animals; *3* – monitoring of the pain threshold in every 30 minutes during 5 hours; *4* – calculation of the analgesic activity comparing to control.

It has been found that on the model of the thermal irritation of paws ("hot plate") sensitivity of mice to pain already decreases by 39.4% in 30 minutes after the beginning of the experiment. In general the analgesic effect lasts about 4.5 hours reaching its maximum in 75.7% ($p < 0.05$) at the point of 2.0 hours. After the change of the thermal irritator by the electric one the picture observed is practically the same – with the maximum of 90.1% ($p \leq 0.05$) during the second hour and further with smooth decline in activity.

On the model of the thermal irritation of the rat's tail ("tail flick") the maximum analgesic effect – 101.0% ($p < 0.05$) already develops in 1 hour after introduction of picolyl-3-amide **12** and retains at ths level during the hour. By the end of testing, i.e. by the 5-th hour, the analgesic activity consistently decreases though its level still remains rather noticeable (32.4%).

When using electrostimulation of the rat's tailhead the pain threshold increases not so rapidly – during the first 30 minutes its growth is only 10.5%. However, further the potency of the analgesic action quickly grows and by the second hour of the experiment it exceeds the control indices by 90.9% ($p < 0.05$), after that it gradually decreases.

A high activity of picolyl-3-amide **12** shown on the models of pains of the central origin allow to suggest about the receptor mechanism of its analgesic effect. To confirm or dispose this assumption we carried out a series of experiments in studying the influence of the lead compound on opioid, adrenergic and dopaminergic receptors. Besides, a possible participation of GABA-ergic links of the central nociceptive system in the mechanism of its analgesic action was checked. All investigations of this series were conducted on the model of the thermal irritation of the rat's tail ("tail flick") according the scheme described above with the only difference that another two groups of animals were added – those taken the known reference drug and its combination with the new substance under research. In all experiments Picolyl-3-amide **12** was introduced orally in the dose of 20 mg/kg as a fine aqueous suspension stabilized by Tween-80. The reference drugs were introduced orally or intraperitoneally in the doses recommended for each of them [67]. When working with combinations of substances at first a reference drug was introduced, then in 20 minutes the lead compound was introduced.

As the experiments showed, analgesic effects of picolyl-3-amide **12** demonstrated by it when taken alone and on background of the preliminary introduction of Naloxone (3.0 mg/kg) differ slightly (Figure 16). Therefore, the lead compound does not have a substantial effect on opioid receptors.

The study of the possible participation of the adrenergic system in the mechanism of the analgesic action of picolyl-3-amide **12** was conducted with the help of α_2-adrenoceptor agonist Clonidine (0.02 mg/kg) and β-adrenergic blocking agent Propranolol (14.5 mg/kg). Analysis of the data obtained testifies that the lead compound in combination with Clonidine losses the most part of its initially high analgesic properties – especially during the first 2.5 hours of the experiment (Figure 17). The same picture can be observed in the case of its combination with Propranolol (Figure 18). It entitles us to believe that picolyl-3-amide **12** exerts its analgesic activity through, at least, partial blocking of central α_2-adrenoreceptors and activation of β-adrenoreceptors.

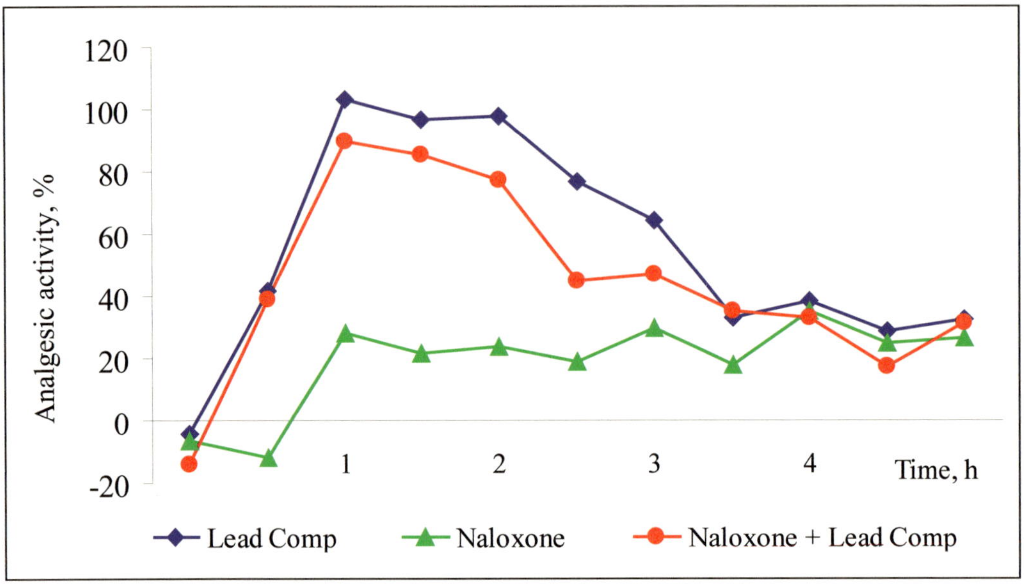

Figure 16. Lead compound & Naloxone

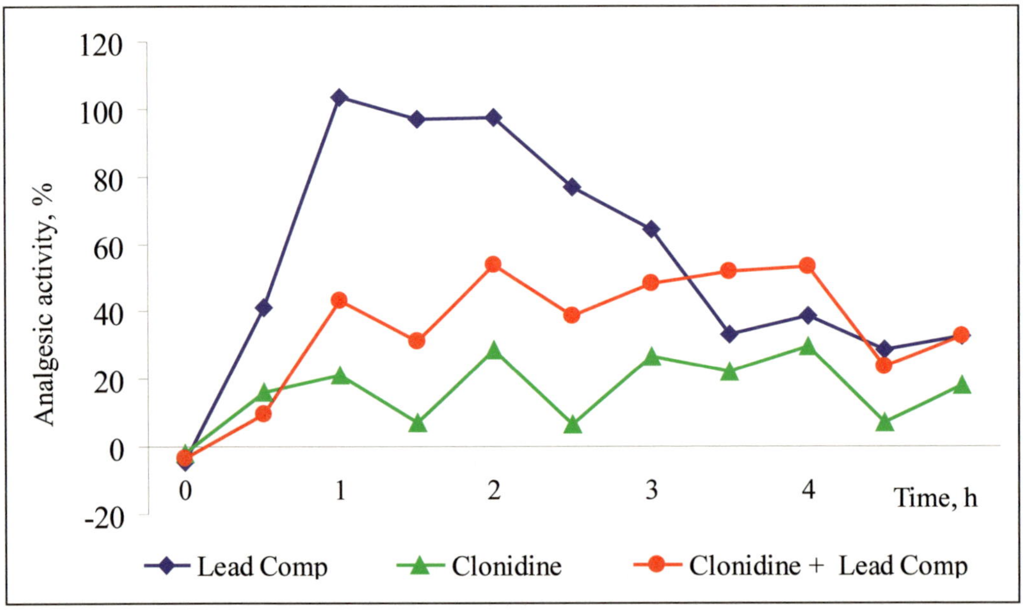

Figure 17. Lead compound & Clonidine

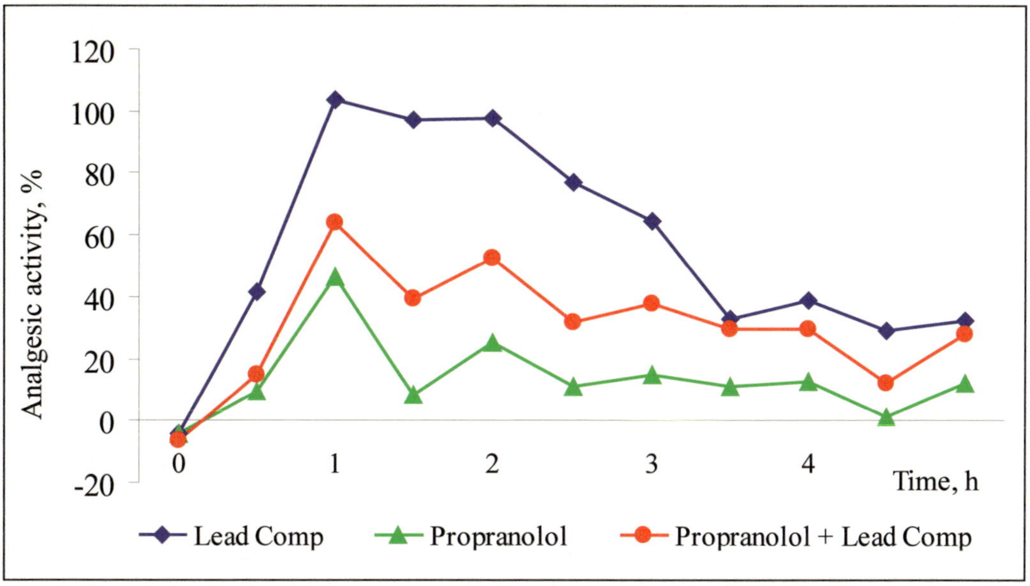

Figure 18. Lead compound & Propranolol

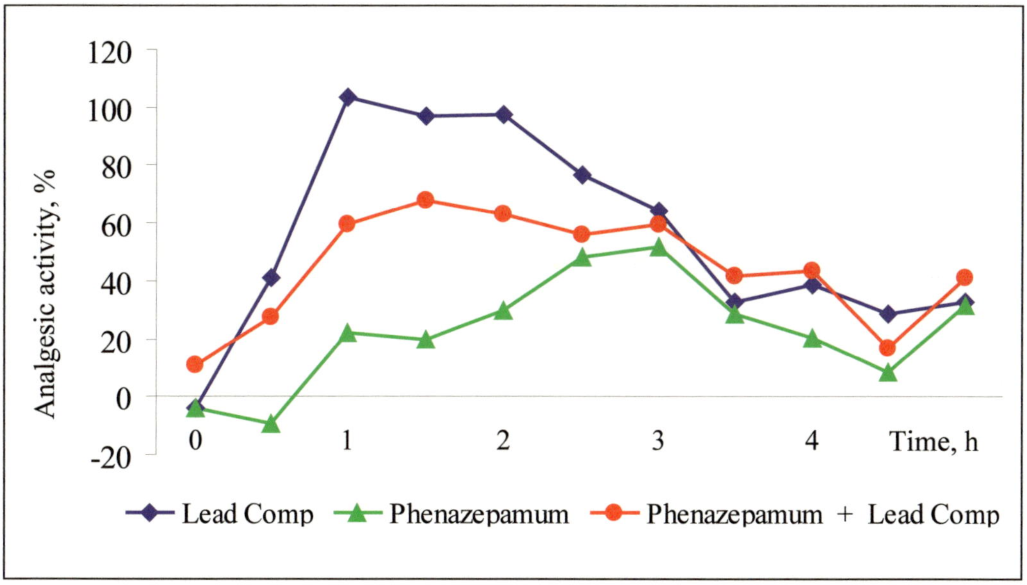

Figure 19. Lead compound & Phenazepamum

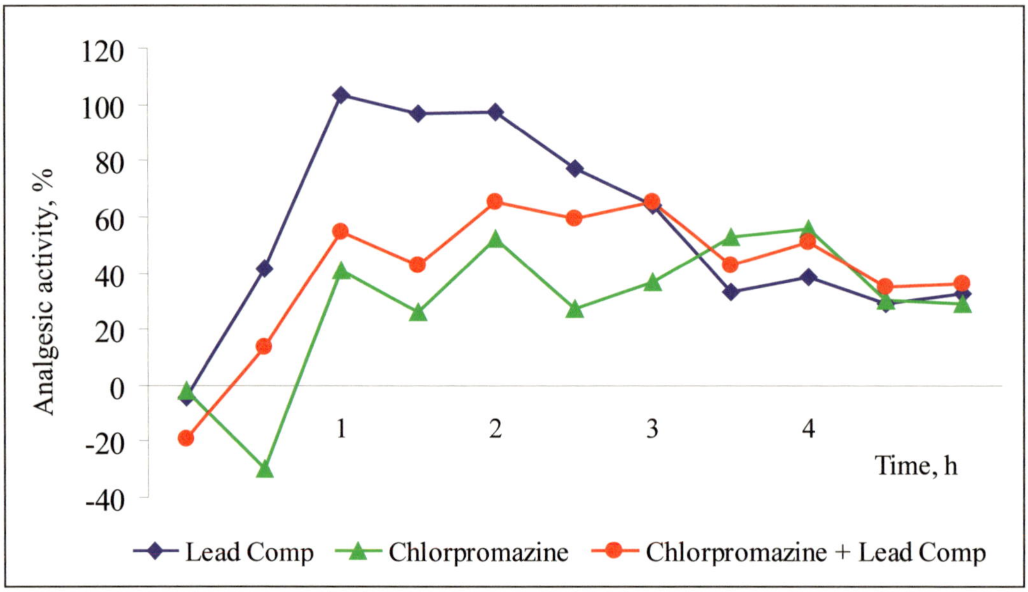

Figure 20. Lead compound & Chlorpromazine

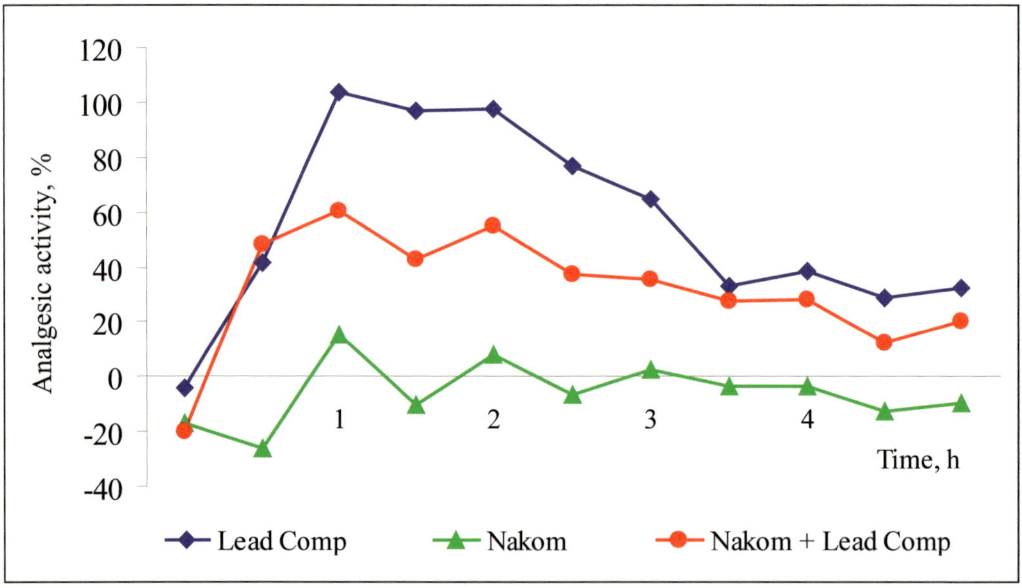

Figure 21. Lead compound & Nakom®

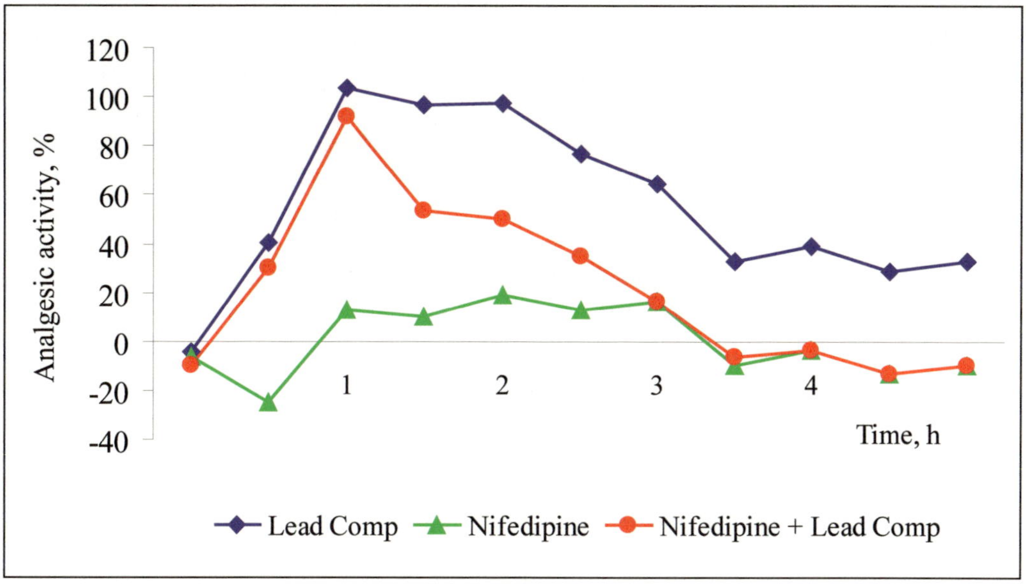

Figure 22. Lead compound & Nifedipine

Differences in analgesic properties of the lead compound, which it exerts with independent introduction and in combination with Phenazepamum (0.19 mg/kg), in general appeared to be not so expressed (Figure 19). Thus, the conclusion can be made about its insignificant effect on the GABA-ergic system.

Participation of picolyl-3-amide **12** dopamine receptors in the mechanism of the analgesic action has been studied with the help of their blocking agent Chlorpromazine (14.0 mg/kg). In this case the effect is more expressed than in the previous test. But in general it appeared to be brief – after gradual increase during the first hour of the experiment it reaches the maximum, retains this level for about 30 minutes, and then begins to fade (Figure 20).

To study the influence of the lead compound on release of dopamine and noradrenaline in the CNS the combined medicinal form Nakom® containing Levodopa, a precursor of dopamine, together with Carbidopa, an inhibitor of its peripheral decarboxylation, was used. If when introduced alone picolyl-3-amide **12** provides a rapid enhancement of the analgesic properties till the maximum value during an hour, on the background of Nakom® (24.0 mg/kg) in 30 minutes after the start of testing the growth of activity is sharply discontinued (Figure 21). By the first hour blocking of the analgesic action of the lead compound achieves approximately 40% and lasts about two hours.

Recently the question about possibilities of creating new pain-killers based on agonists of neuronal nicotinic acetylcholine receptors (*n*AChR) is being actively discussed in scientific literature [68-70]. Epibatidine alkaloid (**30**, Figure 23) isolated from the extract of the Ecuadorean tree frog skin (*Epipedobates tricolor*) became the incentive for development of this approach. In the experiments in mice this compound revealed 200–500 times higher analgesic activity than morphine on various experimental models. It is of great importance that analgesia caused by Epibatidine is not relieved by Naloxone, an opioid receptor antagonist. By its mechanism of action this natural alkaloid appeared to be a powerful agonist of neuronal nicotinic acetylcholine receptors regulating different functions of the nervous system [71]. Therefore, it is not surprising that a lot of attention is paid to synthetic representatives of this group of biologically active substances. The search has been carried out among derivatives of various nitrogen heterocycles [71]. One of the successful findings was 5-(trifluoromethyl)-6-(1-methylazepan-4-yl)methyl-1*H*-quinolin-2-one (**31**), which exhibited a potent agonist activity on several human *n*AChRs [72]. Its structural similarity with 4-hydroxyquinolin-2-ones studied served as a theoretical prerequisite to testing the influence on *n*AChR and picolyl-3-amide **12** offered as a new pain-killer. In this testing a specific nicotinic antagonist Nifedipine being capable to block effectively the analgesic activity of Epibatidine [71] was used. During the first hour Nifedipine (102.2 mg/kg) practically had no effect on the analgesic action of picolyl-3-amide **12** (Figure 22). Then, however, the marked inhibiting effect developed rapidly and preserved till the end of the experiment.

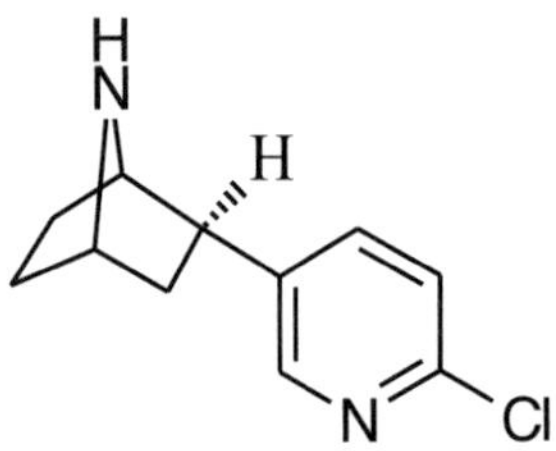

30

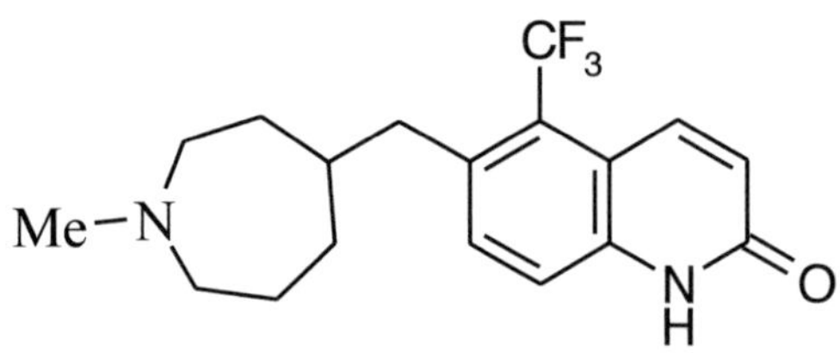

31

Figure 23. Natural (**30**) and synthetic (**31**) agonists of nicotinic acetylcholine receptors

Reviewing the preliminary results of this piece of our work it is worth mentioning the ability of picolyl-3-amide **12** to arrest effectively the pains of central and peripheral origin. By its mechanism of the analgesic action this compound can not be named a selective inhibitor of one type of receptors. Having no effect on opioid receptors picolyl-3-amide **12** reveals its analgesic properties mainly via interaction with the adrenergic system and activation of nicotinic acetylcholine receptors. Other mediator systems, in particular the catecholaminergic one, are involved to much lesser extent. The GABA-ergic link of the central nociceptive system participates little in the mechanism of the analgesic action of the lead compound.

The antipyretic action of the lead compound studied on the model of fever in rats caused by subcutaneous injection of Brewer's yeast suspension [65] is classified as mild. Picolyl-3-amide **12** did not exert any clinically significant anti-inflammatory effect (the paw edema in mice induced by subcutaneous injection of 1% formalin solution [65]).

Taking into account the fact that for many drug of the group of nonnarcotic analgesics the nonselective inhibition of prostaglandin biosynthesis is characteristic we have studied a possible ulcerogenic action of the lead compound by the known method [65]. As it turned out, picolyl-3-amide **12** caused visible changes of the gastric mucosa in the half of experimental mice with a single introduction in very high dose exceeding the therapeutic ones: UD_{50} =1582 mg/kg.

Any new potential drug must comply with current high requirements not only by the specific activity, but safety as well. The study of acute toxicity conducted in white mice has shown that picolyl-3-amide **12** refers to practically nontoxic substances – its median lethal dose (LD_{50}) taken orally is 9527 mg/kg.

Thus, *N*-(3-pyridylmethyl)-4-hydroxy-6,7-dimethoxy-2-oxo-1,2-dihydroquinoline-3-carboxamide (**12**, R = CH_2Py-3) has realistic chances to become a medicine and it is recommended to wide preclinical trials as a promising pain-killer.

7. The latest ideas and findings when creating highly active pain-killers on the basis of 4-hydroxyquinolin-2-ones and related heterocycles

With the beginning of comprehensive preclinical trials of *N*-(3-pyridylmethyl)-4-hydroxy-6,7-dimethoxy-2-oxo-1,2-dihydroquinoline-3-carboxamide the search of new promising compounds, which are suitable for creation of effective analgesics on their basis, does not naturally stop. Using the gathered experience we continued working in this direction attracting mathematical methods in addition to such traditional methods of this sort of investigations as synthetic, physicochemical and pharmacological ones. Besides, to introduce principally new substituents in the quinoline ring, as well as diversification of the objects under study due to heterocycles related in their structure appeared to be very useful and reasonable. In particular, the extremely interesting direction of searching new pain-killers among 4-hydroxyquinolin-2-one derivatives was replacement of carbonyl in position 2 to the sulfo group, i.e. transfer to 4-hydroxy-2,1-benzothiazine 2,2-dioxides.

7.1. QSAR-analysis of the analgesic activity and toxicity of 4-hydroxyquinolin-2-one derivatives

The search of regularities for the "structure – action" relationship in the range of biologically active substances is an important stage on the way of purposeful design of new drugs with the targeted complex of pharmacological properties. In this connection we attempted to generalize the results of the chemical and biological research conducted with the help of QSAR-analysis. For this purpose the dependence of the analgesic activity of various 4-hydroxyquinolin-2-one derivatives on their molecular structure was analyzed according to the definite scheme consisting of some successive steps.

Formation of learning and test samples. The learning sample is formed from 89 compounds of various chemical classes: 4-hydroxy-6,7-dimethoxy-2-oxo-1,2-dihydroquinoline-3-carboxamides (**12**), some *N*-(3-pyridylmethyl)-4-hydroxy-2-oxoquinoline-3-carboxamides (**14**), 4-N-R,R'-aminoquinolin-2-ones (**20e**, **25-27**) and alkyl (4-hydroxy-1-methyl-2-oxo-1,2-

dihydroquinolin-3-yl)acetates (**29**). For external testing of models 17 *N*-(3-pyridylmethyl)-4-hydroxy-2-oxoquinoline-3-carboxamides (**14-16**) and 1-(2-carbamoylethyl)-4-hydroxy-2-oxo-1,2-dihydroquinoline-3-carboxylic acid (**17h**) have been used. The analgesic properties of all compounds have been studied under the same conditions on the model of "acetic acid induced writhing".

Calculation of structural descriptors for all tested compounds. To calculate descriptors two varients of the molecular structure representation – simplex method (Simplex Representation of Molecular Structure or SIRMS) [73] and circulation model (CM) [74] were used. Within the scope of SIRMS the structure is in the form of a set with tetratomic fragments of the fixed composition, topology and symmetry. The values of physical and chemical characteristics of atoms, which are important for displaying a property (lipophilicity, particle charges, etc.), are taken into account when differentiating atoms on simplexes. The structure's descriptor is the number of fragments (simplexes) of a certain type. The circulation model of a molecule is a structure of arbitrary construction in the form of pseudocycle, for which similarity parameters of Cremer-Pople cycle [75] are calculated; they act as descriptors.

Statistical data processing, selection of significant descriptors. During preprocessing of the whole array of descriptors those that do not correlate with the property are excluded. Then analysis of intercorrelating descriptors is carried out. It is evident that pairs of descriptors correlating among themselves contain the same structural information; therefore, one of these descriptors can be excluded. Further selection of only significant descriptors is performed from the rest array with the help of the trend-vector procedure [73].

QSAR models building, their validation and verification with the help of the moving control procedure and test sample. For building QSAR models the method of partial least squares (PLS) [73] was used. Its undoubtful advantage is quantitative interpretability of the "structure – property" dependences obtained. For each group of the descriptors selected (circulation and simplex) two models were obtained. Their approximation possibilities were estimated on the basis of determination coefficients (R^2), statistical stability (Q^2) – with the help of the procedure of external five-fold cross-validation [73]. The predictive capability of models was esrimated on the basis of determination coefficients (R^2_{test}) for test samples and the mean-squared prediction error (S_{test}).

Statistical characteristics of both models are rather high – for simplex descriptors: $R^2 = 0.95$, $Q^2 = 0.75$, $R^2_{test} = 0.86$, $S_{test} = 5.6$; for descriptors of the circulation model: $R^2 = 0.93$, $Q^2 = 0.75$, $R^2_{test} = 0.81$, $S_{test} = 5.1$.

These two models are combined in final consensus QSAR model validated by the external test sample (Table 6) formed from 18 compounds, which have not taken part in model building.

The analysis of the data given in Table 6 shows that the mean forecast error for the analgesic activity is only 8%. Therefore, the predictive force of the QSAR model obtained is quite satisfactory and suitable to use for interpretation, out of experimental screening of compounds previously unstudied and molecular design.

Interpretation of models, estimation of contributions of the physicochemical factors and structural fragments in the analgesic activity. Application of the PLS method allows to

Compound	Analgesic activity, %		Compound	Analgesic activity, %	
	Experimental	Calculated		Experimental	Calculated
6 (R = All)	56	47	**14m**	50	70
12 (R = CH2Py-3)	75	72	**14n**	75	71
14a	64	68	**14o**	74	75
14b	60	69	**14p**	63	72
14g	78	76	**14q**	59	71
14h	54	63	**14r**	58	71
14j	63	64	**15**	45	39
14k	70	74	**16**	81	61
14l	61	73	**17h**	60	66

Table 6. The estimation of the predictive force of the QSAR on the external test set

estimate quatitatively the contribution of each particular descriptor in the biological activity. And since a descriptor is the molecule's fragment taking into account the physicochemical characteristics of atoms, the possibility to estimate their relative importance appears. This information is needed for further estimation of the supposed mechanisms of the activity demonstration, as well as design of new highly active agents.

In the sector diagram (Figure 24) the results of analysis of relative contribution of various physical and chemical factors to the analgesic activity of 1,2-dihydroquinolin-2-ones derivatives are presented.

As seen from the given diagram, the electrostatic factors such as partial charges on atoms, polarizability and lipophilicity have the greatest influence on the analgesic effect. On this basis it can be assumed that the analgesic activity of 1,2-dihydroquinolin-2-ones is mainly determined by their electrostatic interaction with biological targets. The substantial influence of lipophilicity is obviously connected with transmembrane transfer of molecules to the sites of their binding with a receptor.

Similarly in the framework of the symplex approach contributions of individual structural fragments can be calculated and it is possible to determine those that make the maximum positive contribution in the analgesic activity of compounds from the learning sample. However, we think, it is much more interesting to perform computation on totally new and unstudied structures, i.e. to use for the molecular design.

Molecular design of new potentially activepain-killers. With the help of the consensus QSAR model we performed a purposeful design of new promising analgesics of 4-hydroxyquinoline-2-one range. As it is clear from Table 7 where some virtual structures with computed values of their analgesic action are given, the mathematical assessment of the biological activity exceeds greatly the minimal (i.e. 50%) efficiency criterion for the pain syndrome relief. We

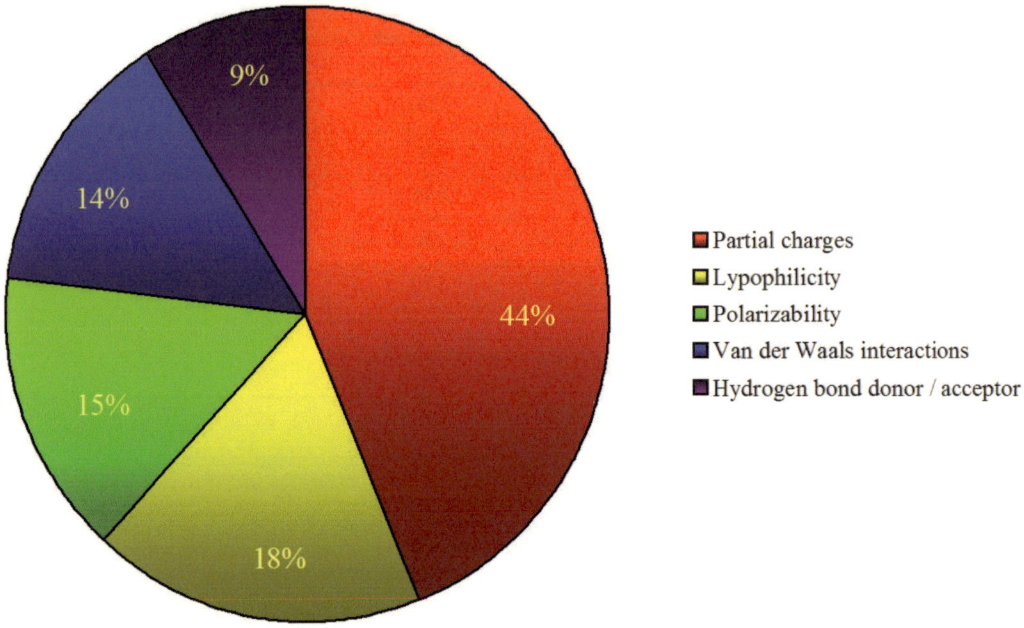

Figure 24. The relative impact of physical and chemical factors on the analgesic activity of 1,2-dihydroquinolin-2-ones

hope the information will be useful for many medical chemists engaged in the problem of effective analgesic agents creation.

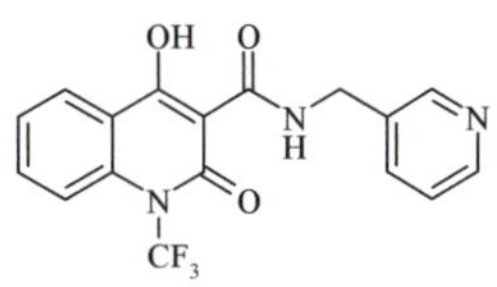 Calculated analgesic activity 70%	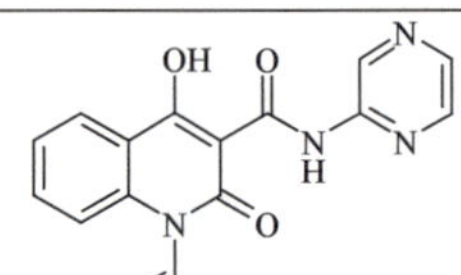 Calculated analgesic activity 78%	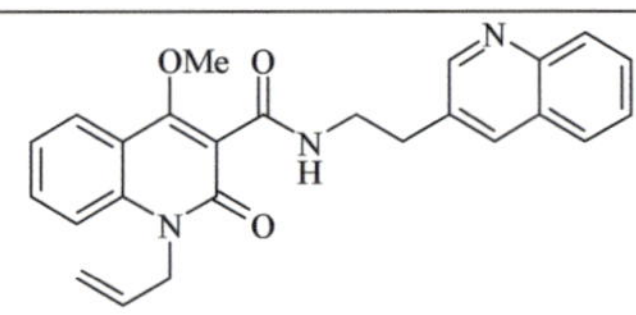 Calculated analgesic activity 77%
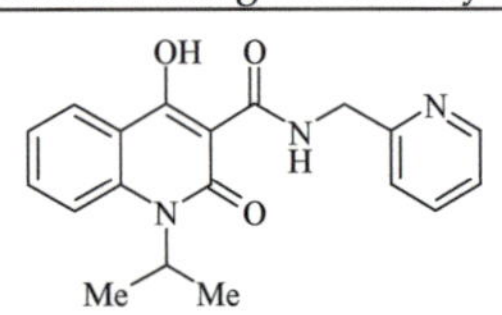 Calculated analgesic activity 77%	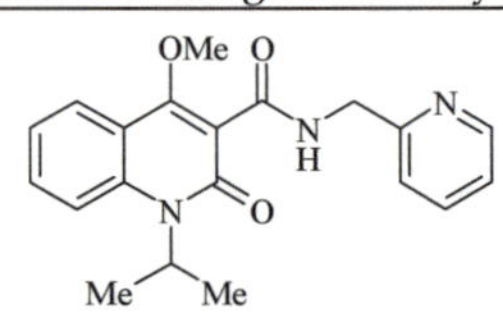 Calculated analgesic activity 75%	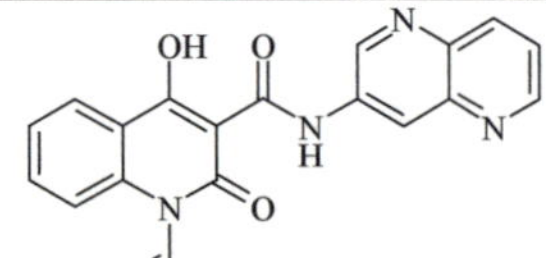 Calculated analgesic activity 80%
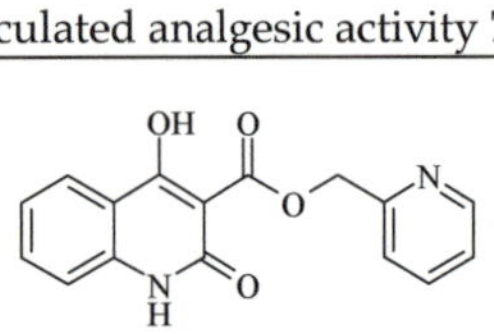 Calculated analgesic activity 72%	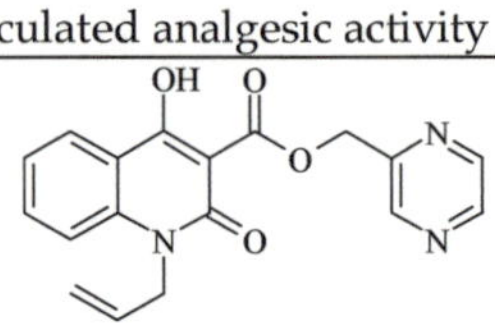 Calculated analgesic activity 76%	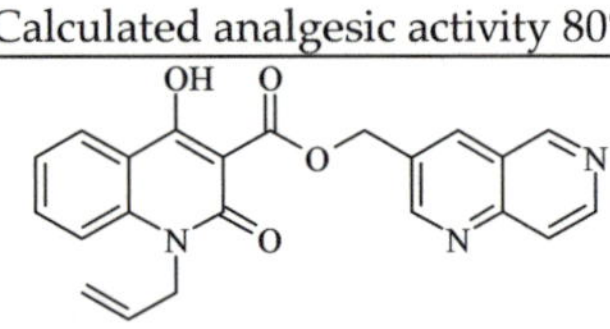 Calculated analgesic activity 77%

Table 7. Virtual quinoline-3-carboxamides and quinoline-3-carboxylates with potentially high activity

Analysis of toxicity and mutagenicity of highly active compounds. Toxicity and mutagenicity are the most important characteristics of any biologically active substance. How powerful specific action a pretender to drug does possess, but without conformance to the current requirements of safety it can never be allowed to medical application. Hence attempts of researchers to manage toxicity and mutagenicity of a new potential drug at the early stages of its development become clearer. Computer prognosis may be quite useful in such cases. For this purpose the already known QSAR models are suitable [73, 75]. One of them allows estimating a possible toxicity of compounds in relation to the model infusoria *Tetrahymena pyriformis,* another one – their mutagenicity within a framework of Ames test. To characterize toxicity the following scale has been suggested: *-2 < low toxic ≤ 0; 0 < moderately toxic < +1; +1 ≤ high toxic*. The results of calculation of mutagenicity are of two classes: *0 – non-mutagenic substances, 1 – mutagenic substances*.

According to the mathematical prognosis the most active pain-killers found among the derivatives of 1,2-dihydroquinolin-2-ones belong to low toxic substances (Table 8). Although calculations confirm our assumption (see section 3.3) about a noticeable increase of toxicity when introducing a bromine atom in the benzene moiety of the quinolone ring, but the presence of the atom is still permitted. But the second bromine atom in the molecule is extremely undesirable – besides enhancement of toxicity it promotes appearance of mutagenicity.

Compound	Toxicity	Mutagenicity	Compound	Toxicity	Mutagenicity
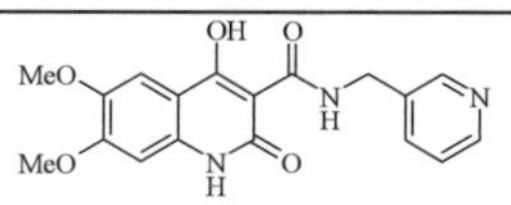	- 1.61	0	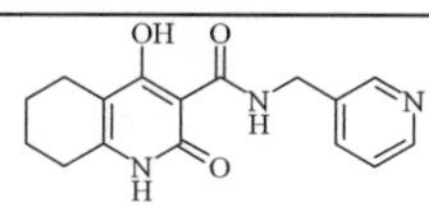	- 1.12	0
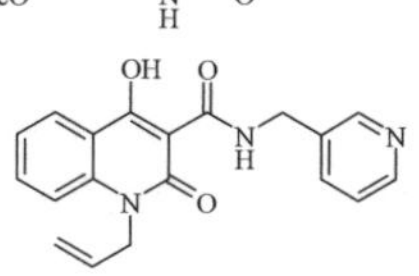	- 0.88	0	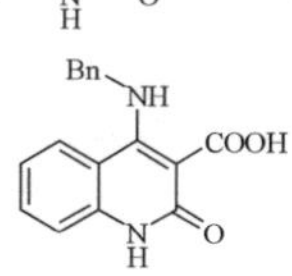	- 1.05	0
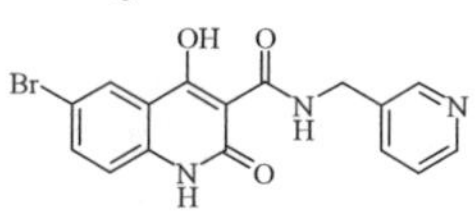	+ 0.15	0	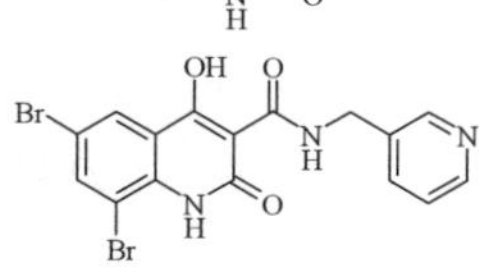	+ 0.23	1

Table 8. Calculated toxicity and mutagenicity of certain 1,2-dihydroquinolin-2-ones

Modeling of active compounds metabolism is one more example of using the obtained QSAR model in chemical and biological research. Modeling itself is performed by another method, of course, – in this case transformation of the most active 1,2-dihydroquinolin-2-ones into virtual metabolites under the influence of the rat liver enzymes has been calculated with the help of QSAR ToolBox 3.0 software [76]. Only after this the QSAR model suggested by us is used; with its help the analgesic properties prediction for all theoretically possible metabolites (Table 9 presents only the small part of them) is performed.

Compound	Possible metabolites		
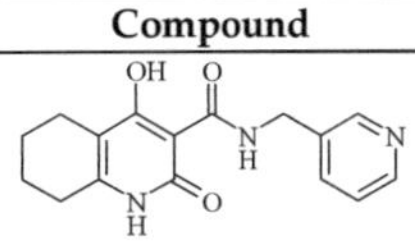 Experimental AA 81%	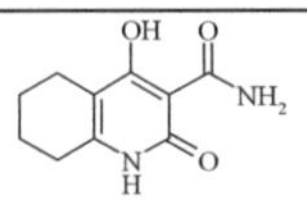 Calculated AA 64%	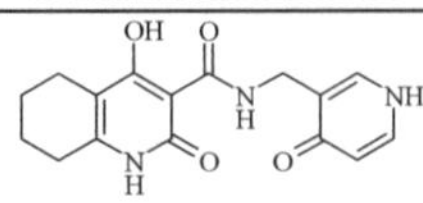 Calculated AA 71%	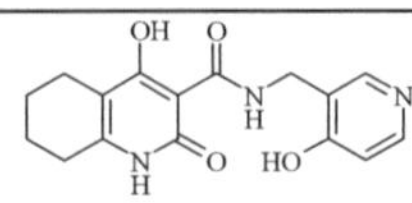 Calculated AA 67%
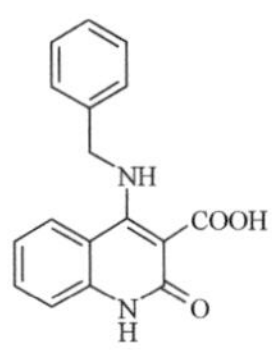 Experimental AA 75%	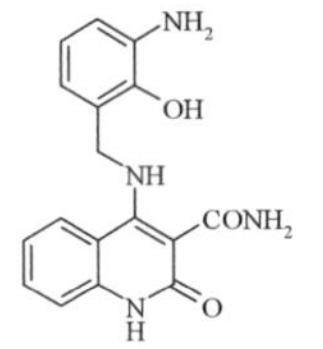 Calculated AA 76%	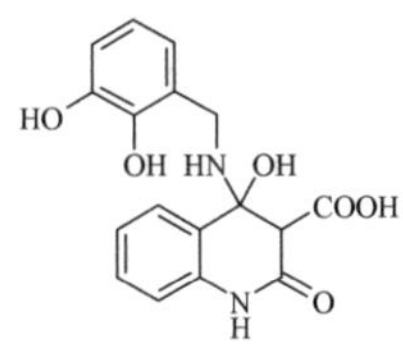 Calculated AA 60%	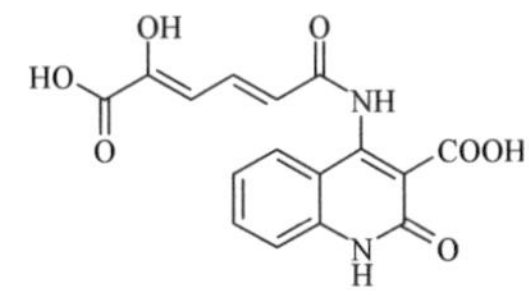 Calculated AA 58%
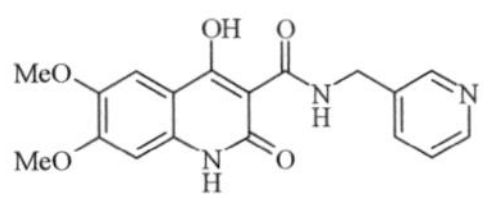 Experimental AA 75%	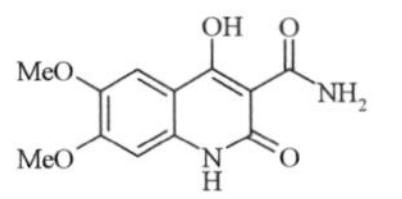 Calculated AA 68%	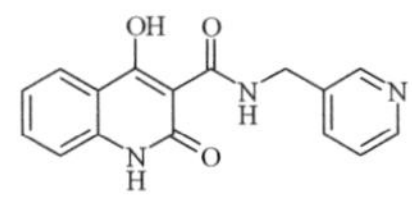 Calculated AA 74%	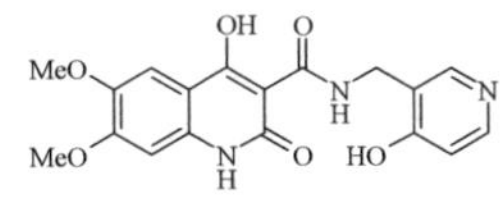 Calculated AA 66%

Table 9. Highly active 1,2-dihydroquinolin-2-ones and their theoretically possible metabolites (AA – analgesic activity)

Such information is rather interesting and important for screening, especially if it is completed by calculations of the possible toxicity and mutagenicity, and not only leading structures, but their virtual metabolites as well. It allows to exclude substances, which are capable to transform into highly toxic or mutagenic products, from candidates to drugs at early stages of screening. Thus, efficiency of the purposeful search of new pain-killers increases significantly.

7.2. 3-(3-R-Carbamoyl-4-hydroxy-2-oxo-1,2-dihydroquinolin-1-yl)propanenitriles and their functional derivatives

Aryl- (hetaryl) propanoic acids and their derivatives have an extremely wide spectrum of biological properties, due to which they have become the base of numerous vital drugs of different pharmacological group [14, 52]. For example, only among NSAIDs permitted to medical application and belonging to nonnarcotic analgesics there are about several dozens of such compounds [46]. Therefore, it is not surprising that further we studied the structures combined two pharmacologically important fragments in one molecule, namely 4-hydroxyquinolin-2-one and propanoic acid. As one of the variants for the practical solution of this task we suggested 3-(3-alkylcarbamoyl-4-hydroxy-2-oxo-1,2-dihydroquinolin-1-yl)propanenitriles (**32**) that are easily avaliable synthetically [77, 78]; as a rule, in the conditions of alkaline hydrolysis they give the corresponding 3-(3-alkylcarbamoyl-4-hydroxy-2-oxo-1,2-dihydroquinolin-1-yl)propanoic acids with good yields (**33**, Figure 25) [78].

The analgesic activity for the synthesized compounds of this great series was measured on the "acetic acid induced writhing" test. The test substances and the reference drug Diclofenac were administered *per os* in the form of a thin aqueous suspension stabilized by Tween-80 in the dose of 5 mg/kg. This dose corresponds to ED_{50} of Diclofenac exactly for the model of "acetic acid induced writhing" [39]. The analysis of the research data obtained shows that the great

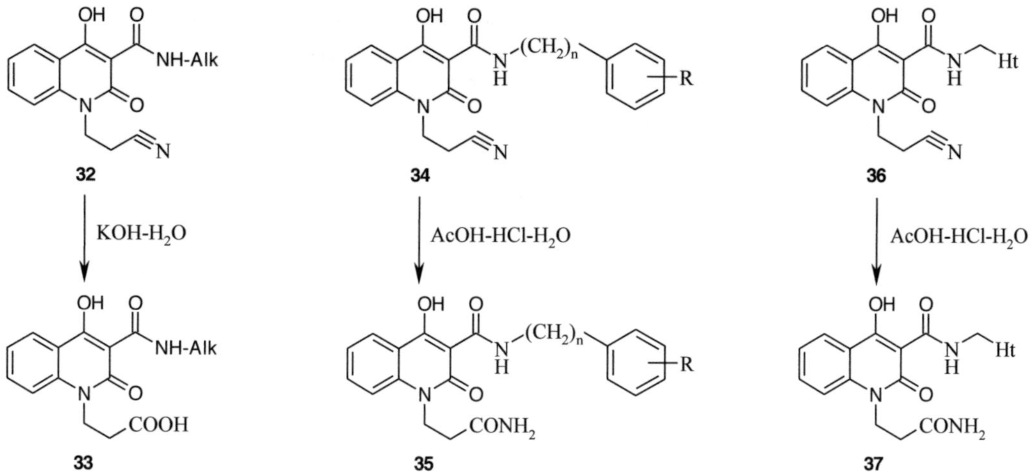

Figure 25. Quinolinyl-propanenitriles **32**, **34**, **36**, quinolinyl-propanoic acids **33** and quinolinyl-propaneamides **35**, **37**

majority of the substances investigated actually reveal the marked and statistically valid ($p \leq 0.05$) analgesic properties.

Thus, from the group of 3-alkylcarbamoyl substituted quinolinyl-propanenitriles **32** some compounds such as propyl- (**32d**), *iso*-butyl- (**32g**), *sec*-butyl- (**32h**), 2-hydroxyethyl- (**32u**), 3-chloropropyl- (**32x**) and 3-methoxypropyl- (**32y**) amides are of immediate interest, their analgesic effect does not yield Diclofenac and even exceeds it (Table 10). In general, transfer from nitriles **32** to the corresponding propanoic acids **33** affects analgesic properties negatively. However, there some positive exceptions – in the case of allylamide **33c**, for example, the transformation mentioned is accompanied with the substantial intensification of activity. If the fact that the synthetic precursor of this compound is also highly active is taken into account, then nitrile **32c** → acid **33c** bunch can be of interest for further more detailed study.

Such approach for studying 3-(3-R-carbamoyl-4-hydroxy-2-oxo-1,2-dihydroquinolin-1-yl)propanenitriles appears to be quite logical and reasonable. However, as a minimum, one important moment was still omitted – intermediate quinolinyl-propaneamides, which form inevitably during trasformation of nitriles into acids, stay out of sight. Meanwhile, interest to these compounds rises many times if it is taken into account that in a living organism metabolism of nitriles can be by different ways, including that by the primary hydration to amides [79, 80]. With regard to the issues in focus it means that the efficiency of any nitrile or amide as a pain-killer increases greatly if their metabolites also reveal analgesic properties. Therefrom the idea appeared to involve by all means the intermediate link – quinolinyl-propaneamides together with initial quinolinyl-propanenitriles and final propanoic acids in the range of the investigations conducted. This allows to select, first of all, those compounds that besides the own high analgesic effect will have a rather active metabolite as promising leading structures from the chain of nitrile → amide → acid.

Compound	Alk	Analgesic activity (decrease in the amount of "acetic acid writhing", %)	
		32 (-$CH_2CH_2C{\equiv}N$)	**33** (-CH_2CH_2COOH)
a	Me	36.3	35.6
b	Et	44.2	28.7
c	All	59.5	73.3
d	Pr	51.0	0
e	*i*-Pr	38.8	40.4
f	Bu	18.6	33.2
g	*i*-Bu	62.1	0
h	*s*-Bu	64.3	10.5
i	C_5H_{11}	38.5	40.7
j	*i*-C_5H_{11}	42.1	20.4
k	C_6H_{13}	47.0	17.9
l	C_7H_{15}	45.3	16.7
m	C_8H_{17}	49.4	22.5
n	C_9H_{19}	42.6	31.3
o	$C_{10}H_{21}$	40.2	16.8
p	*cyclo*-C_3H_5	43.3	0
q	*cyclo*-C_5H_9	40.5	22.9
r	*cyclo*-C_6H_{11}	48.7	15.2
s	*cyclo*-C_7H_{13}	46.4	12.6
t	Adamantan-1-yl	31.1	10.5
u	CH_2CH_2OH	51.2	–
v	$CH_2CH_2CH_2OH$	47.3	–
w	CH_2CH_2Cl	24.9	–
x	$CH_2CH_2CH_2Cl$	63.0	–
y	$CH_2CH_2CH_2OMe$	50.6	–
z	$CH_2CH_2CH_2OPr$-*i*	45.4	–
Diclofenac (5 mg/kg)		52.0	

Table 10. The analgesic activity of alkylcarbamoyl substituted quinolinyl-propanenitriles **32** and the corresponding quinolinyl-propanoic acids **33**

To implement this idea the method of selective hydration of 3-(3-R-carbamoyl-4-hydroxy-2-oxo-1,2-dihydroquinolin-1-yl)propanenitriles to the corresponding propaneamides is required. The task is not so simple than it may seem at first sight since amides primarily formed are usually subjected to hydrolysis much easier than initial nitriles. As a result, it is not always possible to stop the reactions of this type at the stage of amides formation. It is for this reason that the aforementioned alkaline hydrolysis of nitriles **32** to acids **33** is intentionally unsuitable for obtaining propaneamides.

Compound	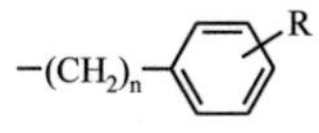	Analgesic activity (decrease in the amount of "acetic acid writhing", %)	
		34 ($-CH_2CH_2C{\equiv}N$)	**35** ($-CH_2CH_2CONH_2$)
a	$PhCH_2$	54.4	–
b	*cyclo*-$C_6H_{11}CH_2$	29.3	–
c	2-$FC_6H_4CH_2$	20.3	38.3
d	4-$FC_6H_4CH_2$	67.1	36.4
e	2-$ClC_6H_4CH_2$	16.5	0
f	4-$ClC_6H_4CH_2$	0	56.0
g	2-$MeC_6H_4CH_2$	39.2	40.9
h	3-$MeC_6H_4CH_2$	18.0	41.1
i	4-$MeC_6H_4CH_2$	0	28.6
j	2-$MeOC_6H_4CH_2$	38.1	–
k	4-$MeOC_6H_4CH_2$	34.8	35.5
l	3,4-$(MeO)_2C_6H_3CH_2$	0	39.2
m	Piperonyl	0	14.7
n	(±) PhCH(Me)	16.1	47.8
o	*S*(-) PhCH(Me)	10.6	46.1
p	*R*(+) PhCH(Me)	21.7	47.0
q	(±) 4-$MeOC_6H_4CH(Me)$	46.6	–
r	*S*(-) 4-$MeOC_6H_4CH(Me)$	17.3	–
s	*R*(+) 4-$MeOC_6H_4CH(Me)$	22.5	–
t	$PhCH_2CH_2$	55.3	–
u	3-$ClC_6H_4CH_2CH_2$	42.6	–
v	4-$ClC_6H_4CH_2CH_2$	23.4	–
w	4-$MeOC_6H_4CH_2CH_2$	64.6	35.7
x	3,4-$(MeO)_2C_6H_3CH_2CH_2$	39.5	20.8
y	$PhCH_2CH_2CH_2$	46.6	
Diclofenac (5 mg/kg)		57.2	

Table 11. The analgesic activity of arylalkylcarbamoyl substituted propanenitriles **34** and the corresponding propaneamides **35**

We succeeded to find the effective method of transformation of 3-(3-arylalkylcarbamoyl-4-hydroxy-2-oxo-1,2-dihydroquinoline-1-yl)propanenitriles (**34**) into the corresponding propaneamides **35** with the help of a simple and available reagent – the mixture of hydrochloric and acetic acids with the low content of water [81]. The method is interesting by the fact that, if required, it allows to perform more profound chemical transformations – for example, hydrolysis of nitriles in amides – only by increasing the reaction duration.

Compound	CH_2-Ht	Analgesic activity (decrease in the amount of "acetic acid writhing", %)	
		36 ($-CH_2CH_2C{\equiv}N$)	**37** ($-CH_2CH_2CONH_2$)
a	Picolyl-2	72.3	47.0
b	Picolyl-3	36.6	10.2
c	Picolyl-4	21.0	31.2
d	Furfuryl	0	–
e	5-Me-furfuryl	59.8	–
f	Tetrahydrofurfuryl	15.4	0
g	Thiophen-2-ylmethyl	0	–
Diclofenac (5 mg/kg)		44.3	

Table 12. The analgesic activity of hetarylalkylcarbamoyl substituted propanenitriles **36** and the corresponding propaneamides **37**

Comparison of analgesic properties of the obtained triad of arylalkylcarbamoylsubstituted propanenitriles, propaneamides and propanoic acids allows to assert that, as a rule, the acid appears to be the least active in the chain of nitrile → amide → acid. Thus, further we focused our efforts on studying only nitriles and amides. It follows from the data given in Tables 11 and 12 that often quinolinyl-propaneamides actually demonstrate higher analgesic properties than their synthetic precursors. Therefore, it is expedient to perform the further search of potential pain-killers in the range of the compounds studied among 1-(2-cyanoethyl)- and 1-(2-carbamoylethyl)-quinolines. Furthermore, with transfer from acids to amides or nitriles acidity decreases essentially, as well as probability of manifestation of the ulcerogenic action being a serious drawback of many modern analgesics.

By the available data from the whole group of quinolinyl-propanoic acids derivatives studied so far, in addition to the abovementioned allyl substituted nitrile **32c**, 1-(2-cyanoethyl)-*N*-(2-pyridylmethyl)-4-hydroxy-2-oxo-1,2-dihydroquinoline-3-carboxamide (**36a**) deserves attention. The basis for this conclusion is a high analgesic activity of not only these nitriles themselves, but of their possible metabolites as well – acid **33c** and amide **37a**, respectively.

7.3. 1-R-4-Hydroxy-2,2-dioxo-1*H*-2λ6,1-benzothiazine-3-carboxamides

Oxicams are an integral part of the range of modern non-steroidal anti-inflammatory drugs with the marked analgesic effect in the range of their biological activities [14, 46, 52]. Piroxicam (**38**, R = 2-Py, Figure 26) became the first commercially successful drug of this group. Later its more effective analogs – Isoxicam (**38**, R = 5-Me-isoxazol-3-yl), Meloxicam (**38**, R = 5-Methiazol-2-yl), etc., appeared at the pharmaceutical market. Today they are widely used by practical medicine in treating numerous rheumatic and autoimmune human diseases under the common name of selective inhibitors of cyclooxygenase-2. It is interesting that isomeric oxicams of 4-hydroxy-1-R-2,2-dioxo-1*H*-2λ⁶,1-benzothiazine-3-carboxamides (**39**), which are different only by reverse mutual arrangement of atoms of nitrogen and sulfur in the thiazine cycle, remain practically completely unstudied at present. The cause of the existing situation is known – it is the absence of effective preparative methods for the synthesis of compounds of this chemical group.

38 **39**

Figure 26. Oxicams (**38**) and isomeric 4-hydroxy-2,2-dioxo-1*H*-2λ⁶,1-benzothiazine-3-carboxamides (**39**)

It should be noted that almost half a century ago some 1-*N*-methyl-substituted carboxanilides **39** were obtained by the reaction of l-methyl-3,4-dihydro-lH-2,l-benzothiazin-4-one 2,2-dioxide with isocyanates in dimethyl sulfoxide solution with the yields from 28 to 100% [82]. However, because of the low yields at the first two stages of obtaining the initial l-methyl-3,4-dihydro-lH-2,l-benzothiazin-4-one 2,2-dioxide this four-step synthetic scheme of 1-methyl-4-hydroxy-2,2-dioxo-1*H*-2λ⁶,1-benzothiazine-3-carboxamides **39** appeared to be unattractive. Furthermore, its application is greatly limited by the necessity of using isocyanates – they are often expensive or almost unavailable reagents, and it significantly complicates the research for purposeful search of "structure – property" regularities. As a result, unfortunately, this undoubtedly interesting work [82] has not got its further development.

Taking these circumstances into account we offer a fundamentally different three-step scheme for the synthesis of the target 1-R-4-hydroxy-2,2-dioxo-1*H*-2λ⁶,1-benzothiazine-3-carboxamides **39** suggesting the initial obtaining of alkyl 1-R-4-hydroxy-2,2-dioxo-1*H*-2λ⁶,1-benzothiazine-3-carboxylates; with their subsequent amidation a practically unlimited and freely available range of various alkyl-, aryl- and hetarylamides can be used.

As was shown earlier, lower alkyl 1-R-4-hydroxy-2-oxo-1,2-dihydroquinoline-3-carboxylates are easily and rapidly amidated by primary and even secondary alkyl-, aryl- and hetarylamines. At the same time for their high reactivity it is necessary their simultaneous presence in the pyridinic part of the molecule of both 4-OH and 2-C=O groups [32]. With the transfer to alkyl 1-R-4-hydroxy-2,2-dioxo-1*H*-2λ⁶,1-benzothiazine-3-carboxylates the powerful acidifying effect of the sulfo group so greatly increases 4-OH-acidity that the ordinary salt formation begins to prevent amidation. By comparison – the salts of alkyl 1-R-4-hydroxy-2-oxo-1,2-dihydroquinoline-3-carboxylates are extremely unstable with amines and rapidly decompose even by carbon dioxide of the air [83]; and, as a rule, they do not cause problems in amidation. On the contrary the similar salts of their 2-sulfo analogs can be readily isolated and characterized. When heating them in the medium of a highly boiling inert solvent they can be transformed with the high yields into the corresponding 1-R-4-hydroxy-2,2-dioxo-1*H*-2λ^6,1-benzothiazine-3-carboxamides **39**. Although for this purpose several hours are needed, whereas in case of 2-carbonyl derivatives the similar procedure takes only 3-5 min.

In general, the method offered appeared to be quite effective and with its help we succeeded in synthesizing a great series of the target alkyl-, arylalkyl-, aryl- and hetarylamides of 1-R-4-hydroxy-2,2-dioxo-1*H*-2λ^6,1-benzothiazine-3-carboxylic acids. To confirm their structure NMR (^{1}H and ^{13}C) spectroscopy, mass spectrometry, and in some cases X-ray structural analysis have been used.

The screening study of analgesic properties of 1-R-4-hydroxy-2,2-dioxo-1*H*-2λ^6,1-benzothiazine-3-carboxamides **39** was performed in white nonlinear male rats using the standard model of "tail flick" thermal irritation [65]. The substances under research and reference-drugs were introduced in the dose of 20 mg/kg orally in the form of a fine aqueous suspension stabilized by Tween-80. The antinociceptive effect was estimated by comparing the duration of the latent period (the time before tail flick) and in one hour after introduction of the substances studied.

According to the results of the pharmacological research among 1-R-4-hydroxy-2,2-dioxo-1*H*-2λ^6,1-benzothiazine-3-carboxamides **39** synthesized the substances, which exceed greatly the known drugs both of oxicam range (Piroxicam and Meloxicam) and other chemical groups (Diclofenac, Ketorolac and even Nalbuphine, narcotic analgesic introduced intraperitoneally) by their analgesic properties have been found. On this basis some of them are recommended for further profound study as new potential analgesics.

Therefore, the results obtained has demonstrated clearly and convincingly that optimization of the known drugs by creation of their close structural analogs differing only by inverse mutual arrangement of atoms or substituents, which we have called "flip-flop drugs" methodology, is rather interesting, productive and promising for the future.

8. Conclusion

Reviewing the preliminary results of the complex research, which is far from its completion as yet, even now it is possible to state with certainty that 4-hydroxyquinolin-2-ones have actually appeared to be practically the inexhaustible source of highly effective pain-killers. One of these compounds – *N*-(3-pyridylmethyl)-4-hydroxy-6,7-dimethoxy-2-oxo-1,2-dihydroquinoline-3-carboxamide – possesses important analgesic properties on various experimental models; it is practically nontoxic, does not have the ulcerogenic action in therapeutic doses, greatly exceeds many currently known medicines by these parameters and thanks to these facts it is recommended to wide preclinical trials. Besides, according to the results of QSAR-

http://dx.doi.org/10.5772/57402

analysis not only relative contributions of some physical and chemical factors and the structural fragments to the analgesic activity of 1,2-dihydroquinolin-2-ones have been determined, but new potentially highly active virtual substances, which are suitable enough for synthesis and further testing, have been suggested. The primary pharmacological screening has also found some promising analgesics, but among 3-(3-R-carbamoyl-4-hydroxy-2-oxo-1,2-dihydroquinolin-1-yl)propanenitriles already obtained and 1-R-4-hydroxy-2,2-dioxo-1*H*-2λ^6,1-benzothiazine-3-carboxamides that are structurally related to them.

Acknowledgements

We sincerely appreciate the help of Doctor of Chemistry A.V. Turov (Taras Shevchenko National University, Kiev, Ukraine) and Candidate of Chemistry S.V. Shishkina (NTC "Institute for Single Crystals" National Academy of Sciences of Ukraine, Kharkov, Ukraine) in studying the structure of the compounds synthesized.

Author details

Igor V. Ukrainets[1], Olga V. Gorokhova[1], Nidal Amin Jaradat[2], Lidiya A. Petrushova[1], Elena V. Mospanova[3], Larisa V. Savchenkova[4], Victor E. Kuz'min[5] and Anatoliy V. Lyahovsky[5]

1 Department of Pharmaceutical Chemistry, National University of Pharmacy, Kharkov, Ukraine

2 Department of Pharmacy, An-Najah National University College of Pharmacy, Nablus, Palestine

3 Department of Organic Substances Technology, Chemical Technologies Institute of the Vladimir Dal' Eastern-Ukrainian National University, Rubizhne, Ukraine

4 Department of Clinical Pharmacology and Pharmacotherapy, Lugansk State Medical University, Lugansk, Ukraine

5 Department of Molecular Structure and Chemoinformatics, A.V. Bogatsky Physico-Chemical Institute NAS of Ukraine, Odessa, Ukraine

References

[1] Goebel JR, Doering LV, Shugarman LR, Asch SM, Sherbourne CD, Lanto AB, Evangelista LS, Nyamathi AM, Maliski SL, Lorenz KA. Heart failure: the hidden problem

of pain. Journal of Pain and Symptom Management 2009; 38(5) 698-707. DOI: 10.1016/j.jpainsymman.2009.04.022.

[2] Alexander EP. History, physical examination, and differential diagnosis of neck pain. Physical Medicine and Rehabilitation Clinics of North America 2011; 22(3) 383-393. DOI: 10.1016/j.pmr.2011.02.005.

[3] Foster NE, Hartvigsen J, Croft PR. Taking responsibility for the early assessment and treatment of patients with musculoskeletalpain: a review and critical analysis. Arthritis Research & Therapy 2012; 14(1) 205. DOI: 10.1186/ar3743. http://arthritis-research.com/content/14/1/205 (accessed 29 February 2012).

[4] Henderson RA, Lachiewicz PF. Groin pain after replacement of the hip: aetiology, evaluation and treatment. Journal of Bone and Joint Surgery. British volume 2012; 94(2) 145-151. DOI: 10.1302/0301-620X.94B2.27736.

[5] Yuxiang L, Lingjun Z, Lu T, Mengjie L, Xing M, Fengping S, Jing C, Xianli M, Jijun Z. Burn patients' experience of pain management: a qualitative study. Burns: Journal of the International Society for Burn Injuries 2012; 38(2) 180-186. DOI: 10.1016/j.burns. 2011.09.006.

[6] Balagué F, Mannion AF, Pellisé F, Cedraschi C. Non-specific low back pain. Lancet. 2012; 379(9814) 482-491. DOI: 10.1016/S0140-6736(11)60610-7.

[7] McGeary DD, McGeary CA, Gatchel RJ. A comprehensive review of telehealth for pain management: where we are and the way ahead. Pain Practice: the official journal of World Institute of Pain 2012; 12(7) 570-577. DOI: 10.1111/j. 1533-2500.2012.00534.x.

[8] Divakaran E. Pain - when it affects the person. Journal of Pain & Palliative Care Pharmacotherapy 2011; 25(4) 372-373. DOI: 10.3109/15360288.2011.625469.

[9] Van der Veek SM, Derkx HH, de Haan E, Benninga MA, Boer F. Social Science & Medicine 2012; 74(2) 112-119. DOI: 10.1016/j.socscimed.2011.10.023.

[10] Bond M. Pain education issues in developing countries and responses to them by the International Association for the Study of Pain. Pain Research & Management : the journal of the Canadian Pain Society 2011; 16(6) 404-406.

[11] Goldberg DS, McGee SJ. Pain as a global public health priority. BMC Public Health 2011, 11(10) 770. DOI:10.1186/1471-2458-11-770. http://www.biomedcentral.com/ 1471-2458/11/770 (accessed 6 October 2011).

[12] Sarzi-Puttini P, Vellucci R, Zuccaro SM, Cherubino P, Labianca R, Fornasari D. The appropriate treatment of chronic pain. Clinical Drug Investigation 2012; 32(1) 21-33. DOI: 10.2165/11630050-000000000-00000.

[13] McGee SJ, Kaylor BD, Emmott H, Christopher MJ. Defining chronic pain ethics. Pain Medicine (Malden, Mass.) 2011; 12(9) 1376-1384. DOI: 10.1111/j.1526-4637.2011.01192.x.

[14] Kleemann A., Engel J., Kutscher B., Reichert D. Pharmaceutical Substances: Syntheses, Patents, Applications of the most relevant APIs; 5th Revised edition. Stuttgart: Thieme; 2008.

[15] Aronson J.K. Meyler's Side Effects of Analgesics and Anti-inflammatory Drugs; 1st edition. San Diego: Elsevier Science; 2009.

[16] Sewell RA, Halpern JH, Pope HG Jr. Response of cluster headache to psilocybin and LSD. Neurology 2006; 66(12) 1920-1922. DOI: 10.1212/01.wnl.0000219761.05466.43.

[17] Sarbani Pal, Shylaprasad Durgadas, Suresh Babu Nallapati, Khagga Mukkanti, Ravikumar Kapavarapu, Chandana Lakshmi T. Meda, Kishore V.L. Parsa, Manojit Pal. Novel 1-alkynyl substituted 1,2-dihydroquinoline derivatives from nimesulide (and their 2-oxo analogues): A new strategy to identify inhibitors of PDE4B. Bioorganic & Medicinal Chemistry Letters 2011; 21(21) 6573-6576.

[18] Alam MM, Shaharyar M, Hamid H, Nazreen S, Haider S, Alam MS. Synthesis of novel 8-hydroxyquinolin based 1,3,4-oxadiazoles and S-substituted 1,2,4-triazole derivatives and evaluation of their anti-inflammatory, analgesic, ulcerogenic and antimicrobial activities. Medicinal Chemistry 2011; 7(6) 663-673. DOI: 10.2174/157340611797928334.

[19] Son MH, Kim JY, Lim EJ, Baek DJ, Choi K, Lee JK, Pae AN, Min SJ, Cho YS. Synthesis and biological evaluation of 2-(arylethynyl)quinoline derivatives as mGluR5 antagonists for the treatment of neuropathic pain. Bioorganic & Medicinal Chemistry Letters 2013; 23(5) 1472–1476. DOI: 10.1016/j.bmcl.2012.12.056.

[20] Diaz JL, Christmann U, Fernández A, Luengo M, Bordas M, Enrech R, Carro M, Pascual R, Burgueño J, Merlos M, Benet-Buchholz J, Cerón-Bertran J, Ramírez J, Reinoso RF, Fernández de Henestrosa AR, Vela JM, Almansa C. Synthesis and Biological Evaluation of a New Series of Hexahydro-2H-pyrano[3,2-*c*]quinolines as Novel Selective σ1 Receptor Ligands. Journal of Medicinal Chemistry 2013 May 9;56(9):3656-65. DOI: 10.1021/jm400181k.

[21] Bouzidi N, Deokar H, Vogrig A, Boucherle B, Ripoche I, Abrunhosa-Thomas I, Dorr L, Wattiez AS, Lian LY, Marin P, Courteix C, Ducki S. Identification of PDZ ligands by docking-based virtual screening for the development of novel analgesic agents. Bioorganic & Medicinal Chemistry Letters 2013; 23(9) 2624-2627. DOI: 10.1016/j.bmcl.2013.02.100.

[22] Furlotti G, Alisi MA, Apicella C, Capezzone de Joannon A, Cazzolla N, Costi R, Cuzzucoli Crucitti G, Garrone B, Iacovo A, Magarò G, Mangano G, Miele G, Ombrato R, Pescatori L, Polenzani L, Rosi F, Vitiello M, Di Santo R. Discovery and pharmacological profile of new 1H-indazole-3-carboxamide and 2H-pyrrolo[3,4-*c*]quinoline deriv-

atives as selective serotonin 4 receptor ligands. Journal of Medicinal Chemistry 2012; 55(22) 9446-9466. DOI: 10.1021/jm300573d.

[23] Rajanarendar E, Nagi Reddy M, Rama Krishna S, Rama Murthy K, Reddy YN, Rajam MV. Design, synthesis, antimicrobial, anti-inflammatory and analgesic activity of novel isoxazolyl pyrimido[4,5-b]quinolines and isoxazolyl chromeno[2,3-d]pyrimidin-4-ones. European Journal of Medicinal Chemistry 2012; 55 273-283. DOI: 10.1016/j.ejmech.2012.07.029.

[24] Ukrainets IV, Sidorenko LV, Davidenko AA, Yarosh AK. 4-Hydroxy-2-quinolones. 174. Hydrochlorides of [(alkylamino)-alkyl]amides of 1-allyl-4-hydroxy-6,7-dimethoxy-2-oxo-1,2-dihydro-quinoline-3-carboxylic acid – a new class of opioid receptor antagonists. Chemistry of Heterocyclic Compounds 2010; 46(4) 445-451.

[25] Ukrainets IV, Mospanova EV, Davidenko AA, Shishkina SV. 4-Hydroxy-2-quinolones. 180. Synthesis, chemical reactions, and analgesic activity of 1-allyl-4-hydroxy-6,7-dimethoxy-2-oxo-1,2-dihydroquinoline-3-carboxylic acid alkylamides. Chemistry of Heterocyclic Compounds 2010; 46(9) 1084-1095.

[26] Ukrainets IV, Mospanova EV, Jaradat NA, Bevz OV, Turov AV. 4-Hydroxy-2-quinolones. 204. Synthesis, bromination, and analgetic properties of 1-allyl-4-hydroxy-6,7-dimethoxy-2-oxo-1,2-dihydroquinoline-3-carboxylic acid arylalkylamides. Chemistry of Heterocyclic Compounds 2012; 48(9) 1347-1356.

[27] Ukrainets IV, Sidorenko LV, Gorokhova OV, Shishkina SV, Turov AV. 4-Hydroxy-2-quinolones. 118. Synthesis, structure, and chemical properties of 2-bromomethyl-5-oxo-1,2-dihydro-5H-oxazolo-[3,2-*a*]quinoline-4-carboxylic acid and its ethyl ester. Chemistry of Heterocyclic Compounds 2007; 43(5) 617-628.

[28] Ukrainets IV, Tkach AA, Grinevich LA, Turov AV, Bevz OV. 4-Hydroxy-2-quinolones. 154. Pyrimidin-2-ylamides of 1-R-4-hydroxy-2-oxo-1,2-dihydroquinoline-3-carboxylic acids. Synthesis, structure, and properties. Chemistry of Heterocyclic Compounds 2009; 45(5) 567-579.

[29] Ukrainets IV, Grinevich LA, Tkach AA, Bevz OV, Slobodzian SV. 4-Hydroxy-2-quinolones. 168. Synthesis, chemical and antitubercular properties of 1-R-4-hydroxy-2-oxo-1,2-dihydroquinoline-3-carboxylic acid pyrazin-2-ylamides. Chemistry of Heterocyclic Compounds 2009; 45(9) 1058-1068.

[30] Ukrainets IV, Bevz OV, Mospanova EV, Savchenkova LV, Yankovich SI. 4-Hydroxy-2-quinolones. 202. Synthesis, chemical and biological properties of 4-hydroxy-6,7-dimethoxy-2-oxo-1,2-dihydroquinoline-3-carboxylic acid alkylamides. Chemistry of Heterocyclic Compounds 2012; 48(2) 320-326.

[31] Jönsson S, Andersson G, Fex T, Fristedt T, Hedlund G, Jansson K, Abramo L, Fritzson I, Pekarski O, Runström A, Sandin H, Thuvesson I, Björk A. Synthesis and biological evaluation of new 1,2-dihydro-4-hydroxy-2-oxo-3-quinolinecarboxamides for

treatment of autoimmune disorders: structure-activity relationship. Journal of Medicinal Chemistry 2004; 47(8) 2075-2088.

[32] Ukrainets IV, Sidorenko LV, Svechnikova EN, Shishkin OV. 4-Hydroxy-2-quinolones. 130. The reactivity of ethyl 4-hydroxy-2-oxo-1,2-dihydroquinoline-3-carboxylates. Chemistry of Heterocyclic Compounds 2007; 43(10) 1275-1279.

[33] Tsuji K, Spears GW, Nakamura K, Tojo T, Seki N, Sugiyama A, Matsuo M. Synthesis and antinephritic activities of quinoline-3-carboxamides and related compounds. Bioorganic & Medicinal Chemistry Letters 2002; 12(1) 85-88.

[34] Collin X, Robert JM, Duflos M, Wielgosz G, Le Baut G, Robin-Dubigeon C, Grimaud N, Lang F, Petit JY. Synthesis of N-pyridinyl(methyl)-1,2-dihydro-4-hydroxy-2-oxoquinoline-3-carboxamides and analogues and their anti-inflammatory activity in mice and rats. The Journal of Pharmacy and Pharmacology 2001; 53(3) 417-423.

[35] Bevz OV, Yankovich SI, Mospanova YeV, Ukrainets IV, Savchenkova LV. Synthesis and analgetic activity of 4-hydroxy-6,7-dimethoxy-2-oxo-1,2-dihydroquinoline-3-carboxylic acid hydroxy-, alkoxy- and cycloalkylamides. [in Ukrainian]Visnik Farmatsii 2011; No. 4(68) 45-48.

[36] Mospanova YeV, Ukrainets IV, Bevz OV, Savchenkova LV, Yankovich SI. The search of new analgesics among 4-hydroxy-6,7-dimethoxy-2-oxo-1,2-dihydroquinoline-3-carboxylic acid benzylamides. [in Russian]. Zhurnal Organicheskoi i Farmatsevticheskoi Khimii 2012; 10(2) 50-53.

[37] Mospanova YeV, Ukrainets IV, Bevz OV, Savchenkova LV, Yankovich SI. The search of new analgesics in the range of 4-hydroxy-6,7-dimethoxy-2-oxo-1,2-dihydroquinoline-3-carboxylic acid pyridylamides. [in Ukrainian]. Visnik Farmatsii 2011; No. 2(66) 29-31.

[38] Mospanova YeV, Ukrainets IV, Bevz OV, Savchenkova LV, Yankovich SI. Halogen substituted anilides of 4-hydroxy-6,7-dimethoxy-2-oxo-1,2-dihydroquinoline-3-carboxylic acid. Synthesis and biological properties. [in Russian]. Zhurnal Organicheskoi i Farmatsevticheskoi Khimii 2011; 9(3) 56-59.

[39] Singh PP, Junnarkar AY, Rao CS, Varma RK, Shridhar DR. Acetic acid and phenylquinone writhing test: a critical study in mice. Methods and Findings in Experimental and Clinical Pharmacology 1983; 5(9) 601-606.

[40] Wagener M, Lommerse JP. The quest for bioisosteric replacements. Journal of Chemical Information and Modeling 2006; 46(2) 677-685. DOI: 10.1021/ci0503964.

[41] Villar HO, Hansen MR. Computational techniques in fragment based drug discovery. Current Topics in Medicinal Chemistry 2007; 7(15) 1509-1513. DOI: 10.2174/156802607782194725.

[42] Devereux M, Popelier PL. In silico techniques for the identification of bioisosteric replacements for drug design. Current Topics in Medicinal Chemistry 2010; 10(6) 657-668. DOI: 10.2174/156802610791111470.

[43] Wirth M, Zoete V, Michielin O, Sauer WH. SwissBioisostere: a database of molecular replacements for ligand design. Nucleic acids research 2013; 41(D1) D1137-1143. DOI: 10.1093/nar/gks1059.

[44] Zefirova ON, Zefirov NS. On the history emergence and development of the concept bioisosterism. [in Russian]. Reports of Moscow State University. Series 2, Chemistry 2002; 54(4) 221-226.

[45] King F.D. Medicinal Chemistry: Principles and Practice. Cambridge: Royal Society of Chemistry; 2002.

[46] Sigidin Ya.A., Shvarts G.Ya., Arzamastsev A.P., Liberman S.S. Drug Therapy of the Anti- inflammatory Process (Experimental and Clinical Pharmacology of Anti-inflammatory Medications). [in Russian]. Moscow: Meditsina; 1988.

[47] Ukrainets IV, El Kayal SA, Gorokhova OV, Sidorenko LV, Alexeeva TV. Synthesis and antituberculosis properties of 1-R-4-hydroxy-2-oxo-1,2-dihydoquinoline-3-carboxylic acids picolylamides. [in Ukrainian]. Visnik Farmatsii 2005; No. 1(41) 10-14.

[48] Bernshtein J. Polymorphism in molecular crystals. Oxford: Clarendon Press; 2002.

[49] Zefirov NS, Palyulin VA, Dashevskaya EE. Stereochemical studies. XXXIV. Quantitative description of ring puckering via torsional angles. The case of six-membered rings. Journal of Physical Organic Chemistry 1990; 3(3) 147-154.

[50] Ukrainets I, Golik N. Polymorphism of the new quinolone diuretic Carboquinol. In: proceedings of the XVth International Conference "Heterocycles in Bio-organic Chemistry", 27-30 May 2013, Riga, Latvia. Riga: Ieguldījums Tavā Nākotnē; 2013.

[51] Ukrainets IV, Davidenko AA, Mospanova EV, Sidorenko LV, Svechnikova EN. 4-Hydroxy-2-quinolones. 176. 4-R-2-Oxo-1,2-dihydroquinoline-3-carboxylic acids. Synthesis, physico-chemical and biological properties. Chemistry of Heterocyclic Compounds 2010; 46(5) 559-568.

[52] Mashkovskii M.D. Drugs. [in Russian]. Moscow: RIA Novaya Volna, Umerenkov; 2009.

[53] Ukrainets IV, Mospanova EV, Davidenko AA, Shishkina SV. 4-Hydroxy-2-quinolones. 192. Relationship of structure and analgesic activity of 4-amino-2-oxo-1,2-dihydroquinoline-3-carboxylic acids and their derivatives. Chemistry of Heterocyclic Compounds 2010; 46(11) 1371-1379.

[54] Kaneko T. Troglitazone (CS-045): a new antidiabetic agent. Hormone and Metabolic Research 1997; 29(5) 203-213.

[55] Thacker HP. S-amlodipine – the 2007 clinical review. Journal of the Indian Medical Association 2007; 105(4) 180-182.

[56] Kubinyi H. In Looking ups of the New Compounds-leaders for Creation of Drugs [in Russian]. Russian Chemical Journal 2006; L(2) 5-17. http://www.chem.msu.su/rus/journals/jvho/2006-2/5.pdf

[57] Yurovskaya MA, Kurkin AB. Some aspects of the relationship chirality and biological activity. [in Russian]. In: proceedings of the International Scientific Conference "Advances synthesis and complex formation", 18-22 April 2011, Moscow. Russian Federation: Peoples' Friendship University of Russia; 2011.

[58] Fernandes BJ, Silva CM, Andrade JM, Matthes AC, Coelho EB, Lanchote VL. Pharmacokinetics of cyclophosphamide enantiomers in patients with breast cancer. Cancer Chemotherapy and Pharmacology 2011; 68(4) 897-904. DOI: 10.1007/s00280-011-1554-7.

[59] de Sousa DP, Nóbrega FF, Santos CC, de Almeida R.N. Anticonvulsant activity of the linalool enantiomers and racemate: investigation of chiral influence. Natural Product Communications 2010; 5(12) 1847-1851.

[60] Raffa RB, Friderichs E, Reimann W, Shank RP, Codd EE, Vaught JL, Jacoby HI, Selve N. Complementary and synergistic antinociceptive interaction between the enantiomers of tramadol. The Journal of Pharmacology and Experimental Therapeutics 1993; 267(1) 331-340.

[61] Shishkin OV, Pichugin KYu, Gorb L, Leszczynski J. Structural non-rigidity of six-membered aromatic rings. Journal of Molecular Structure 2002; 616(1-3) 159-166.

[62] Ukrainets IV, Mospanova YeV, Baumer VN. The crystalline structure of 2-oxo-4-(phenylethylamino)-1,2-dihydroquinoline-3-carboxylic acids as the factor that determines their analgetic activity. [in Russian]. Zhurnal Organicheskoi i Farmatsevticheskoi Khimii 2012; 10(1) 66-71.

[63] Ukrainets IV, Mospanova EV, Savchenkova LV, Yankovich SI. 4-Hydroxy-2-quinolones. 195. Synthesis of novel, potential analgesics based on 4-(hetarylmethyl)amino-2-oxo-1,2-dihydroquinoline-3-carboxylic acids. Chemistry of Heterocyclic Compounds 2011; 47(1) 67-73.

[64] Ukrainets IV, Mospanova EV, Davidenko AA, Tkach AA, Gorokhova OV. 4-Hydroxy-2-quinolones. 179. Synthesis, structure and anti-inflammatory activity of 4-hydroxy-1-methyl-2-oxo-1,2-dihydroquinoline-3-ylacetic acid and its derivatives. Chemistry of Heterocyclic Compounds 2010; 46(8) 947-956.

[65] Vogel H.G., editor. Drug Discovery and Evaluation: Pharmacological Assays. Berlin: Springer; 2008.

[66] Ukrainets IV, Shishkina SV, Shishkin OV, Davidenko AA, Tkach AA. Ethyl 2-(4-hydroxy-1-methyl-2-oxo-1,2-dihydroquinolin-3-yl)acetate. Acta Crystallographica Section E 2009; E65, o968.

[67] Mokhort M.A., Yakovleva L.V., Shapoval O.M. Search and experimental study of pharmacological substances, which are offered as non-narcotic analgesics. In: Stefanov O.V. (ed.), Preclinical Investigations of Medicinal Agents: Methodological Recommendations [in Ukrainian]. Kiev: Avitsena; 2001, p. 307-320.

[68] Gotti G, Carbonelle E, Moretti M, Zwart R, Clementi F. Drugs selective for nicotinic receptor subtypes: a real possibility or a dream? Behavioural Brain Research 2000; 113(1-2) 183-192.

[69] Arias HR. Localization of agonist and competitive antagonist binding sites on nicotinic acetylcholine receptors. Neurochemistry International 2000; 36(7) 595-645.

[70] MacPherson RD. The pharmacological basis of contemporary pain management. Pharmacology & Therapeutics 2000; 88(2) 163-185.

[71] Tolstikov G.A., Dembitskii V.M., Tolstikova T.G., Shults E.E. Epibatidine and problem of non-opioid analgesics. In: Kartsev V.G. (ed.) Selected Methods for Synthesis and Modification of Heterocycles. Vol. 1. [in Russian]. Moscow: IBS PRESS; 2003. p. 418-449.

[72] Young TG, Broad LM, Zwart R, Astles PC, Bodkin M, Sher E, Millar NS. Species Selectivity of a nicotinic acetylcholine receptor agonist is conferred by two adjacent extracellular β4 amino acids that are implicated in the coupling of binding to channel gating. Molecular Pharmacology 2007; 71(2) 389-397.

[73] Kuz'min V.E., Artemenko A.G., Muratov E.N., Polischuk P.G., Ognichenko L.N., Liahovsky A.V., Hromov A.L., Varlamova E.V. Virtual screening and molecular design based on hierarchical QSAR technology. In: Puzyn T., Cronin M., Leszczynski J. (eds) Recent Advances in QSAR Studies. New York: Springer; 2009. p.127-172.

[74] Leonenko II, Egorova AV, Ognichenko LN, Lyahovsky AV, Alexandrov DI, Ukrainets IV, Kuzmin VE, Antonovych VP. QSPR analysis luminescent properties complexes Eu (III) and Tb (III) amides with 2-oxo-4-hydroxyquinoline-3-carboxylic acid. Objects and Methods of Chemical Analysis 2011; 6(1) 38-49.

[75] Sushko I, Novotarskyi S, Körner R, Pandey Anil Kumar, Cherkasov A, Jiazhong Li, Gramatica P, Hansen K, Schroeter T, Müller K-R, Lili Xi, Liu Huanxiang, Yao Xiaojun, Öberg T, Hormozdiari F Dao Phuong, Sahinalp C, Todeschini R, Polishchuk P, Artemenko A, Kuz'min V, Martin TM, Young DM, Fourches D, Muratov E, Tropsha A, Baskin I, Horvath D, Marcou G, Muller C, Varnek A, Prokopenko VV, Tetko IV. Applicability Domains for Classification Problems: Benchmarking of Distance to Models for Ames Mutagenicity Set. Journal of Chemical Information and Modeling 2010; 50(12) 2094-2111. DOI: 10.1021/ci100253r.

[76] OECD Quantitative Structure-Activity Relationships Project. http://www.qsartoolbox.org (accessed 3 June 2013).

[77] Ukrainets IV, Gorokhova OV, Andreeva XV, Sim G. Synthesis, structure and analgesic activity of 1-(2-cyanoethyl)-4-hydroxy-2-oxo-1,2-dihydroquinoline-3-carboxylic acid hydroxy-alkylamides and their derivatives. International Journal of Pharmacy and Pharmacology 2012; 1(3) 034-040.

[78] Ukrainets IV, Andreeva KV, Gorokhova OV, Kravchenko VN. 4-Hydroxy-2-quinolones. 221. Synthesis, structure, and biological activity of 3-(3-(alkylcarbamoyl-4-hydroxy-2-oxo-1,2-dihydroquinolin-1-yl)propanoic acids. Chemistry of Heterocyclic Compounds 2012; 48(12) 1809-1816.

[79] Brady D, Beeton A, Zeevaart J, Kgaje C, van Rantwijk F, Sheldon RA. Applied Microbiology and Biotechnology 2004; 64, (1) 76-85. DOI: 10.1007/s00253-003-1495-0.

[80] Faber K. Biotransformations in Organic Chemistry, Heidelberg: Springer; 2011.

[81] Ukrainets IV, Gorokhova OV, Andreeva KV. Transformation of 3-(3-arylalkylcarbamoyl-4-hydroxy-2-oxo-1,2-dihydroquinolin-1-yl)propanenitriles into amides and acids. Russian Journal of Organic Chemistry 2013; 49(6) 867-871.

[82] Lombardino JG. Preparation of some 4-hydroxyl-l-methyl-1*H*-2,l-benzothiazine-3-carboxanilide 2,2-dioxides. Journal of Heterocyclic Chemistry 1972; 9(2) 315-317.

[83] Ukrainets IV, Sidorenko LV, Golovchenko OS. 4-Hydroxy-2-quinolones. 132. Synthesis, chemical, and biological properties of 1-R-4-hydroxy-2-oxo-1,2-dihydroquinoline-3-carboxylic acids 2-nitrobenzylidenehydrazides. Chemistry of Heterocyclic Compounds 2007; 43(11) 1434-1439.

Chapter 3

The Evolving Role of Opioid Treatment in Chronic Pain Management

Hans Hansen, Carl E. Noe and Gabor B. Racz

Additional information is available at the end of the chapter

http://dx.doi.org/10.5772/58818

1. Introduction

Opioids for chronic pain management have become increasingly controversial, yet many patients continue to be treated with high doses for prolonged periods of time. The misconception between patients and providers alike is that these drugs can be taken without consequences. This liberalized thinking is far from the clinical practice of just two decades ago. Opioids have been destigmatized, and the origins can be traced to industry and a few thought leaders that have since retracted their belief that opioids may be prescribed without negative consequences.

During the 1990's chronic and cancer pain was recognized as being undertreated worldwide. The result was to soften prescribing resistance, particularly in the United States. As a result, many states in the U.S. passed intractable pain treatment acts to protect physicians from disciplinary action when prescribing opioids for non-cancer pain, as well as cancer pain. Unfortunately, that liberalization of opioid prescribing has been associated with a parallel increase in prescription opioid overdoses and deaths. Over the past decade, opioid overdose risk has become such a serious risk factor that Naloxone rescue units have been developed for home use. This rampant failing of safe prescribing habitry has resulted in a ready supply of opioids and a willingness of the consumer to seek these drugs.

Healthy Americans issued a report in October 2013 stating:

"Drug overdose deaths exceed motor vehicle-related deaths in 29 states and Washington DC. Misuse and abuse of prescription drugs costs the country an estimated $ 53.4 billion a year in lost productivity, medical costs and criminal justice costs, and currently only one in 10 Americans with a substance abuse disorder receive treatment." [1] Clearly, the indiscriminate

INTECH
open science | open minds

© 2015 The Author(s). Licensee InTech. This chapter is distributed under the terms of the Creative Commons Attribution License (http://creativecommons.org/licenses/by/3.0), which permits unrestricted use, distribution, and reproduction in any medium, provided the original work is properly cited.

use of opioids has overwhelmed practical and safe prescribing methods, and regulatory agencies have been slow to respond to this opioid prescription epidemic.

This chapter will review recent studies on the subject of opioid prescribing, misuse, and abuse, and present arguments both for and against opioid therapy for chronic pain. Prescribing providers are encouraged to evaluate patients for risk factors of opioid abuse prior to initiating opioid therapy and during treatment. This is good medical practice. Additionally, it is stressed to prescribers to limit opioid doses and duration of drug exposure to further decrease the potential for adverse outcome. [2] Therefore, it is important to educate providers and patients about alternatives to opioids, including non-pharmacologic treatment, and introduce this multimodality concept.

Pain is subjective, and must be addressed from the patients' point of view. Most physicians struggle with pain as a diagnosis because there are few tools available to verify its existence. The value of advanced therapies, such as diagnostic interventions, help characterize the diagnosis, and opioids are rarely a first treatment step in the clinical treatment of chronic pain. Medical specialists are encouraged to improve sharing information about analgesic modalities and alternative interventions that may help an individual patient limit their opioid dose. Advanced therapies, such as interventional options, may not be known to midlevel providers who care for many patients with chronic conditions. Exhausting conservative measures to reduce the opioid load is necessary to optimize best clinical outcome and reduce risk in a clinical pain practice.

Opioid prescribing became an easy and time efficient method to treat pain in non-palliative care settings over the past two decades. The Federation of State Medical Boards endorsed opioids as a legitimate treatment option. [3] Like any clinical therapy, some patients seem to do very well with chronic opioid therapy while others do not. The overdose and diversion problems associated with increased opioid prescribing have recently called for enhanced regulatory activity from a public health perspective. Rethinking prescribing habits is different than relating new therapies in the traditional care model. Opioids are expected by patients, and as a society, expectations of relief are considered a "right", resistance to change is met with varying degrees of resistance. These layers of complexity in the clinical setting place the burden on the provider to secure a course of care that is compassionate, yet safe and effective.

Over the past 20 years, the prevalence of chronic pain and selecting the proper treatment has remained a consistent challenge for providers and patients alike. Advances in the treatment of chronic pain have primarily centered on pharmacologic management, therapy, and interventional tools. Positive outcomes are often associated with a multimodality approach, but the financial challenges of the healthcare system may limit access to these sophisticated treatment options. Long considered a fifth pathway, proper treatment of pain is necessary, but will be unlikely to support a priority position in the healthcare hierarchy of the future. With the emergence of innovative healthcare payment programs and strong government influence, priority will be given to chronic life-threatening disease states, and followed by those with progressive disabling afflictions. Chronic pain, which is often

http://dx.doi.org/10.5772/58818

a cruel and disabling state, is not a life-threatening entity. In this rapidly evolving health-care delivery system, the pain care provider will be challenged to render effective care, increase the quality of life of those in pain, and minimize risk and cost. Not surprisingly, it is expected that with rising healthcare costs, opioid use will be considered cheap, and a first choice. Escalating opioid use, however, has a direct relationship with adverse consequences. The rapidly increasing supply of opioids in the United States underscores this observation.

DRUGS	1998	1999	2000	2001	2002	2003	2004	2005	2006	2007	2008	2009	2010	12-year % change from 1998 to 2010
Nonmedical Use of Psychotherapeuitics[2, 3]	5.759 (2.6%)	9,220 (4.2%)	8,761 (3.9%)	11,102 (4.9%)	14,795 (6.3%)	15,163 (6.4%)	14,849 (6.2%)	15,346 (6.3%)	16,482 (6.7%)	16,280 (6.6%)	15,166 (6.1%)	16,006 (6.4%)	16,031 (6.3%)	178%
Pain Relievers	--	6,582 (3.0%)	6,466 (2.9%)	8,353 (3.7%)	10,992 (4.7%)	11,671 (4.9%)	11,256 (4.7%)	11,815 (4.9%)	12,649 (5.1%)	12,466 (5.0%)	11,885 (4.8%)	12,405 (4.9%)	12,213 (4.8%)	85% From 1999
OxyContin®	--	--	--	--	--	--	1,213 (0.5%)	1,226 (0.5%)	1,323 (0.5%)	1,422 (0.6%)	1,459 (0.6%)	1,677 (0.7%)	1,869 (0.7%)	54% From 2004
Tranquilizers	1,940 (0.9%)	2,728 (1.2%)	2,731 (1.2%)	3,673 (1.6%)	4,849 (2.1%)	5,051 (2.1%)	5,068 (2.1%)	5,249 (2.2%)	5,058 (2.1%)	5,282 (2.1%)	5,103 (2.0%)	5,460 (2.2%)	5,581 (2.2%)	188%
Stimulants3	1,489 (0.7%)	2,291 (1.0%)	2,112 (0.9%)	2,486 (1.1%)	3,380 (1.4%)	3,031 (1.3%)	3,254 (1.4%)	3,088 (1.3%)	3,791 (1.5%)	2,998 (1.2%)	2,639 (1.1%)	3,060 (1.2%)	2,887 (1.1%)	94%
Sedatives	522 (0.2%)	631 (0.3%)	611 (0.3%)	806 (0.4%)	981b (0.4%b)	831 (0.3%)	737 (0.3%)	750 (0.3%)	926 (0.4%)	864 (0.3%)	621 (0.2%)	811 (0.3%)	907 (0.4%)	56%
Marijuana and Hashish	18,710 (8.6%)	19,102 (8.6%)	18,589 (8.3%)	21,086 (9.3%)	25,755 (11.0%)	25,231 (10.6%)	25,451 (10.6%)	25,375 (10.4%)	25,378 (10.3%)	25,085 (10.1%)	25,768 (10.3%)	28,521 (11.3%)	29,206 (11.5%)	56%

DRUGS	1998	1999	2000	2001	2002	2003	2004	2005	2006	2007	2008	2009	2010	12-year % change from 1998 to 2010
Cocaine	3,811 (1.7%)	3,742 (1.7%)	3,328 (1.5%)	4,186 (1.9%)	5,902 (2.5%)	5,908 (2.5%)	5,658 (2.4%)	5,523 (2.3%	6,069 (2.5%)	5,738 (2.3%)	5,255 (2.1%)	4,797 (1.9%)	4,449 (1.8%)	17%
TOTAL ILLICIT DRUGS1	23,115 (10.6%)	25,402 (11.5%)	24,535 (11.0%)	28,409 (12.6%)	35,132 (14.9%)	34,993 (14.7%)	34,807 (14.5%)	35,041 (14.4%)	35,775 (14.5%)	35,692 (14.4%)	35,525 (14.2%)	37,957 (15.1%)	38,806 (15.3%)	68%

--Not available

Note: 2002 to 2010 data is based on 2010 National Survey on Drug Use and Health Survey Report. a Difference between estimate and 2010 estimate is statistically significant at the 0.05 level. b Difference between estimate and 2010 estimate is statistically significant at the 0.01 level.1 Illicit Drugs include marijuana/hashish, cocaine (including crack), heroin, hallucinogens, inhalants, or prescription-type psychotherapeutics used nonmedically. Illicit drugs other than marijuana include cocaine (including crack), heroin, hallucinogens, inhalants, or prescription-type psychotherapeutics used non-medically. The estimates for nonmedical use of psychotherapeutics, stimulants, and methamphetamine incorporated in these summary estimates do not include data from the methamphetamine items added in 2005 and 2006.

2 Nonmedical use of prescription-type psychotherapeutics includes the nonmedical use of pain relievers, tranquilizers, stimulants, or sedatives and does not include over-the counter drugs.

3 Estimates of nonmedical use of psychotherapeutics, stimulants, and methamphetamine in the designated rows include data from methamphetamine items added in 2005 and 2006 and are not comparable with estimates presented in NSDUH reports prior to the 2007 National Findings report. For the 2002 through 2005 survey years, a Bernoulli stochastic imputation procedure was used to generate adjusted estimates comparable with estimates for survey years 2006 and later.

Source: Substance Abuse and Mental Health Services Administration. Results from the 2010 National Survey on Drug Use and Health: Summary of National Findings. http://www.samhsa.gov/data/NSDUH/2k10NSDUH/2k10Results.pdf [170]. Access date 2/22/2012

Table 1. Types of illicit drug use in the past year among persons aged 12 and older: numbers in thousands from 1998 to 2010 (12 years)

There is good evidence that opioids are effective, and the Institute of Medicine (IOM) does promote pain treatment with these agents, but the rapidly increasing availability of drug does

http://dx.doi.org/10.5772/58818

seek justification. Opioids in the U.S. are a popular choice to treat painful complaints, with use rising from 96mg of morphine equivalents per person in 1997 to 710mg per person in 2010. The staggering opioid availability is equivalent to 7.1kg of opioid for every 10,000 people [4]. This begs the question, is there a proportionate growth in pain and suffering? Have we undertreated pain as a legitimate affliction for decades, or are we pressured to a more aggressive care model?

Gram for gram, the U.S. consumes more opioids than any other country in the world. Despite increasing availability and distribution, limited evidence exists that effective chronic pain treatment is a reduced cost to society, or improves function. There is an abundance of evidence, however, that with this increased availability and use, increased morbidity and mortality escalates in an almost parallel fashion [5].

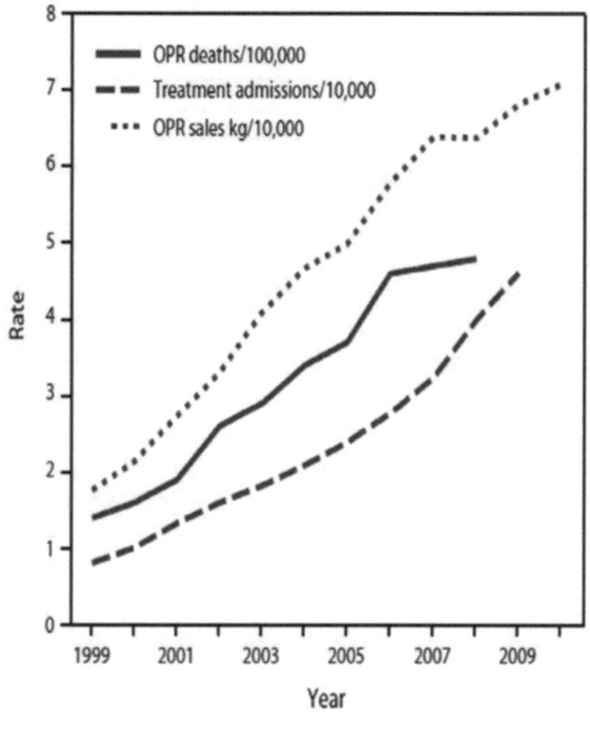

Unintentional opioid overdoses have exceeded heroin and cocaine deaths combined. Opioids contribute to 1 death every 36 minutes [6-10]. The societal impact is more complex than most providers realize. For every death, 9 patients are admitted for substance abuse treatment and 161 for abuse and dependence, with an estimated cost burden of $20 billion [11]. Heroin has recently reemerged in certain areas of the country, presumably as opioid availability decreases. Novel combinations of fentanyl and heroin are a fatal combination.

Nonmedical use of opioids for recreational purposes is now considered an epidemic in the U.S. [12]. The inevitable catastrophe of reckless prescribing and aberrant consumer behavior

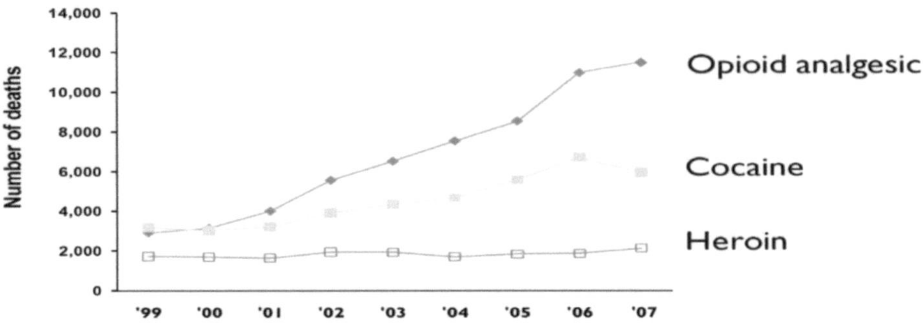

is measured by unexpected adverse consequences. This high risk behavior can result in disastrous outcomes. For every 50 people who take recreational opioids, the result is an unexpected death [13]. First observed a decade ago when emergency department visits due to opioid poisoning rose by almost five-fold, regulatory agencies remained silent. The response to this crisis has remained feeble. The perception that pain is undertreated, promoted by special interest groups and pharma, has led to an explosion of prescriptions and supply slowly being recognized as a major healthcare challenge.

According to the ARCOS data provided by the Drug Enforcement Administration, major classes of opioids have increased substantially in total grams of distribution despite the readily available data linking adverse outcome to availability [14]. In the early 1990s opioid analgesics, led by morphine, Fentanyl, Oxycodone, and Hydrocodone had significant increases in use. From 2004-2011 Hydrocodone use increased by 73%, morphine 64%, methadone 37%, and Fentanyl 35%. Sales of opioids quadrupled between 1999 and 2010 [15]. Hydrocodone is the number one dispensed prescription in the U.S., and the U.S. is the world leader in its consumption [16]. The most remarkable increase in use and availability was buprenorphine. Buprenorphine is indicated for the treatment of addiction and dependency, and in some cases, pain. This is the irony of controlled substance management. To control risk, the provider must be educated and vigilant in techniques to avoid dependence, misuse, abuse, and diversion. The flawed concept of dependency and addiction presents itself with buprenorphine. Buprenorphine is a substitute drug of dependency, and not surprisingly, abuse is on the rise.

The Drug Abuse Warning Network (DAWN) exists to provide information to governmental agencies about emergency department visits related to opioid poisoning. Even codeine, which is reported to have a decrease in prescriptions this decade, increased in misuse. Hydromorphone led the way with the highest increase between 438%, followed by Oxycodone, Fentanyl, Hydrocodone, and Methadone. Prescription opioids revealed in DAWN data mention an increase in adverse events 4% in 1996 data to 20% in 2011 [17]. Not surprisingly, patients seeking detoxification also increased during this period. With the increasing liberalization of laws surrounding marijuana, a drug of abuse that should be treated no differently than any other molecule of abuse and misuse. This drug has also realized an increase in adverse outcomes. Marijuana is considered a safe and benign drug by a vast majority of Americans, but like any abusable substance, has risk. Unlike every other drug, the legislation of marijuana for medical or recreational purposes was not the doing of the FDA, but by the voter. Marijuana is a drug of consequences. It is abusable, associated with psychometric impairment and addiction. Prior to functional executive brain maturation at age 25, irreversible impairment of IQ may occur. Definable benefits to medical application are being studied. Bone healing, neuronal protection after stroke, and seizure management may benefit from a medical application. Smoking the drug to obtain THC is unmeasured and variable. Liquid variants may be superior. As the THC potency continues to be engineered and enhanced in the weed, the medical value may be diminished. THC concentration has increased from 2% in the 1970s to 8% and rising [18]. Interestingly, although highly habituating, patients seeking detoxification from cocaine have decreased.

The use of controlled substances for recreational purposes or diversion was not realized as a problem to its full extent until 1996. Prior to 1996, the DAWN and ARCOS data did not reveal any particular trend in abuse, misuse, or diversion. During that same period of time, medical use of opioids was increasing rapidly, but no particular trend divulged the urgent need for increased scrutiny of these agents. Most believed that the increased use of opioids was responsible for improved treatment of chronic pain. The opposite appears to be evident. Despite mounting evidence that chronic opioid therapy does not improve quality of life, their use continues to rise [19]. Further underscoring this irony is the persistent lack of evidence supporting chronic use, and the abundance of evidence that reveals these agents are risky, and in certain patient populations, dangerous. Efforts at educating the medical community are in place, but persistent widespread use is continuing to promote misuse, abuse, and diversion. The group most willing to prescribe controlled substances is also the provider with the least amount of time to assess risk, and apply principles of adherence monitoring. Primary care physicians are responsible for the largest population of patients chronically exposed to controlled substances. It surprises many that the vast majority of opioid prescriptions are from general practitioners, family medicine, and internists. Anesthesiologists and physical medicine, traditionally associated with pain clinics, are responsible for only about 6% of total prescriptions combined [20].

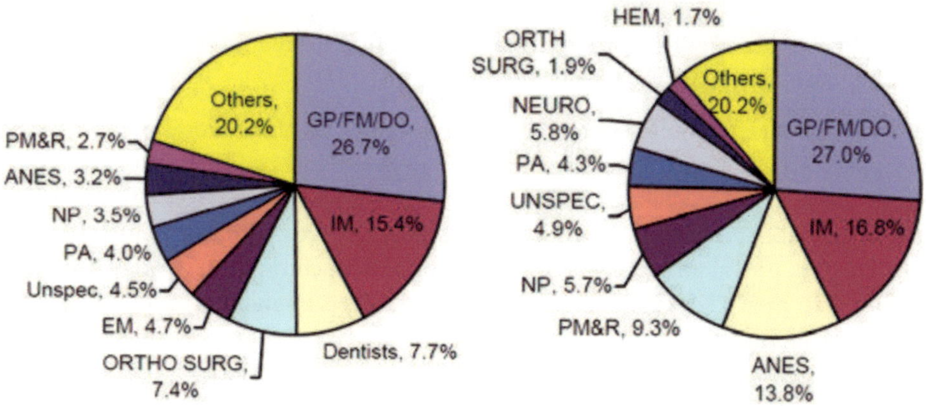

2. Epidemiology

Epidemiology is the study of factors that determine or influence a pattern in prevalence of disease or a condition in populations [21]. Healthcare spending accounts for 16% of the gross domestic product and is continuing to climb, with expectations approaching 25% of the GDP by 2025 [22]. Chronic illnesses are a major cost driver, with projected increases from 133 million in mid-2000, to 171 million in 2030 [23]. The healthcare burden of chronic non-malignant pain is enormous, and a major cost driver in chronic disease. More than ¼ of Americans suffer from daily pain at a cost of almost $60 billion in lost productivity in the U.S. alone [24]. Those of lower socioeconomic status experience pain more often. Individuals making $30,000 or less a year spend nearly 20% of their life in moderate to severe pain. This directly contrasts to households earning more than $100,000 a year, which experienced pain at 8% of their life or less. Those that did not finish high school feel twice as much pain as college graduates. A number of proposed reasons for this discrepancy can be presumed. Those with lower socioeconomic status tend to have more labor-intensive work, and fewer conveniences. The type of work performed is less ergonomically appealing, and those with lower socioeconomic status tend to have more drivers of poor well health characteristics, such as tobacco consumption. It is not surprising that pain medications are a first choice in those suffering from pain, because they are easily obtainable. Americans spend approximately $2.6 billion in over-the-counter pain medications alone and $14 billion on analgesics as a class [25].

The burden of pain is also felt psychologically. Over a quarter of patients believe they will always have pain and there is no solution, and their doctor rarely understands how they feel. Up to 1/3 of chronic pain patients have reported they received little, if any, relief from treatments or therapies. The prevalence of pain in the American population is substantial, with 4 out of 10 Americans saying they experience pain daily, which rises in the aging population approaching 60% in those aged 65 and older. 9 out of 10 Americans say they experience pain some time each month, which would increase utilization of healthcare services to be directly related to these incidences of pain. In fact, despite the prevalence of pain, nearly two-thirds see a doctor only when they cannot stand the pain any longer [26].

Pain remains one of the most frequent chief complaints in the primary care office, with 40% of primary care visits seeking relief, and 20% of those are chronic pain visits. In primary care practices, almost 15% of patients require pain medication or treatment. Up to 20% of patients in a primary care setting are on chronic opioid therapy [27].

Loss of work is a major problem related to pain. Almost 55% of the work force reports having pain the past 2 weeks and of that, almost 15% experience lost productivity due to pain. One percent of the work force is absent from work one or more days a week, with headache and back pain being the most common complaint. Migraines are estimated to affect 30 million a year, with overall prevalence in the U.S. population approaching 15%. Women are three times more likely than men to develop migraines, with peak year's incident age 25-45 [28]. Osteoarthritis, low back, and neck pain is another substantial percentage of the American population suffering from pain. 16% of the U.S. population, or almost 45 million, report pain directly related to osteoarthritis [29]. The incidence of low back pain peaks about the sixth decade of life, and 50% of Americans report some episode of back pain. Neck pain occurs about half as often as low back pain, and effects 10% of the general population [30].

3. Anatomy, neurobiology, and nociceptive systems

"The affective motivational aspect of pain originates in the periphery and suffering is not merely a matter for neocortex, it is profoundly more ancient and primitive biogenetically and is reflected in fiber tracts and neural networks throughout the nervous system." [31]

Pain is "an unpleasant sensory or emotional experience associated with actual potential tissue damage or described in terms as such tissue damage" [32].

Pain is a personal experience, and is a perception of abnormality that relies on descriptors. It is a sensory event of the peripheral and central nervous system, and is only partially defined by the initiating or traumatic event. The effects of pain at any level projects changes to the central nervous system that increase the likelihood of neurobiological changes, within nociceptive systems. The inciting pain generator becomes less relevant over time, as pain is promoted neurobiologically. As more recent understanding of these nociceptive systems evolves, it is better understood that pharmacologic manipulation is often necessary to modulate chronic pain states.

Acute pain is a symptom of a disease and is usually self-limited. It is provoked by tissue injury, not just stimulation, and is usually associated with abnormal functioning of somatic structures. This event could be secondary to emotional responses, autonomic, or a psychological stimulation and response. It has a biological function to alert and warn the individual, and also withdraw for healing and resting. Chronic pain however, sometimes can become the disease itself. It persists beyond the usual course of the acute disease. Chronic pain persists beyond tissue healing and usually is experienced over three months, or some combination therein, associated with impaired function and quality of life indices. Like many other chronic conditions such as hypertension and diabetes, treating chronic pain requires its own set of paradigms and treatment strategies. If the patient has an uncontrolled pain condition, what would normally be an eventful recovery could lead to persistent pain, and often requires chemical therapy or interventions in a multimodality approach to control the pain. Chronic pain is provoked by a chronic pathological process and can result from a dysfunction in the central nervous system. The nervous system evolves into a hypervigilant state, or "wind up", and in turn activates central nervous system elements that may provoke psychological and depressive conditions. Autonomic and neuroendocrine responses may be absent, and it is here that chronic pain is felt to alter biological function [33]. The central nervous system is being remodified to recognize the neurobiological changes that chronic pain evokes. As many of these pain pathways are intimately related with the limbic system and primitive brain structures, associated mood and behavioral changes occur. The interrelationship between the primitive brain and higher cognitive function eventually signals the prefrontal cortex that an abnormal sensation is felt. The patient is then motivated to dampen these systems, and when persistent pain is untreated, impaired restorative sleep capacity is observed, anxiety is detected, and situational depression emerges from these pain states. This further withdraws the patient from active lifestyle, and other somatic complaints develop as comorbidities.

4. Nociception

A nociceptor is normal if it hurts. The anatomic pathway, spinal thalamic tract, is activated by a peripheral nociceptor, transmitted to the dorsal horn in the spinal cord, which then progresses the signal contralaterally through the spinal thalamic tract to the brain and limbic structures. The dorsolateral funiculus, a modulating descending pathway, dampens the effect of pain at the juncture of the first and second order neuron. The second order neuron resides in a well laminated architecture, the "rexed lamina," located in the dorsal horn of the spinal cord. Here it begins, here it is modulated. At the cellular level, opioid receptors at the second order neuron, which is in the dorsal horn of the spinal cord, diminish the impact of the nociceptor stimulus.

There are two types of nerves that are relevant to pain processes. Acute pain is a fast, electric-like pain that is transmitted by A-delta nociceptors. Dull, aching, throbbing, phylogenetically primitive pain is transmitted by the C-fiber nociceptor. At the cellular level, a process of transcription and gene induction elaborates algogenic mediators of pain. The algogenic mediators may be nitric oxide, cholecystokinin (CCK), substance P, and prostanoids, to name a few. Substance P sensitizes the CNS at the receptor site, where N-methyl-D aspartate (NMDA) receptors promote activation of ion channels in pain promoting areas.

Pain signaling, from outside in, cutaneous muscle and visceral tissues initiate high threshold chemical, mechanical, or thermal stimuli to activate neurophysiologic pathways through electrophysiological activity, and engages the second ordered neuron at the rexed lamina. Both sodium and calcium influx leads to release of calcium intracellular stores, and decreased nociceptor thresholds. When this occurs long term, the transcriptive events at the neuron may become sensitized. This is the beginning of the origination of pain, outside in, toward the spinal cord. The role of algogenic mediators of pain may lead to a number of descriptive pain states at this level, such as hyperpathia, hyperalgesia and allodynia. The type 1 and 2 A-delta fibers are small (1.1 to 5-micrometers in diameter), myelinated, and rapidly conducting (at 5 to 30 meters per second). This is a sharp electric pain. The quick retraction from a hot ember, or stubbing a toe. C-fibers, are the smaller (.25 to 1.3 micrometer diameter) unmyelinated slow fibers, (0.5 to 2 meters per second) that give a poor characterization of pain. These are the "second pain" transmitters that quantify pain poorly. C-fibers are considered polymodal, and are activated by mechanical, chemical or thermal mechanisms. The vague abdominal discomfort in the viscera is an example of C-fiber mediated pain, leading to vague descriptors of pain that are poorly localized in the gut. The odd finding that abdominal pain sometimes activates a discomfort in other parts of the body may be explained by the convergence of afferent activity at the second order neuron from different structures. Visceral stimulation has often been observed to incite pain in the shoulder. When adrenergic receptors are activated, peripheral autonomic dysfunction, and sympathetically driven pain may emerge. Ultimately, these sympathetic changes are manifested in pseudomotor changes, and are revealed as the progressive alterations in the periphery, such as seen in complex regional pain syndrome (CRPS).

Once converged at the dorsal horn, the A-delta and C-fibers synapse at laminae 1-2, 2A, and 5. At the dorsal horn, a complicated and coordinated activation of many of the important cascade elements that promote pain occur. Glutamate activation of the AMPA receptor induces a sodium current and depolarization, with sustained activation of the NMDA receptor. Proteins and synaptic elements are influenced by brain derived neurotrophic factor (BDNF), inducing cellular translational events. The cascade of neurogenic inflammation is begun at the C-fiber with release of substance P, CGRP, and the resultant algogenic mediators of pain. The A-delta and C-fiber synapse with the wide dynamic range nociceptive fibers and increase the sensation of pain by a process of "summation" which amplifies pain. With repetitive noxious input, the WDR neuron is engaged in "wind up" and remain sensitized.

Ultimately, the spinothalamic tract interacts with higher centers directly approximated with many important nuclei, and deep brain structures. The "personality of pain" is directly affected by the transmission of brain through these intermediary relationships. Serotonin and norepinephrine is intimately related to these pathways. Some serotonin receptors seem to be upregulated with persistent pain stimulation. Dopamine and dopaminergic pathways in the primitive brain structures are directly affiliated with the emotional and behavioral aspects of pain. At many points through the periphery to the dorsal root ganglion, rexed lamina, as well as ascending and descending pathways, opioids have a strong influence on analgesia and the behavioral aspects of pain. Once pain is interpreted by the higher conscious state, memory and behavioral influences are introduced. Pain is a global experience, with limbic system engagement, prefrontal cortex, and primitive brain structures motivating an individual to seek relief.

Of the four types of pain – somatic, visceral, sympathetic, and neuropathic pain – somatic and visceral are nociceptive pains. Neuropathic and sympathetic are non-nociceptive. The nociceptive pain from stimulated receptors is normal if it hurts. The non-nociceptive pain rises from central nervous system and peripheral nervous system dysfunction. There are no pain receptors in this type of pain, and therefore it is caused by a dysfunctioning nociceptive system. Somatic pain, or more commonly musculoskeletal pain, is sharp and well localized. The type of pain that would be termed nociceptive or visceral are opioid responsive. Choosing the type of medication treatment for different types of pain requires an understanding of the type and described pain.

5. Scope of problem

The Institute of Medicine has published a report that reveals 116 million Americans suffer from pain that persists from weeks to years [34, 35]. The estimated financial impact is up to $635 billion per year in the U.S. [36-38]. It would seem logical that treating pain with an opioid strategy would diminish this staggering number, when in fact there is very little evidence that the desired relief and productivity is returned with these agents. Contrary to intuition, evidence suggests the alarming trend in misuse, abuse, and diversion overwhelms most potential benefits of chronic opioid use, and might argue against chronic exposure. As regulatory restrictions relaxed in the 90s, the trend to prescribe opioids increased alarmingly. Based on the patients self-report of pain, this subjective report is frequently the only tool provider's use to initiate treatment deemed chronic in nature. It was erroneously assumed that the humane approach to addressing a chronic pain condition was to prescribe an ever increasing load of opioids and adjunctive medication. Evidence is lacking in non-cancer pain that pain conditions improved as the dose escalated. Opioid-induced hyperalgesia, endocrine disorders, and the potential for poisoning highlight the better conservative course of care, supporting a more conservative contemporary decision making. The current trend in chronic pain care does not seem to reflect this approach.

The National Survey on Drug Use and Health (NSDUH), under the sponsorship of The Substance Abuse and Mental Health Services Administration (SAMHSA) is distributed to Americans from age 12 and older. Not surprisingly, marijuana is the most commonly used substance with 17 million current past month users, followed by pain relieving drugs. SAMHSA 2012 identified marijuana as the leading drug of abuse in first time users aged 12 and older. Marijuana is considered a gateway drug, and increasingly destigmatized. A staggering 38 million in 2010 used illicit drugs, which is 15% of the American population. Nonmedical use of psychotropic therapies from 1998 to 2010 exceeded marijuana, and is ten times that of cocaine [39].

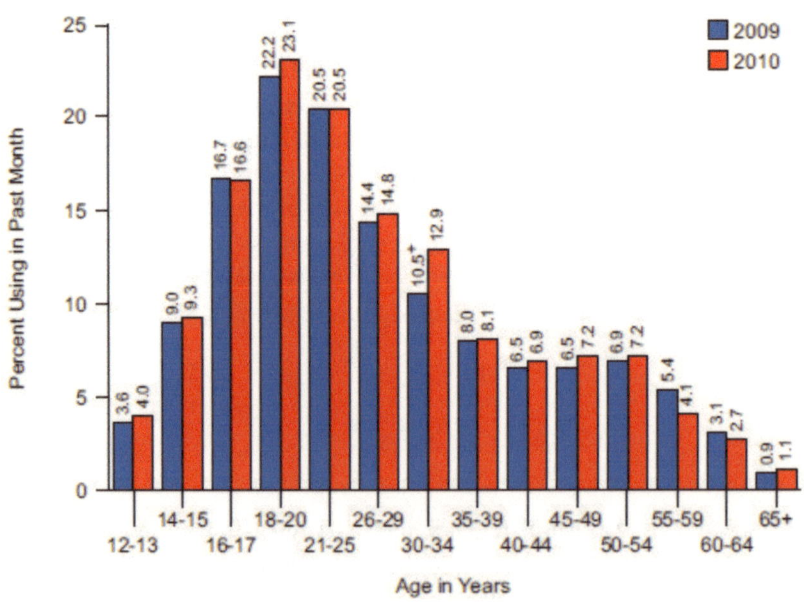

+ Difference between this estimate and the 2010 estimate is statistically significant at the .05 level.

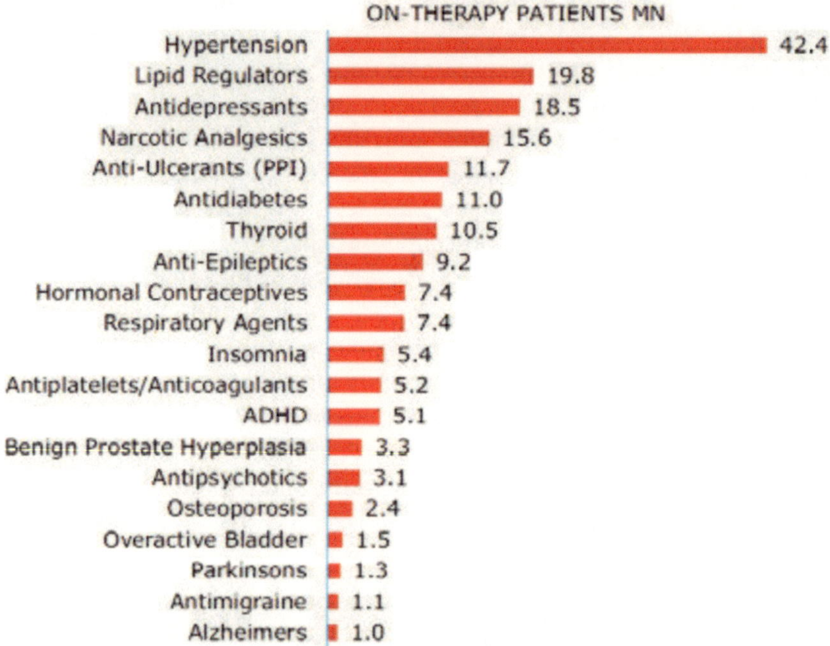

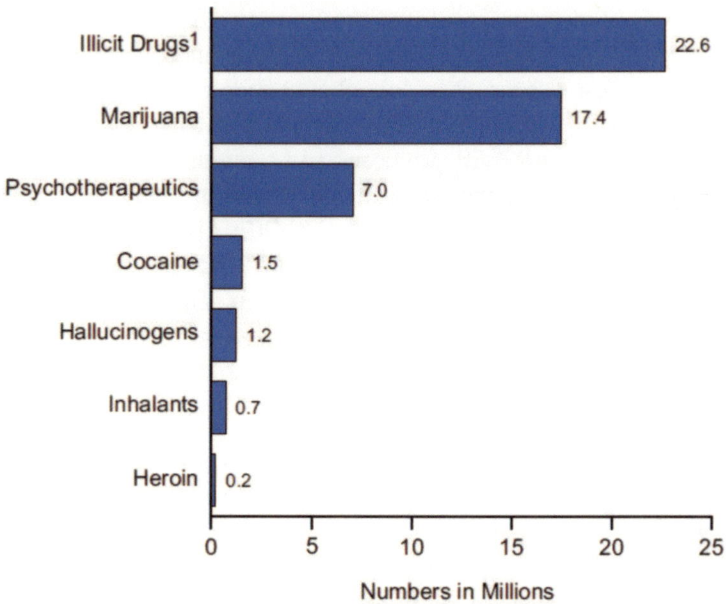

[1] Illicit Drugs include marijuana/hashish, cocaine (including crack), heroin, hallucinogens, inhalants, or prescription-type psychotherapeutics used nonmedically.

The prevalence of those complaining of pain is staggering, estimated to be upwards of 100 million Americans (IOMPPT). Conversely, the incidence of diabetes registers at 25.8 million, heart disease 16.3 million, cardiovascular accidents 7 million, and all cancers combined at 11.9 million (ADA, AHA, ACA) [40]. With the prevalence of pain affecting roughly 1 in 4 Americans, there is little question why a suffering individual would seek any form of therapy, including opioids, to treat chronic nonmalignant pain. Most unfamiliar with interventional pain medicine or other options to treat their pain feel that there is only a pharmacologic solution. This multimodality approach is often underutilized to reduce opioid use. If it comes from a doctor, patients believe opioids must be safe. A report by Russell Portanoy and Kathleen Foley in 1986 opened the door to the subsequent belief that opioids are safe and have little consequences. The paper titled "Chronic Use of Opioid Analgesics and Nonmalignant Pain: Report of 38 Cases" opined that opioid maintenance therapy can be a "safe, salutary, and more humane alternative to options of surgery or no treatment for those patients with intractable nonmalignant pain and no history of drug abuse" [41]. Further supported by the historical facts that opioids have been used for thousands of years, and referenced in ancient writings, the use of opioids found a natural segway into a cost-effective and humane prescriptive environment. The first steps of an epidemic were born.

All but uncontrolled until the Harrison Act of 1914, there was little regulatory restriction on narcotics (controlled substances) in the United States. After the occupation of the Philippines in 1912, and the resultant Hague Treaty, the American response to the concern of British domination of Chinese opium trade resulted in enhanced law enforcement that had very few options to curb opioid use and the potential for misuse [42]. The rest of the world was not quick to adopt or enforce regulation, and until 1961 there were no regulations that addressed worldwide production and distribution of narcotics. The Controlled Substance Act of 1970 was a first step to address these concerns when "no relief or cure is possible, or none has been found after reasonable efforts to legitimize opioid/controlled substances prescriptive purposes." Steadily over the past few years, with advocacy and patients' bill of rights, medical societies support, and the generation of a perceived fifth pathway of pain control in the community, opioid use escalated. The National Vital Statistics Office has seen a steady rise in opioid prescriptions. Available opioids have realized a threefold rise from the late '90s. If pain relievers and tranquilizers were mixed together, as often is the case, the combination would significantly exceed marijuana use. Cocaine and heroin use remain far behind. This underscores the quadrupled death rate from 1999 to 2010. The patients really haven't changed that much, but the exposure to opioids has. [43]

Technology has given us the opportunity to identify and track prescriptive habitry, as well as patient behaviors. With any sharing of sensitive medical information, controls should be in place to assure that the proper individuals have access to the data, and HIPAA integrity is enforced. One of the major questions posed by recent efforts of accumulating patient data electronically is the question of narcotic misuse patterns by the patient, and the potential for inappropriate distribution by pharmacies and physicians. Patient data systems throughout the United States address these questions in different manners. Some embrace the access of law enforcement, others strictly prohibit information exchange to only providers, unless the power of the subpoena is in place. Both have pros and cons. Furthermore, physicians, extenders, dentists, pharmacies and others that prescribe are not required to access this database. The question of poor standard of care is introduced when the potential for harm exists. An overly relaxed due diligence by the prescriber or dispenser is to ignore this important technology.

In 2005, George Bush signed into place the National All Scheduled Prescription Electronic Reporting (NASPER) program which would cross state lines and provide a database to reduce cross state seeking and opioid distribution activity [44]. NASPER remains to be funded, and was ahead of its time when introduced. The current climate of opioid of misuse, abuse, and diversion underscores the need for such a program. The American College of Physicians supports NASPER, as well as other organizations, such as the founding organization of this piece of legislation The American Society of Interventional Pain Physicians (ASIPP).

Americans consume a remarkably large percentage of opioids prescribed worldwide. As a leading country in consumption, the United States only makes up 4.6% of the world's population. The U.S., however, consumes 80% of the world's available opioids. The most common opiate prescribed is hydrocodone, which the United States consumes 99% of the world's distribution of this drug. 34.2 million Americans greater than age 12 can claim use of opioid for nonmedical use at some time in their life [45]. Nonmedical use of opioids is staggering. According to DAWN data, 425,000 emergency department visits in 2010 were a direct result of nonmedical use of opioids [46]. With more than 39,000 Americans dying from drug poisoning in 2009, over 14,000 of those were from prescription opioids. But that is just a small component of the problem. For each one death there were 10,000 admissions for abuse, 32 emergency department visits for misuse or abuse, 130 who abused the drug or are addicted, on top of 825 nonmedical users for recreational purposes [47]. With such ready availability and willingness to use opioids perceived as "safe", the stigma of controlled substances is removed. In the medicine cabinet, the risk of street drugs is not a factor. Cocaine, heroin, even marijuana has a supplier for distribution of unknown character, and the drug is always of unknown origin and purity. Not so with controlled substances, regulated by the FDA. The danger, however, is real. Each passing year for the past fifteen, the opioid death rate, opioid treatment admissions, and kilograms sold is in parallel progression with the availability.

Opioid analgesic deaths exceeded cocaine and heroin deaths at an ever-increasing rate since 1999. Cocaine deaths are actually decreasing. Recently, heroin deaths have increased, but still remains one-sixth that of opioid analgesics. Methadone is one of the cheapest and readily available opioids, and is one of the leading drugs responsible for opioid fatalities. Methadone is just 3% of opioid prescriptions in the United States but is associated with >30% of deaths from opioids [48]. This staggering relationship could be attributed to methadone's unpredictable metabolism and half-life, and the numerous drugs that interact with methadone metabolism and excretion.

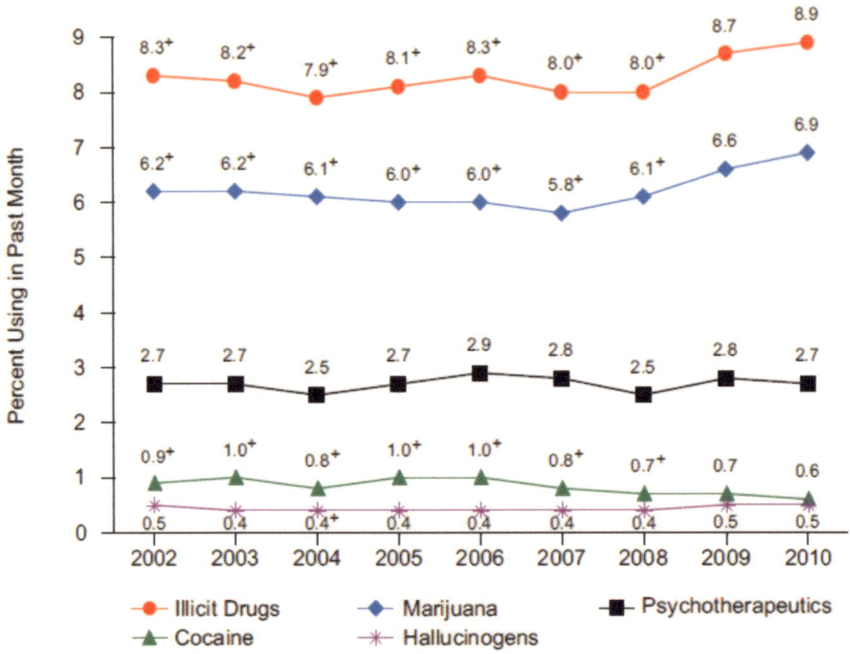

+ Difference between this estimate and the 2010 estimate is statistically significant at the .05 level.

6. The evidence

The diversity of chronic pain conditions is extensive. Pain complaints range from headache pain, spine pain, abdominal pain, myofascial pain, to extensive undefined widespread discomfort. Chronic nonmalignant pain is rarely a single diagnosis. There is evidence that controlled substances are helpful to control symptoms, improve function, and quality of life. There is good evidence that opioids are strong analgesics, and have a role in chronic pain management.

There is also extensive evidence that controlled substances are responsible for misuse, abuse, and diversion. Particularly concerning is the concept of diversion. The DEA introduces a mixed message to prescribers treating those with pain. First, the DEA is responsible for the availability of the drug and will acknowledge that the physician is best prepared and trained to determine whether opioids are indicated. The DEA will further point out that the physicians are at risk for providing these medications, and may be unwittingly providing controlled substances to inappropriate recipients. The word recipient is used over patient as often is the case of those seeking drugs for distribution. These diverters are neither a patient, nor have a truly justifiable chronic pain condition that would warrant controlled substances. If a physician is a partner in diversion, knowingly or not, law enforcement has the option to prosecute.

- SS 841 knowingly or intentionally distributing or dispensing a controlled substance

- No legitimate medical purpose for the prescription in that the same was not issued/filled in the usual course of professional practice or was beyond the bounds of medical practice
- The conviction will be upheld even if the government does not present compelling evidence that the doctor prescribed with malicious motive or the desire to make a profit
- Abbreviated or no medical history of physical examination is probative on the question of whether a legitimate medical purpose exists

Prescribing to an individual with a nefarious purpose, even if you are unaware, may implicate the prescriber and result in a legal action. The provider does not have to know, or profit from the encounter. It simply has to happen. So the benefits of analgesia and improved function and quality of life are now weighed against the abuse risk, misuse, and addiction threat. The epidemic of chronic pain, its treatment with opioids, and the parallel morbidity and mortality compels the prescriber to utilize all tools available to ensure that the proper prescription is given to the proper individual for the proper purpose. The implications of this standard are far reaching. Increased scrutiny can now be placed on individuals who prescribe beyond their scope of care. An example might be an ophthalmologist providing diet pills to his mistress [49]. To the busy family practice physician that has not exercised proper caution, and only performs a brief history or physical that does not support opioid use in the documentation, the risk/reward benefit does not fall in the practitioner's favor. It is not necessarily the intention to provide substandard care, but time pressures are very real and patient needs and demands can be extensive. A patient or individual that is persistent in aggressively obtaining controlled substances knowingly does so against the physician's common daily practice paradigm. Most physicians are ill-equipped to confront a patient that exhibits inappropriate pain behaviors and drug seeking activity. In some cases, a level of fear and bullying is injected into the practice from a patient that is highly motivated to obtain a controlled substance. Evidence exists that a physician is most likely to be non-confrontational, and accommodating, to diminish conflict. This would include writing a prescription as the most expeditious and safest way to remove this patient burden. Deyo, et al reported 61% of patients with low back pain in primary care settings were on opioids at one point in the course of care [50]. Almost 20% of these were long-term users in the primary care setting. Primary care physicians are the most common prescriber of opioids, followed by surgical specialties. Primary care providers are also the source of most immediate-release opioid prescriptions. Despite limited evidence that effective chronic pain care therapy is enhanced with short-acting opioids, these highly abusable agents are commonly prescribed [51]. Numerous guidelines also point out that long-term exposure to opioids is of questionable benefit, with only small to moderate improvements in most pain states. By contrast, evidence exists that poor patient selection is a leading cause of adverse outcome when opioids are utilized to treat painful disorders [51].

Another concern regarding controlled substances, opioids in particular is the milligram dosing the patient is exposed to. A group in Washington State recommends the dosing equivalent not exceed 120mg of Morphine [52]. Proponents of education emphasize proper prescription habits to realize establishment of medical necessity, which isn't always obvious. Once need is established, identifying the risk of misuse, abuse, and diversion, and utilizing strategies to mitigate risk is good medical practice.

Another important concept is acknowledging the multimodality approach to dealing with pain, and subsequently reducing the opioid load. It has been demonstrated that interventional techniques do address this concern and can reduce or eliminate the need for controlled substances.

The typical patient referred to a pain management physician either comes from a surgical referral or a primary care. As stated earlier, primary care is responsible for most opioid prescriptions and often patients expect that opioid therapy will remain stable and be continued at the current dosing. Over time, the patient develops a number of expectations as to entitlement of these drugs. Frequently referred to as "my hydros" or "my Oxys" for example, a high level of anxiety is demonstrated when patients are educated about dose reduction, and exit strategies from opioid-based therapy. This is an "opioid" stress test. Aberrant personality behaviors can be confrontational, and emotional. Sometimes threats are made, and retaliation may use the anonymity of social media, criticizing the physician in the numerous online rating services, and even reporting the provider to the medical board. These retaliatory activities are a demonstration of inappropriate illness behaviors, and reveals that the patient was a poor choice for long-term opioid therapy. There is some truth to the belief that a good pain management provider, with skill at controlled substance management, will have poor ratings in social media and other physician rating services. The sad but true irony is that patients read these online ratings, and make ill-conceived judgments about the individual provider, or the care they have been rendered, owing more credibility to the rating sites than the patient/physician relationship. This is a new form of physician slander, and there is virtually no response that a physician can muster to defend their reputation. There is good evidence this retaliation occurs.

Patients with non-cancer pain treated in the non-specialist's office are often referred without benchmarks. Benchmarks are understanding the benefit risk ratio of opioids and treatment strategies at 3, 6, 9, and 12 months. These benchmarks should be straight forward and easy for the patient to realize, with documentation to the medical record in the form of function and quality of life indices. The patient might describe his/her benchmarks as simple as walking ¼ mile at 3 months four times a week, or even consider advanced lifestyle changes. Within these benchmarks, the concept of the exit strategy is defined. This eliminates the misunderstanding that opioids are an indefinite life treatment expectancy. There is no barrier to communication, and documentation in the medical record is an aid to better understand treatment efficacy and direction, demonstrating progression or regression over time.

With the initiation of opioids, there is a true and defined legitimate medical need, carried by a diagnosis, supported by diagnostics, and usually physical exam findings. As subjective as chronic pain can be, there are many tools available that document function and quality of life indices, and ultimately the true effectiveness of a treatment profile. If opioids render little help in improving movement forward in these benchmarks, or if benchmarks are never even considered, it is difficult to justify continued opioid exposure. If the risk/reward benefit of opioids is poorly documented, and the patient makes very little progress with poor lifestyle choices, ultimately opioids are of little positive value. A patient may be unable or unwilling to make an effort to change modifiable features in their health profile, and therefore it makes

http://dx.doi.org/10.5772/58818

little sense to continue what is most likely a failed treatment paradigm. The multimodality tools available, such as cognitive behavioral therapy, interventional techniques, durable medical items, and advancing forward functional enhancements should have a tangible result. If the goal of the patient is just to obtain a pill, it is unreasonable to expect significant improvement at 3, 6, 9, or 12 months, and may signal inappropriate illness behaviors. There are exceptions to each treatment plan. It is reasonable to allow flexibility with pain complaints as there are multiple factors involved in the complex nature of chronic pain, where the diagnosis rarely stands as a singular complaint. The goal however, is to be clear with the patient that there is a plan. Consequences exist for the provider and for the patient if the plan is not realized, and efforts to move forward ultimately fail. The patient comes to the physician for thoughtful care, not just obtaining a prescription every month.

6.1. Recent studies supporting opioid therapy

Different combinations of opioids can add energy to effectiveness in the properly chosen patient. A recent long term (52 week) study revealed sustained relief with 2 different opioid preparations in patients with chronic non-cancer pain.[53] This study did not include a placebo group but it did demonstrate sustained pain relief over a longer period of time than previous studies. Another randomized trial of two opioids versus placebo has shown superior pain relief with both active analgesics for chronic knee pain. [54] Newer agents are associated with less drug liking, and the potential for abuse. Tapentadol has been reported to be superior to oxycodone for osteoarthritis pain in terms of worker productivity and cost. Tapentadol is available in 50 mg, 75 mg and 100 mg doses. The starting dose is 50-100 mg every 4-6 hours. The maximum daily dose is 600 mg/day. [55] The abuse-resistant technology, Intac®, reduces the diversion potential as well. Buprenorphine transdermal has been compared to oxycodone over a 12-week period. A higher dose of buprenorphine (20 micrograms/hour) has been demonstrated to be superior to oxycodone and low dose buprenorphine (5 micrograms/hour). [56] Buprenorphine/naloxone sublingual film comes in 2mg/0.5 mg. 4 mg/1 mg, 8 mg/2 mg and 12 mg/3 mg doses. It is important to note that naloxone does not reverse non-opioid associated respiratory depression and sedation that might occur with barbiturates, alcohol, or benzodiazepines.

6.2. The growing argument against chronic opioid therapy

Numerous recent studies have reported several problem areas react with chronic oral opioid therapy. [57] Overdoses have increased significantly and are related to high doses and prolonged duration of treatment. Opioids for arthritis pain have been associated with increased risk of fractures [58, 59]. The reason for this association is unknown. The DAWN data teaches us that chronic opioid therapy is associated with increased emergency room visits. Increasing opioid dosing has also been associated with increased risk of trauma in automobile accidents. [60]

Among our military veterans, post-traumatic stress disorder and opioid therapy have been associated with poor outcomes in veterans with chronic pain. [61]

CLINICAL VIGNETTE. A 33 year old male arrives in the clinic late, claiming "car trouble." The individual has been asked to produce medications for a pill count, and a urine drug screen is planned. This is a part of normal clinic operations. A previous attempt at having the individual arrive for a pill count was thwarted when a family member died and services were attended out of state.

Pain described is sharp electric-like pain, in a non dermatomal distribution, right leg predominant. Some left arm pain, and some paracervical discomfort is evident. Further descriptors of the pain are vague and nonphysiologic. Pain is migratory, and often associated with back pain and headaches. There is no neurological deficit and no focality.

This type of vague pain pattern reveals no specific characteristics which a diagnostic platform can evolve. Often these pains are described as "myofascial or fibromyalgic." A type of pain that is poorly characterized and exaggerated, often inconsistent with examination findings. In this particular case, according to the patient the only that helps the pain is Oxycodone, and a specific dose is requested, "30s".

When treating any type of pain, a diagnosis must precede a clinical pathway. In this particular case, the only treatment that helps is an opioid-based pain medication in a young individual, with very poorly characterized pain. Because it is migratory, and nonspecific, an interventional procedure would have limited value. Allowing for age, and the lack of specific diagnostic findings, suggests this pain is better treated with non-narcotic medication alternatives. The pain described shares some characteristics of neuropathic pain and somatic character. A generalized pain treatment plan would include medications that would have minimal habituation potential, and poor drug "liking." Gabapentin or Pregabalin would be a good choice and could potentially diminish the central nervous system contribution assisting the myofascial component, and carries minimal risk of misuse, abuse, or diversion. Drugs such as Gabapentin and non-narcotic medication alternatives are also a good stress test. A patient that is seeking for a specific drug therapy is challenged to try something new, and this care is clinically sensible with less risk. If aberrancies evolve, the stress test would be positive.

Evidence suggests the alarming trend in abuse, misuse, and diversion overwhelms the most powerful benefit from chronic opioid use, and argues against chronic exposure. As regulatory restrictions were relaxed in the '90s, the trend to prescribe opioids has increased alarmingly. Based on the patients self-report of pain, it is frequently the only tool we have to identify of chronic nature. The humane approach when addressing a chronic pain condition was felt to prescribe ever increasing milligram equivalents of opioids, as well as other adjunctive medication. Evidence is lacking in non-cancer pain that pain conditions and function treated with opioids actually improve when chronic in nature. Opioid induced hyperalgesia (OIH), endocrine disorders, and potential poisoning highlight the better course of care that stress non-narcotic options and minimize opioid exposure [62]. Specifically, an exit strategy should exist when opioids are prescribed. If this is not always practical, benchmarks are usually a strong predictor of positive or negative outcome.

Obesity, depression, multiple symptoms and etiologies of chronic pain are predictors of poor long-term outcomes for patients with chronic pain who are continued on chronic opioid therapy. [63]

Additional risk factors related to poor outcomes for chronic pain patients have been reported and include opioid use, older age, female gender, anti-social personality, government disability, and severe disability at initial evaluation and not working at discharge. [64] Furthermore, opioid prescription for longer than 7 days has been reported as a risk factor for long-term disability in workers with acute back pain. [65] The threshold to prescribe opioids in the primary care setting is low, particularly with vague diagnosis states and external pressures. Those that are treated with opioids for chronic pain often request ever increasing doses.

A 52-week study showed no major outcome difference between patient groups treated with a stable opioid dose regimen versus an escalating opioid dose regimen. This suggests that higher doses are not associated with additional benefit. Notably, 27% of the subjects in this study were discharged due to misuse. [66]

Several studies have demonstrated significant analgesia with opioids for chronic pain, the magnitude of pain relief is 20-30 %. However, 20-30% improvement is the same range as the response to tricyclic antidepressants, gabapentinoids, duloxetine and tramadol. The functional improvement associated with this analgesia is variable. Functional improvement is associated with rehabilitation treatments such as interdisciplinary care; however, interdisciplinary treatment is often not associated with pain relief. A weakness of many opioid studies is the duration of therapy. The longest randomized, placebo controlled trials are weeks in duration rather than months or years, which is often the duration of treatment with opioids used in chronic pain. Also, patients are excluded from studies if they have psychiatric problems including addiction.

Diversion of prescribed opioids is a known problem, particularly among younger patients. No validated risk assessment tool exists and no failsafe way to prevent diversion has been found that resolves or eliminates this risk. The risk of addiction is real. In a study of patients in treatment for opioids, 39% reported being addicted to prescription opioids before switching to heroin. [67]

Addiction and abuse are related problems that are often overlooked. The acute care setting of a primary care office is a high risk environment to avoid this consequence.

7. Clinical vignettes

A patient presented to a pain center reporting a history of chronic pain secondary to brachial plexus avulsion. He fully availed himself to all diagnostic and treatment modalities that failed. The final treatment recommendation was a dorsal root entry zone radiofrequency ablation. When advised that no guarantee of pain relief was made, he elected to continue opioid treatment. He requested a letter supporting the prescribing of opioid for his condition. He used the letter to secure prescriptions from multiple physicians.

Lesson learned – urine drug screens may not detect multiple prescribing sources.

A patient with complex regional pain syndrome reported relief from 6-4 mg Hydromorphone tablets every four hours. He stated he could get more relief from 7 tablets. A urine drug screen showed marijuana and it was learned that he had obtained opioids from 150 physicians and was eventually indicted on criminal charges related to selling prescription drugs. Then the patient was reported to be deceased. When law enforcement officers go to his home, the patient answers the door.

Lesson learned-urine drug screening is a useful part of an initial evaluation of patients who report current opioid use.

A new patient was admitted to the hospital with a history of pancreatitis. The patients' medical history included being treated by a physician in another state with Hydromorphone 4 mg and took 2400 pills per month in addition to high doses of long acting oxycodone. The prescription was confirmed by a phone call to the dispensing pharmacy. The patient was treated with an intravenous PCA pump and used minimal doses without any withdrawal symptoms or pain escalation.

Lesson learned-The street value of prescription opioids is significant and physicians must develop "street smarts" in order to avoid being duped into prescribing for patients who are taking enough opioid to have a positive urine drug screen but selling the rest of their prescription as a means of financially supporting themselves. Quantitative and qualitative drug testing on admission is important before opioids are administered by the emergency room or hospital.

8. Adherence monitoring and the concept of accountability

As with any treatment plan, there are heralding moments in a patient's course of care that requires definitive action. Medical decision making in chronic pain is not always straight forward. There is a strong subjective interpretation of the complaint, and the supportive evidence of disease is not always visible. When the provider defines the need to initiate opioid therapy or controlled substance management, any one of a number of findings could be entered into a complex differential diagnosis. Often patients with pain suffer from situational anxiety depression, and poor restorative sleep patterns. Comorbid disease states are the norm and not the exception. Home and lifestyle intrusions involve many members of the patients surrounding environment, with a psychosocial component that is often as complex as the painful entity being treated. Formal and informal risk stratification may involve opioid risk tools, historical precedent such as criminal history or misuse, abuse and diversion history, and is documented at early stages in a patient's encounter. The medical history or the Physician State Drug Monitoring Programs (PDMP) might reveal a story of multiple prescribers, multiple prescriptions, and pharmacies [68-72]. These red flag incidences underscore the need for the previously mentioned "plan". Benchmarks that affect the patients function and quality of life status act as a strong director of care and compliance, as well as the willingness to be actively involved in wellness to modifiable features and health profile. Adherence monitoring tracks conformity and a patient's willingness to follow principles and policies of controlled substance management. Ongoing adherence monitoring is time consuming and labor intensive. Often the patient is introduced to the practice from primary care offices that are overwhelmed by the opioid load and patient behavior, and given just enough medicine until the patient arrives for the appointment. The false belief that this is less risky from an administrative position adds further complexity to the first encounter. The patient expects that prescriptions will be written. The provider must establish a relationship from in-depth historical investigation which can take time. The appropriate patient for opioid therapy, or one that is at high risk, requiring an elevated level of adherence monitoring, is decided early in the relationship. These are a new set of rules for the patient, underscored by a patient care agreement, understood by the patient, with no barrier to communication. This accountability and expectation requires the patient/physician relationship to grow in trust, and these actions should not be seen as an intimidation, but more of a "universal precaution" [73]. As much as we have employed universal precautions for blood borne pathogens, we apply these principles to opioid risk intolerance. Every patient that receives controlled substances is at risk for misuse, abuse, and diversion. The unique patient population of an individual practice will best define what benchmarks are needed, what precautions need to be taken, and when the patient is held to task. Also in place are positive reinforcement scenarios, to help the patient understand that this is a part of what is routinely done in the clinic, and necessary. A process of resolution is in place if the patient deviates from the treatment plan, or presents a challenge with aberrancies or red flags in controlled substance management. As previously mentioned, an opioid exit strategy may be introduced from the very beginning of the relationship so that there are no misunderstandings. Particularly true in painful states such as fibromyalgia, and vague musculoskeletal complaints such as "low back pain", opioids are not always the best choice. Other adjunctive medications and non-narcotic options will decrease the opioid load, and many times increase relief cycling and compliance.

The process of adherence monitoring is a directed care approach to ensure that the patient receives the medication needed, in the dose necessary for therapeutic benefit, and that legitimate need is met. The components of legitimate medical need, or necessity, are a community standard, and not set by the DEA, or other regulatory agencies. Most agree that legitimate need is intuitive, but nonetheless requires careful documentation.

Another principle of adherence monitoring is defining the diagnosis. Within the expected activities of a history and physical, the formulation of a diagnosis evolves. In those that suffer from chronic pain, the diagnosis may be very straight forward such as a herniated nucleus pulpolsus (HNP), or as vague and challenging as interstitial cystitis, abdominal pain, myofascial pain, or headaches. The patient usually has pain that can't be seen, touched, felt, or measured and challenges the definition of legitimate medical need. Functional assessments, impairment of activities, and the life experiences are documented to support clinical assumptions. When opioids are introduced, the diagnosis often defines the length of exposure to an agent and the expected opioid load. An HNP may be considered correctable or not, and a headache may be cyclical or transient, and very real but invisible problems such as a traumatic brain injury or cluster migraine have driven some to suicide. Whatever the diagnosis, the record will reflect a level of support for that diagnosis that further legitimizes the need for opioid therapy. Risk is also assigned early, simply as low, medium or high defined by individual practitioners tolerances and training. If the patient experiences surgery, such as those that have isolated discogenic pathology, an exit strategy from opioids might be sooner than the individual that has a recurrent or persistent painful disorder such as CRPS. Individualized therapy requires documentation that exceeds a line or two of "I think it therefore it is". Once opioid therapy is initiated, as diagnosis directed, adherence monitoring begins.

Adherence monitoring is a complicated process of laboratory assessment, physical pill counts, database interrogation, and good judgment. Ultimately, the provider and patient realize a safer care environment.

9. Drug testing

There are four commonly utilized forms of drug testing – urine drug screening, specific drug analysis, blood, hair sampling, and saliva testing. Drug detection periods can be in the minutes to hours in blood, and similar with saliva. Urine is detected sometimes within minutes, and lingers for many days. Sweat is similar, whereas hair might be detected hours through months. Drug testing is not screening. Screening is a word that does not define necessity, which is required for testing. The purpose of adherence monitoring, including drug testing, is to strengthen the patient/physician relationship built on trust. Another purpose of urine drug testing is to identify if the patient is taking medication prescribed, or not prescribed, and as directed. Of the choices, urine drug screening is considered the gold standard. The results are a product of the dose, metabolites, type of test used, characteristics of the drug, cutoff levels, and the frequency of use.

Drug	Duration
Amphetamine	2 – 4 Days
Methamphetamine	2 – 4 Days
Barbiturate	2 – 30 Days
Benzodiazepine	Up to 3 Days
Cocaine	1 – 3 Days
Heroin/Morphine	1 – 3 Days
Marijuana – Chronic	30 – 70 Days
Marijuana – Occasional	1 – 3 Days
Methadone	2 – 4 Days, maybe longer (150 hours)
PCP – Chronic	Up to 30 Days
PCP – Occasional	2 – 7 Days

Table 2. Duration for a positive screen

Metabolites also play an important role in urine drug testing. The recent use of genetic testing plays an important role in metabolite assessment. The importance of not only identifying the current drug in testing, but its metabolite, is now realized as an impact item of adherence monitoring. Transformation has occurred in healthcare that is just now being more defined in clinical personalized care. Previously the pathology, physiology, as well as chemistry have helped us understand disease. Today, the complexity of metabolic progression of clinical drug therapy can require a suitable drug that can be individualized. With the model of genomics and personalized care model, we can now follow the best course of care with specific agent selection. If an individual's hepatic metabolism does not support a 2D6 pathway, another agent might be more desirable, utilizing another p450 enzyme pathway. The concept of pseudoaddiction has been reborn. Pseudoaddiction was introduced in the late '80s, based on the flawed concept that individual reports of increased pain may occur because the patient is under dosed [74, 75]. Now with the revelation of genetic metabolic variability, it can be demonstrated that a chosen agent may be an inferior ineffective choice. Testing may suggest that it is not that the drug is underdosed as with pseudoaddiction, but there is a poor metabolic progression to activity of the chosen agent. For example, Hydrocodone is metabolized to normorphine, norhydrocodone, hydrocodol, Hydromorphone, and hydromorphol. Oxycodone is metabolized to noroxycodone, Oxymorphone, oxycodols, and oxides. Some of these metabolites are clinically active and potent, such as Hydromorphone in the case of hydrocodone. If the metabolic pathway does not exist to metabolize hydrocodone to its metabolite, such as a weak 2D6 response, the efficacy of that drug will be significantly diminished. The rate of drug metabolism may also be identified. Poor metabolizers to rapid metabolizers of a drug might affect the chosen agent and its clinical activity. Over the next few years genetics will help us tailor courses of therapy that are individualized, and help us improve patient care.

Urine drug screening and adherence monitoring is necessary to manage controlled substance therapy, and diagnose misuse, abuse, and diversion. We test patients to monitor adherence, support patient advocacy, uncover diversion, and addiction. We choose who to test as a process of adherence monitoring, coupled with informed consent. Patients tend to declare themselves during the course of treatment. Those that are resistant to certain drug or treatment profiles, push specific drug requests. Any patient with aberrant behavior, or in recovery, would be a high risk individual requiring enhanced monitoring. These tests are indicated when the physician detects a clinical indication to do so to support decision making. Often, the clinician will utilize a point of care sample, but confirmation usually follows if there is a red flag question or unclear detection of a drug. Poorly identified drugs in point of care include Methadone, Fentanyl, Oxycodone, and Tapentadol. Also GHB, anabolic steroids, designer drugs, inhalants, and hallucinogens are difficult to detect. Point of care tests are based on competitive antibodies and the drug saturates the antibody. Point of care is desirable due to the rapid turnaround time, cost, and portability, but often requires a qualitative assay. Gas chromatography liquid and mass spectrometry (GC-MS) is a common form of confirmation, but is expensive and can take a number of days. Some point of care detection sensitivities are very accurate, such as cocaine, with a primary metabolite benzoylecgonine. There is low cross reactivity with other substances, and is considered very reliable at point of care. Less so are nonspecific opioids, as well as synthetic opioids. When assessing a urine test, positive results require close analysis.

There are many cross reactants, and positive results do not always mean an illicit substance has been ingested. For example, a morphine positive urine drug screen may also result from a metabolite of codeine, which is morphine. The reverse is not true. Also seen is the possibility of positive THC, when the patient has a prescription for Marinol. To ensure the validity of a specimen, which can be tampered by dilution and adulterants, adding verification with creatinine, pH and temperature are applied. High volume ingestion of water, such as two quarts, might produce a negative result with the cutoff level being diluted to a negative result. Even the internet offers tools to pass a drug test. Most are adulterants and oxidants.

Drug	Screening cut-off concentrations ng/mL urine	Confirmation cut-off concentrations ng/mL	Urine detection time	Immunoassay (I) Chromatography (C)
Hydrocodone	300	50	1 – 2 days	I & C
Oxycodone	100	50	1 – 3 days	I & C
Morphine	300	50	3 – 4 days	I & C
Methadone	300	100	5 – 10 days	I & C
Hydromorphone	300	100	1 – 2 days	I & C
Meperidine	300	100	1 – 2 days	I & C
Codeine	300	50	1 – 3 days	I & C
Benzodiazepines	200	20 – 50	Up to 30 days	I
Barbiturates	200	100	2 – 10 days	I & C
Marijuana	50	15	1 – 3 days for casual use; up to 11 weeks for chronic use	I & C
Cocaine	300	50	1 – 3 days	I & C
Amphetamine	1,000	100	2 – 4 days	I & C
Methamphetamine	1,000	100	2 – 4 days	I & C
Heroin*	10	25	1 – 3 days	I & C
Phencyclidine	25	10	2 – 8 days	I & C

*6-MAM, the specific metabolite is detected only for 6 hours.

Table 3. Urine drug testing: Typical screening and confirmation cut-off concentrations and detection times for drugs of abuse.

Adherence monitoring with urine testing is just one technique. Pill counts also reveal compliance. Depending on the personality of the patient, motivating features of their personality, and their apparent risk – mild, moderate, or high risk – different delivery systems might even be considered. The common and erroneous belief that a patch system is a significant improvement in safety is not borne out in the reality of pain care. These patches can be utilized nefariously, and have street value. It is recommended that spent patches associate with an accountability system, such as placing them in an envelope, or on a piece of paper with each patch dated, and returned to the clinic for inspection. In the case of Fentanyl, there is significant Fentanyl left in the patch after three days. Patients who say that their patch does not work after "two days" might be given more patches, with the increased potential for diversion. If diversion is not suspected or borne out when a properly dosed drug is ineffective, the argument for genetic testing could be made. Poor or rapid metabolism is possible, and alters the effectiveness of the chosen agent. Those at high risk, such as those that are on Medicaid or disabled, have a history of substance abuse, bipolar, borderline personality, chaotic lifestyle, and alcoholism, and those that exaggerate symptom response, require significant adherence monitoring. Drug testing may be more frequent than two times a year, as are pill counts and other adherence monitoring techniques. Plans must be in place with written agreements that include informed consent and therapeutic boundaries understood by the patient, family members, and relevant individuals, such as those with power of attorney. There are some patients that controlled substances just are not safe enough to give, or will be misused, in which the clinical course of care begs another form of treatment such as interventional medicine, manual medicine, or other pharmacologic manipulations. Those that have deviations from the patient care agreement, adulterance of the urine, misuse, abuse, or divert, should be introduced to a pathway in their best interest. Simply discharging the patient is unacceptable. Offers to afford the patient care in another arena are considered good medical care, and referrals to psychiatry, addiction medicine, methadone clinics, and other community services are strongly urged. The process of abandonment cannot be ignored. The reality of those that use controlled substances is that most make mistakes. This does not mean that they are bad people, or do not have a legitimate medical illness that can be treated by other means.

10. PDMP

The prescription database management systems or programs (PDMP) that are seen in nearly all 50 states identify the origin of the prescription, the physician, and the details of the prescription such as number of pills, refills, and date. Utilizing this information, the practitioner will then determine if the patient is utilizing medication properly, if violation of patient care agreement is evident, and ensure that compliance is in place.

10.1. Communication

Pain care in modern medicine is an expectation that has even been assigned its own vital sign. Unlike a number of years ago, care providers are becoming more enlightened regarding the necessity and societal need for pathways of relief in those that are impaired by pain. Methods and techniques of pain treatment are as varied as the providers that care for these individuals. A full spectrum of care is available today, from manual therapy to interventional medicine, and pharmacologic strategies have many choices. Occasionally the clinician is challenged to provide adequate care, but lacks the availability of the proper therapeutic option. Chronic pain care by its very nature will be treated by multiple specialties, each offering its own solution. The Code of Ethics published in the American Medical Association 1847 "from the age of Hippocrates to the present time, the annals of every civilized people contain abundant evidence of the devotedness of medical men to the relief of their fellow creatures from pain and disease" [76]. By the very nature of pain and its associated diagnosis, cross specialty cooperation is necessary to obtain the best outcome. It is therefore, the duty of a care provider to offer pain care and relieve suffering. Edwards, in Pain and the Ethics of Pain Management 1984 stated "there is a duty to do all that can be done within the limits of current medical knowledge and available resources to relieve all the pain and suffering which can be alleviated" [77]. Herein lies the problem. Not all chronic pain disease states can be clearly defined, unlike other medical disease states. Pain is really the reflection of an individual's own subjective interpretation that has a number of biopsychosocial influences.

Chronic pain care is also constrained by the financial and medical/legal environment. From a regulatory perspective, the pain care provider may find road blocks to address an individual's pain. Fear of reprisal or a negative peer opinion will often lead to under treatment of pain. Other providers don't find an interest in treating pain because of the vagarity of an individual diagnosis and lack of diagnostic tools available to assess the patient that has pain. Pain is one of the most common complaints in a physician's office, and is often the lowest point of focus. Pain is more than a symptom; it is also reflective of a disease state or illness, and is rarely a singular disease entity. Comorbidity should be expected. This further complicates the treatment pathway and promotes polypharmacy. The patient develops a "personality of pain" responsible for inflicting emotional, and neuropsychiatric impairment. This psychological decay further leads to decline in function. The complexity of the pain diagnosis can change the identity of an individual that diminishes the feeling of wellness from every aspect of an individual's life. Situational depression and anxiety are deleterious problems in the patient suffering from pain, and are often a comorbidity. Magnified by the lack of cohesion in pain care, these different facets of pain diagnosis often go untreated, diminishing the potential effectiveness of a prescribed treatment course. It is not that a certain medication pathway, or interventions "don't work", it is more likely that the individual patient is not treated as a whole. This fragmented care is costly to the patient and society.

Over the past ten years the prevalence of chronic pain has remained a consistent challenge for providers and patients. The advances in treating pain primarily revolve around pharmacologic management, interventional tools, and musculoskeletal therapy. The realities of our evolving healthcare delivery systems may continue to limit access to this already under treated population. Now considered a fifth pathway, pain itself will be unlikely to support a priority position in the healthcare hierarchy. With innovative payment programs such as ACOs, and the remnants of managed care, priority will be given to chronic life-threatening disease states, and then followed by those with progressive disabling afflictions. Chronic pain, which is many times disabling, is not a life-threatening entity. The pain provider will be challenged to render effective care, increasing function and quality of life, and minimizing risk in the new order. With rising healthcare costs opioid use has increased. Escalating opioid use has a direct relationship with adverse consequence. Considered inexpensive, opioid therapy is actually quite costly. The potential for abuse events and long-term use may be significantly higher than adjunctive or interventional options.

Clinical Vignette. A new patient complains of low back pain. He was referred for medication management. Payer source is Medicaid, he does not work, and the MRI reveals modest degenerative changes. He is a smoker, and recently divorced. The exam reveals nonphysiologic findings and otherwise unremarkable.

At initial visit, an intake questionnaire suggested possible use of a controlled substance that was supplied by a family member, and a urine drug sample is obtained. Within the sample, nonspecific opioid at point of care was found, and was positive for THC.

The patient is requesting a pain prescription, and is persistent as to the need to obtain "Oxys" so he can go look for a job. He has been on these before and that is the only thing that works, specifically defining the medication needed that doesn't have Acetaminophen, which upsets his stomach.

A number of issues arise with this vignette, specifically the lack of a clear pain diagnosis. A diagnosis is a necessary component of the controlled substance management plan, and necessary to the medical record. Low back pain is a common complaint, but it is just that, a complaint or a symptom, not a diagnosis. The exam rendered very few clinically relevant findings and the supportive imaging was not remarkable. The patient is specific on the type of medication wanted, in its pure form, and has a chaotic home life. The original history did not bring forward the use of hydrocodone, which was extracted after the point of care testing found unexpected opioids, and THC, illegal substances evident. This is a red flag encounter. A number of inconsistencies and elements of inappropriate seeking behaviors are evident. This coupled with the lack of clear diagnosis, the willingness to take someone else's medication, is counterproductive to establishing a firm patient/physician relationship built on trust. Even the fact that the individual is on a government assistance program increases the risk of misuse.

The clinical scenario would suggest to many providers that this patient needs to be discharged from the clinical environment. This might be a common approach, but it is not the best approach. An individual that has red flags is an individual that requires adherence monitoring and advanced care. With the epidemic of opioid prescription drug deaths, it is this type of individual that does need an intervention. Simply dismissing this individual places the patient and community at risk. This individual will doctor shop, going from practice to practice until they are satisfied, and likely return to that provider with increased requests. The chaotic lifestyle will usually evolve into expectations of a prescription when pills are lost or stolen.

The use of controlled substances for recreational purposes was not realized to the full extent until the era of the late '90s. Prior to 1996, DAWN and ARCOS data did not reveal a particular trend of abuse, misuse, or diversion. That same period of time medical use was increasing rapidly, but there were no particularly revealing trends that divulged the urgent need for increased scrutiny of these agents. Some believe that the increased use of opioids is enhanced realization that chronic pain is undertreated. Recently, however, the trend is more alarming. Even though there is a slight reduction in opioid use overall, misuse has increased.

As with any treatment, the risk/reward benefit is carefully considered prior to initiating therapy. In the case of this vignette, or any scenario where opioid management is considered, the conscious decision to prescribe or not prescribe is based on clinical support. The expectation is that opioids will increase function and quality of life, but that does not always seem to be the case. Despite evidence that opioids do not improve quality of life and may actually increase disability, the use of opioids and controlled substances for the subjective complaints of pain remain robust. Further underscoring this irony is that chronic opioid use lacks evidence supporting use, an abundance of evidence exists that these agents are risky and in certain patient populations, dangerous. Despite remedial efforts at educating the medical community, widespread opioid use promotes misuse, abuse, and diversion. In the case of low back pain, a physician that is pressured in the primary care office for time, and a patient's insistence on obtaining a controlled substance, it is often easy to prescribe and avoid confrontation. Our society is becoming increasingly tolerant of previously forbidden drugs. We are entering into the marijuana era, where states assess the tolerance for recreational use, and legalize the drug for sale and distribution. Patients will then perceive, as many do now, that marijuana is an innocent drug. Marijuana is, however, a drug of abuse. Impairment is a side effect of the drug, just as alcohol and benzodiazepines. Despite states opinions, marijuana is illegal at the federal level. Most providers have entered into an agreement with the Drug Enforcement Administration that they will prescribe by community standard, and will withhold prescriptions when illegal drugs are used. At the federal level, marijuana remains a schedule I drug, where no medical use is defined. Those that prescribe have a DEA certificate that is federal, not controlled by the state, which establishes a legal and ethical question between patient and provider. If a patient perceives marijuana as part of their necessary routine, is it legal and ethical for a physician to prescribe a controlled substance? This question has not been answered.

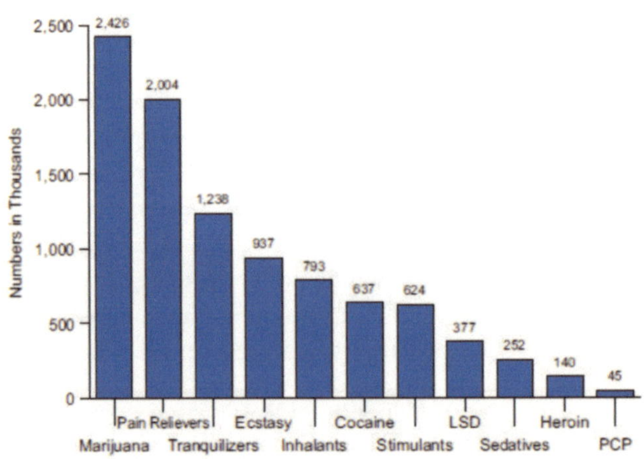

Note: The specific drug refers to the one that was used for the first time, regardless of whether it was the first drug used or not.

Again the risk/reward benefit should be considered foremost in a medical practice. The common denominator of the provider and the patient is the healing interaction in the clinical construct as understood by the patient and clinician equally. When one of the parties, in the case of the vignette, is outside of the expected clinical norm, care options are limited, such as opioid use. Controlled substance management is the most likely choice to be eliminated when aberrancies are noted. Many care options in chronic pain medicine are discretionary, and believe that a patient's pain is "real." Pain is subjective, with physiologic and psychologic comorbidities, and requires the provider to acknowledge the difficulties of treating those in pain. The prescribing physician and the patient enter a cooperative agreement. Each understands expectations and boundaries.

11. Regulatory agency pressure

Regulatory agencies such as state medical boards in the United States, the US Food and Drug Administration, as well as law enforcement agencies are under pressure to crack down on over-prescribing and "pill mills". The Physicians for Responsible Opioid Prescribing (PROP) have recommended changes in the labeling indication for opioids [78]. They have recommended limiting the labeling indication for opioids to limit the duration of opioid therapy to 90 days and limiting the dose to 100 mg/day of morphine equivalents. This expert group also recommends limiting opioid to severe pain rather than moderate pain. These recommendations do not apply to end of life care. The consequences of labeling changes such as these would make chronic opioid therapy an "off-label" use and many physicians would be reluctant to continue prescribing chronic opioid therapy that is considered "off label". If the FDA adopts the recommendation of the petition, signed by experts, it would create a new and unfavorable environment for practitioners and patients. Access to pain care would be reduced.

11.1. Clinical situations as an Alternative to Chronic Opioid Therapy

Clinical Vignette. A rancher takes three hydrocodone per day for osteoarthritis of the knees for years. His orthopedic surgeon wants to wait a few more years before replacing his knees. The patient does not drink alcohol or use other controlled substances, and he continues to work cattle on his ranch. He breaks his own horses.

Some patients do well with opioids, and do not require escalating doses. Without significant dose escalation, they retain a high level of function. In this particular individual, the diagnosis is clear, there have been no discernable side effects, and he is able to continue with his activities of daily living, enjoying a high level of function despite his arthritis.

An elderly patient with spinal stenosis has a history of gastrointestinal bleeding felt to be triggered by anti-inflammatory agents, and reports no significant relief with non-narcotic medication alternatives, including maximum dose of acetaminophen. She has been intolerant of tricyclic antidepressants and gabapentinoids. She is unable to afford non generic therapy. Hydrocodone is intolerably constipating, but she is able to function with Tramadol, and is being treated in an interdisciplinary environment.

This particular patient is an individual that has failed non-narcotic options, but has a spine that may be treated with an interventional approach. She may be a candidate for caudal lysis of adhesions, or the recently introduced minimally invasive lumbar decompression (MILD) procedure, or both before proceeding with further spinal surgery. Certain patient populations are felt to be poor candidates for opioid therapy or unable to tolerate the side effects. Patients with chaotic lifestyles, post-traumatic stress disorder, and certain types of anxiety and depression lead to misuse and potential abuse. Habituation and lack of efficacy are significant problems with opioids. Opioids have been reported to interfere with the treatment of anxiety, and may lead to an actual decline in quality of life, and promote pain and disability. Other groups with obesity, multiple symptom etiologies, and vague pain complaints that do not have a clear substantiated diagnosis are also less attractive candidates for opioid therapy. Risk items might include older age, female, antisocial personality, government disability, severe disability initial evaluation, not working at discharge, and previous history of misuse, abuse, and DWI. As might be expected, the longer a person is out of work the less likely they are to return. Opioids prescribed for longer than 7 days have been reported a risk factor for long-term disability in workers with acute back pain. The 52 week study showed no major outcome differences between patients treated with stable opioid regimen versus escalating opioid dose regimen. Higher doses are not always associated with additional benefits, and the potential of introducing opioid-induced hyperalgesia is another item of concern when utilizing opioids in chronic therapy. This 52 week study had a dropout rate of 27% due to misuse, which is very consistent with a number of other studies that reveal opioids are misused by 20-25% in various patient populations. A retrospective study found no correlation between opioid dose and pain severity in patients with chronic pain who took opioids for an average of 704 days. These patients were treated with higher doses in response to elevated pain complaints, and it was observed that patients on lower doses reported less pain. Conclusions are difficult to discern between the potential for hyperalgesia, versus dosing resistance.

A unique population that is emerging as a significant opioid use category is pregnancy. Of the 1.1 million pregnant women enrolled in Medicaid, 23% filled an opioid prescription in 2007. This is up almost 19% from 2000, according to a recent study published in Obstetrics and Gynecology [79]. It is estimated that 1 in 5 women use opioids during pregnancy. Another study revealed 500,000 privately insured women found 14% were dispensed opioid pain killers at least once during their pregnancy. The rate of opioid prescriptions was the highest in the south and the lowest in the northwest. In the study, of the women enrolled in Medicaid, 41.6% of pregnant women in Utah were prescribed opioids, and Oregon had the lowest at 9.5%. This regional discrepancy does not reflect differences in pain states, but the willingness of the provider to prescribe opioids. Opioids do not have a sufficient number of studies to demonstrate safety in this population. Increasing use of opioids during pregnancy may lead to neonatal abstinence syndrome. It is likely that society expects some type of medication be utilized for pain relief when acetaminophen is not effective. Possibly explaining the increased use is that opioids are one of the few choices other than medication for relief during pregnancy.

Diversion of prescribed opioids remains a rising problem with the young people. Among persons aged 12 older who used pain relievers nonmedically, 55% report they received the drug for free from a friend or a relative, while another 11% bought the drug from a friend or a relative. 7 million, 2.7% of the population, persons aged 12 or older used prescription-type drugs nonmedically in the past month.

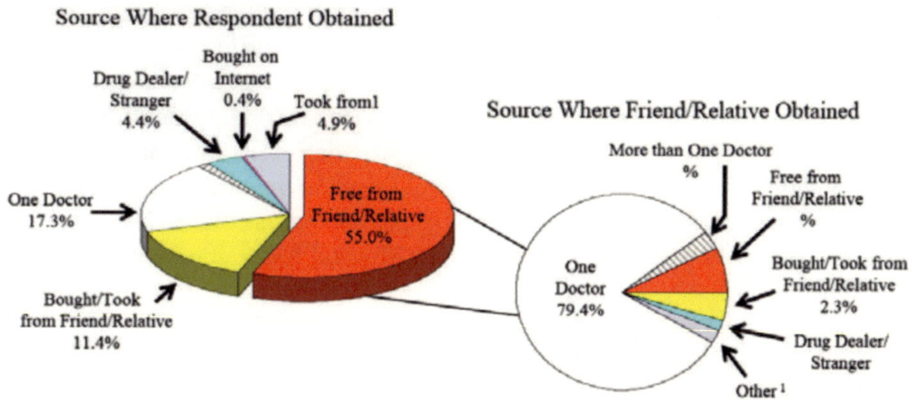

5 million of these used pain relievers. There is no validated risk assessment tool that exists to clearly identify and prevent diversion. Chronic pain may be the complaint, but in one study almost 40% of those addicted to prescription medications eventually switched to heroin [79,80].

12. Overdoses

Overdoses occur, and are a feared complication of controlled substance management. Overdoses on opioids alone are relatively uncommon. Usually overdoses occur with polypharmacy, other offending agents usually being benzodiazepines, or barbiturates. Barbiturates, mixed with alcohol, is a combination with opioids that is extremely hazardous. Although opioids are the most common drug class associated with overdose, the combination of opioids with benzodiazepines and other psychotropic drugs are associated in up to 10% of overdoses. A study in 2006 of West Virginia overdoses was found to be associated with nonmedical use and diversion of opioids, only 44% of victims had been prescribed the found drug.

13. Informed consent

Informed consent is not an optional endeavor in the clinical setting. It is a process, in which there is a communication, established clearly, with no barriers to communication between the physician and the patient. Many times the patient is not the one that would be the necessary recipient of informed consent, such as in the event of a patient rendered insensible, under the context of a court order, or power of attorney. Informed consent is an interrelationship between the patient, physician and society. It is a process that involves many steps, and the physician is ultimately held responsible for breakdown in informed consent.

The process of informed consent is both a legal and clinical action and is a process of protecting the communication lines, and avoids misrepresentation of understanding, and ultimately communication failure. It assumes the physician is an educator to the patient, family, and medical community, and requires that all aware are in acceptance, and aware of potential risks and benefits to a particular treatment or therapy. Informed consent is a necessary element of controlled substance management. Poor communication resulting in altered expectation of the family and patient is a leading factor in the generation of lawsuits. Informed consent reduces this risk and assumes that standard of care between a reasonable prudent physician, nurse, physician's assistant, nurse practitioner, or other provider exists, that has similar training. Under similar circumstances these providers would react to medical issues that establish the standard. A physician has a duty to disclose to his patient the risk of injuries that might result from proposed course of treatment. The American Medical Association guidelines define the physician should

- disclose the patient diagnosis if known
- the nature of proposed treatment or procedure
- the risks and benefits of proposed treatment or procedure
- alternatives
- the risks and benefits of alternative treatment
- the risks and benefits of not receiving or undergoing the treatment.

These guidelines are not requirements, but this list effectively establishes a standard of care by which a physician's disclosures are measured. In general, a physician does not need to advise a patient of every conceivable risk but only the substantial risks must be disclosed. That might be what a physician would reasonably know to be a part of the treatment course, and allowing the patient to decide whether they would want to consider moving forward. Informed consent may be verbal, but documentation establishes a better pathway to defend a dispute. Care must be taken that the individual who is providing informed consent is adequately trained to understand the importance of this task. The patient should have a clear understanding of the implications of informed consent, and ample time to ask questions, and engage in dialogue that addresses the patient's concerns.

Many guidelines now recommend obtaining separate and specific informed consent for opioid treatment. Warning patients of addiction risks as well as overdose and diversion are important. The Federation of State Medical Board rules state:

"Informed consent documents typically address:

- The potential risks and anticipated benefits of chronic opioid therapy.
- Potential side effects (both short-and long-term) of the medication, such as constipation and cognitive impairment.
- The likelihood that tolerance to and physical dependence on the medication will develop.
- The risk of drug interactions and over-sedation.

- The risk of impaired motor skills (affecting driving and other tasks).
- The risk of opioid misuse, dependence, addiction, and overdose.
- The limited evidence as to the benefit of long-term opioid therapy.
- The physician's prescribing policies and expectations, including the number and frequency of prescription refills, as well as the physician's policy on early refills and replacement of lost or stolen medications.
- Specific reasons for which drug therapy may be changed or discontinued (including violation of the policies and agreements spelled out in the treatment agreement)."

14. Opioid agreements

An opioid agreement is sometimes called "a contract." The opioid contract implies a legal component, so better terminology is an "agreement" between the prescriber and those receiving the controlled substances. The opioid agreement, or controlled substance agreement, is an understanding between all parties that there will be one source of prescribed medication that is of controlled nature, and one dispensing pharmacy. There can be some practical adjustments, but the reality is that it is necessary to have this document in place so there is no barrier to communication.

Opioid agreements encourage patients to avoid dose escalations, multiple prescribers and pharmacies, and inform patients of opioid tapering and discontinuation of opioid may occur if necessary.

The Federation of State Medical Board rules state:

"Treatment agreements outline the joint responsibilities of physician and patient and are indicated for opioid or other abusable medications. They typically discuss:

- The goals of treatment, in terms of pain management, restoration of function, and safety.
- The patient's responsibility for safe medication use (e.g., by not using more medication than prescribed or using the opioid in combination with alcohol or other substances; storing medications in a secure location; and safe disposal of any unused medication).
- The patient's responsibility to obtain his or her prescribed opioids from only one physician or practice.
- The patient's agreement to periodic drug testing (as of blood, urine, hair, or saliva).
- The physician's responsibility to be available or to have a covering physician available to care for unforeseen problems and to prescribe scheduled refills."

14.1. Sample Opioid Agreement

The following agreement relates to my use of controlled substances including, but not limited to "narcotics/opioids," to treat chronic pain. I will be provided with the prescriptions only if I understand and agree to the following:

_____1. I understand that, depending on the drug and dose, I can become physically dependent on the medication and can develop withdrawal symptoms if the medication is stopped suddenly or the dose reduced rapidly. Although the risk is small there is a chance of developing an addiction to controlled substances if I am placed on them to help control my pain.

_____2. Controlled substances can cause sedation, confusion, or other changes in mental state and thinking abilities. I understand that the decision to drive while I am taking controlled substances is my own decision, and I agree not to be involved in any activity that may be dangerous to me or someone else such as driving or operating any dangerous equipment, working in unprotected heights or being responsible for another individual who is unable to care for himself or herself if I am in any way sedated, feel drowsy or am not thinking clearly.

_____3. I will not use any illegal substances including, but not limited to, marijuana and cocaine. I will not drive while impaired with alcohol or other substances.

_____4. The Receiving Controlled Substance Policy regarding the dispensing of controlled substances requires that I be seen regularly and I agree to make and keep my appointments. I will advise my doctor of all other medicines and treatments that I am receiving.

_____5. If the medication requires adjustment, an appointment must be made to see the doctor. No adjustments will be made over the telephone. My careful planning is required. I understand that medication refills and adjustments are done during office appointments. I must stay with the prescribed dosing so that I do not run out of medication early. I understand that the Refill Policy is NOT to prescribe early. I agree that I will use my medication exactly as prescribed and that if I run out early, I may go without medication until the next prescription is due, possibly resulting in withdrawal symptoms.

_____6. I understand that the prescriptions are my responsibility once they are placed in my hand and that if anything happens to my prescription (lost, stolen, or accidentally destroyed), I may NOT receive a replacement from my physician. I am expected to file a police report if my medication is stolen. I will be prepared to bring in a copy at my next REGULARLY scheduled visit.

____7. My physician will prescribe whatever medication he/she is comfortable with and thinks is best; he/she is not under any obligation to prescribe any specific medications.

____8. I am aware of the possible risks and benefits of other types of treatments that do not involve the use of opioids. The other treatments discussed include: injections, therapy, and surgery (if indicated).

____9. I agree to come to (Insert Facility Name) with my medication on the same day that I am called and submit to a pill count, and/or urine or blood screening to detect illegal substances or confirm proper use of prescribed medication. The call to come to (Insert Facility Name) can be made either randomly, or if a concern arises. I may be required to bring my unused medication routinely to each office visit. If I do not have insurance or my insurance denies testing, I will be responsible for the cost of the test.

____10. I give permission to (Insert Facility Name) to call any pharmacy or another health care provider at any time, without me being informed, to discuss my past or present use of controlled or illegal substances.

____11. I will not use my pain medication in higher than prescribed amounts for new problems that arise (toothache, surgery, etc.) unless authorized to do so by (Insert Facility Name). I will inform my other doctor(s) of my use of medication for chronic pain, and I will inform (Insert Facility Name) if another physician prescribes controlled substances for the acute problem and I will not mix the medications unless advised to do so by a medical professional either (Insert Facility Name) or the prescribing provider of the acute medication. I understand this is only in acute situations and documentation of the situation must be provided to (Insert Facility Name). My doctor at (Insert Facility Name) is my primary doctor with regard to my pain medications. If there is a medical emergency (e.g. broken leg, surgery requiring post-op pain medication, dental procedures, etc.), another doctor may prescribe pain medication to me, but I will advise the prescribing doctor of my care at (Insert Facility Name) including my binding contract, and authorize the doctor to disclose information to (Insert Facility Name), and I will also notify my doctor at (Insert Facility Name) of the medication and the dosage as soon as the emergency occurs (if after hours, it's my responsibility to call first thing the NEXT business day). It will also be up to my provider at (Insert Facility Name) to determine if it was a true emergency requiring additional medication, if not my contract from this facility may be voided.

____12. (Females only) Because of the risks of certain medications to unborn children, I will inform all physicians, obstetrician/gynecologist and (Insert Facility Name) immediately if I become pregnant or decide to try to become pregnant. I am aware that should I carry a baby to delivery while taking these medicines; the baby will be physically dependent upon opioids. I am aware the use of opioids is not generally associated with risk of birth defects. However, birth defects can occur whether or not the mother is on medicines and there is always the possibility that my child will have a birth defect while I am taking an opioid. I am also aware that opioids may alter my hormones as well.

_____13. (Males only) I am aware that chronic opioid use has been associated with low testosterone levels in males. This may affect my mood, stamina, sexual desire and physical and sexual performance. I understand that my doctor may check my blood to see if my testosterone level is normal.

_____14.My physician can wean me off of controlled substances at any time if he/she feels that it is in my best interest. (Insert Facility Name) will follow relevant laws when weaning me off of my medication. The weaning process can result in withdrawal symptoms. If I am weaned off, (Insert Facility Name) staff may inform my other health care providers as to the reasons for the weaning. (Insert Facility Name) may send me to a detoxification facility if indicated. I understand that (Insert Facility Name) will not be responsible for weaning me off of Methadone if I present with that in my system.

_____15. Abstinence Syndrome (Withdrawal Syndrome): Stopping my opioid, anti-seizure or antidepressant medication abruptly may result in withdrawal symptoms (flu-like symptoms, GI distress, diarrhea, sweating, heart palpitations, and rarely seizures or death). I should wean from my medications rather than stopping them abruptly. It is my responsibility to keep up with the amount of medication I have. I will make my appointments accordingly, before I run out.

_____16.I understand that in general I may be weaned off of my medication or my drug therapy may be terminated at the discretion of my physician if any of the following occur:

a)It is the opinion of my physician that controlled substances are not very effective for my pain and/or my functional activity is not improved.
b)I misuse the medication.
c)I develop rapid tolerance or loss of effect from this treatment.
d)I develop side effects that are significant and detrimental to me.
e)I obtain controlled substances from sources other than my provider at (Insert Facility Name) without informing him or her.
f)Pill counts or test results indicate the improper use of the prescribed medication or the use of other drugs, and/or I fail to submit to such counts/tests on the day that I am called.

g)I am arrested and/or convicted for a controlled or illicit drug violation including drunk driving.

h)Any violation of this agreement.

_____17. I further understand that my drug therapy will be terminated or detoxification in a controlled environment will be required if I give away, sell, distribute and/or transport with the intent to sell or dispense my medication.

_____18.I choose to use ____ Pharmacy, located at ____, for all of my pain medication prescriptions. I will not fill partial prescriptions if my pharmacy does not stock the full quantity of medication. If I change my pharmacy for any reason, I agree to notify my pain physician.

I have read the above Agreement, understand the Agreement, have had all my questions concerning this Agreement answered to my satisfaction, and I agree to abide by the terms of this Agreement if I am placed on controlled substances (including, but not limited to narcotic analgesics). I have received a copy of the Agreement. By signing this form voluntarily, I give my consent for the treatment of my pain with narcotic/opioid pain medicines.

____________________	____________________
Patient	Date
____________________	____________________
Physician	Date
____________________	____________________
Witness	Date

15. Screening questionnaires

The screening questionnaires available for controlled substances are often referred to as opioid risk tools, or ORTs. A number of these exist online, and can be referenced for use. Some are validated and some are not, but they are typically used to identify the risk of addiction, abuse, depression, anxiety, potential for diversion, and overdose among others. Also, comorbid diseases such as depression may be screened for. The usefulness of these tools is not known. They do not identify illegal use, abuse, or diversion.

16. Opioids and delivery systems

A number of synthetic and semi-synthetic opioids are utilized to control pain. The patch delivery system, uniquely associated with Fentanyl, has now been adopted with buprenorphine. Newer molecules such as Tapentadol utilize ascending and descending central nervous system pathways for pain control. Hydrocodone and Oxycodone are among the most commonly used opioids in the United States, and morphine is still considered the gold standard, of which the potency and efficacy of the opioids are measured. Methadone is a synthetic opioid that is inexpensive and long-acting. Methadone has been used for years to prevent patients in recovery from relapsing and using heroin and other street-borne opioids. Methadone clinics typically require patients to come to the clinic daily to receive a daily dose which prevents

http://dx.doi.org/10.5772/58818

overdose. Methadone is associated with its own unique problems including cardiac arrhythmias, and the interaction that it has with many drugs through hepatic metabolic pathways. This makes the half-life of Methadone variable, introducing the drugs unpredictability to the pain care community. Methadone is considered a drug of enhanced risk in this regard. If used at all, Methadone doses should be initiated at low levels and monitored closely.

17. Fentanyl

Fentanyl is an opioid of choice in patients with renal failure or allergy to morphine. Transdermal patch preparations have been associated with less constipation compared to oral opioids, and the delivery system assists in adherence if pills are problematic. However, the steady state of fentanyl may not occur until 12 hours after a dose change so it is not a good sole agent in acute pain settings where dose adjustments need to be made frequently. Even small doses have been associated with respiratory depression and death. Recently, Fentanyl has gained street popularity by mixing with heroin.

Transdermal fentanyl is now available in a lower dose of 12 micrograms per hour. Fentanyl oralets are available in 100 microgram preparations and fentanyl oral film is also available for oral mucosal administration. The buccal absorption is utilized in cancer pain therapy, and onset is rapid.

17.1. Opioid conversion

Patients may need opioid conversion to another opioid for a number of reasons. Sometimes cost is a factor, or rotation to another agent for metabolic reasons such as tolerance and metabolic inefficiency. Multiple opioid conversion charts exist and are of limited value. The emergence of genetic testing has demonstrated that unique patient characteristics do influence the effectiveness of opioids. Incomplete cross-tolerance may exist between different opioids and care should be exercised when converting high doses of opioids. Particular care is exercised with methadone and transdermal patches of fentanyl since a steady state is not reached quickly with these drugs. Dose escalations should be made after several days of treatment rather than changed on a daily basis. Patients are likely to retain previous prescriptions of opioids and may use old prescriptions of long acting opioid to supplement new prescriptions. Some patients may need hospitalization for opioid management and drug holidays, or formally detoxed.

17.2. Other drugs

Ketamine, buprenorphine, butorphanol and other classes of drugs may also be abused or misused along with opioid agonists. Many of these drugs are not detected by routine drug screening, and physicians should welcome information from the patients' family members or friends about the patient's drug and alcohol use.

18. Clinical vignette

A patient with mesothelioma repeatedly escalated their analgesic and called for early refills. The doses exceeded recommended doses and the patient was repeatedly counseled. The patient would not comply and the medication was discontinued. The medication was ketorolac. The behavior was indistinguishable from opioid addiction. This patient eventually died and was managed with other treatments but none were as effective as the intravenous NSAID administered by the patient via a port.

Lesson learned-pseudo-addiction is a real condition and some patients are not able to cope with pain and comply with treatment recommendations. NSAID and acetaminophen abuse are significant problems.

18.1. Intrathecal opioid

Intrathecal opioid infusions have been used to limit oral opioid consumption and control patients who self-escalate doses of opioids. There is little data to support the notion that spinal opioids prevent addiction; however, in a randomized trial of intrathecal opioid versus oral opioid for cancer pain management, patients treated with intrathecal opioid had a 6 month survival rate of 52-59% compared to 32% in the oral opioid group. [81] This suggests that intrathecal opioid may have a safety benefit related to controlled dosing.

18.2. Clinical vignette

A patient had an outpatient trial of intrathecal morphine but did not disclose that they were seeing a psychiatrist who was prescribing benzodiazepines. The patient had a respiratory arrest the morning after the injection.

Lesson learned-intrathecal opioid injections may not have a peak effect until the next day. Patients may need to be hospitalized for trials with intrathecal opioids, especially morphine or other opioids which may have a delayed peak effect.

The Wiley catheter may be used for intrathecal opioid trials and has been associated with a lower incidence (3% versus 10% with larger catheters) of spinal headache in obstetrical patients. [82]

Patients, who respond to a test dose of 0.5 mg of morphine or less, tend to maintain responses to intrathecal opioid. Other factors of success include female gender, age over 65 and a diagnosis of peripheral neuropathic pain. Patients with cervical pain and visceral pain tend to require more rapid dose escalations. [83]

Patients, who respond only to higher doses during a trial, require more dose escalations, conversations to alternative opioids, including oral opioids, and the addition of additional agents such as bupivacaine. Lower daily doses of morphine, as a single agent, may be associated with less risk for granuloma formation, which has been a significant problem with long term intrathecal opioid therapy. Meperidine has been associated with pump malfunctions and should be avoided.

Popular opioid conversion ratios of 100:10:1 for intravenous to epidural to intrathecal may vary significantly in clinical application, and conservative doses should be used to avoid overdoses. Morphine concentrations of 20mg/ml and doses of 0.25mg/day are ideal.

19. Interventional pain management as an alternative to chronic opioid therapy

Procedural interventions to treat pain are attractive options to avoid known and unknown risks of chronic drug exposure. Frequently, interventions assist in diagnosis of the painful state and reduce the opioid load. Also, the cost of some drug therapy is substantial and comparable to procedures over time. Some patients report prolonged periods of pain improvement following interventional procedures.

An example of a useful interventional procedure is epidural lysis of adhesions after years of chronic low back and leg pain. Patients sometimes retain years of improved function and quality of life after this procedure.

20. Interdisciplinary treatment as an alternative to chronic opioid therapy

Interdisciplinary pain management, as an alternative to continuing chronic opioid therapy, has been offered to patients over the past year in our practice. The interdisciplinary program included 8 half day sessions over a 4 week period. Each half day session included 1 hour of cognitive behavioral therapy as a part of a structured sequence of sessions. Theories of pain, relaxation techniques, cognitive restructuring, stress management, pacing, pleasant activity scheduling, anger management, assertiveness training, sleep hygiene, and planning for flare-ups included in the curriculum of care. Each half day session also includes 1 hour of psycho-educational group therapy to complement the individual cognitive behavioral therapy. 1 hour of physical therapy for general conditioning, specific range of motion and strengthening is also an integral part of the program. Physician visits are scheduled during these half day sessions for medication management and limited interventional pain management.

45 patients completed the interdisciplinary treatment program and were able to reduce or eliminate opioids. At the same time, functional improvement was made across multiple measures. Figure 1 shows average pain in previous week. Patients' median pain score dropped approximately 35% after the interdisciplinary treatment.

Figure 2 shows a drop in median opioid dose from low to none. In this analysis, 1=no opioid, 2=low opioid dose (1-40mg per day of oral morphine equivalents), 3=moderate opioid dose (40-100 mg per day of oral morphine equivalents), 4=high dose opioid (greater than 100 mg per day of oral morphine equivalents).

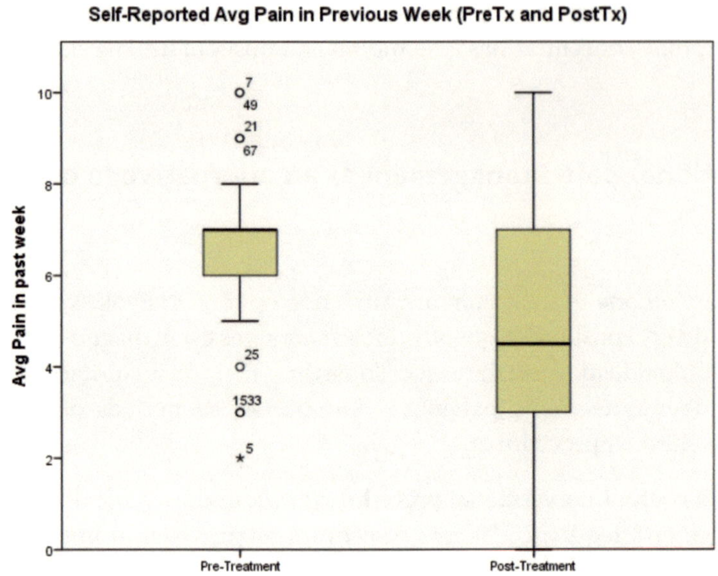

Figure 1. Visual analogue pain scores

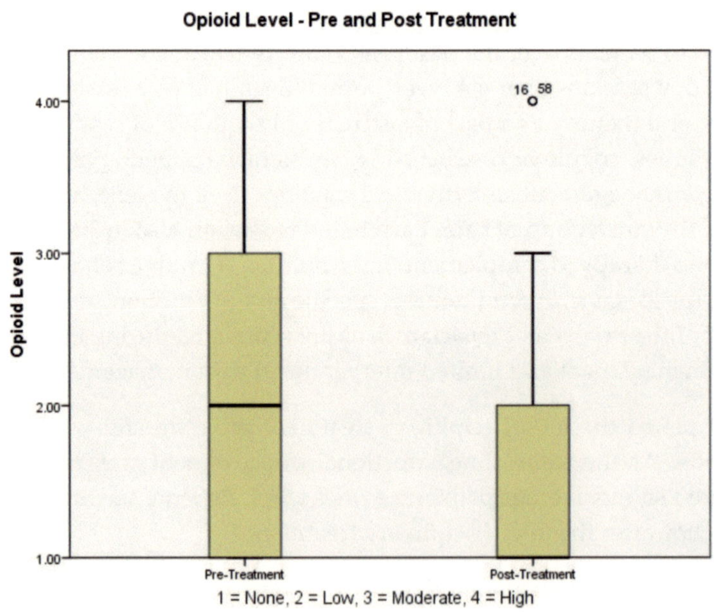

Figure 2. Opioid doses

Figure 3 shows a reduction in pain interference after interdisciplinary treatment.

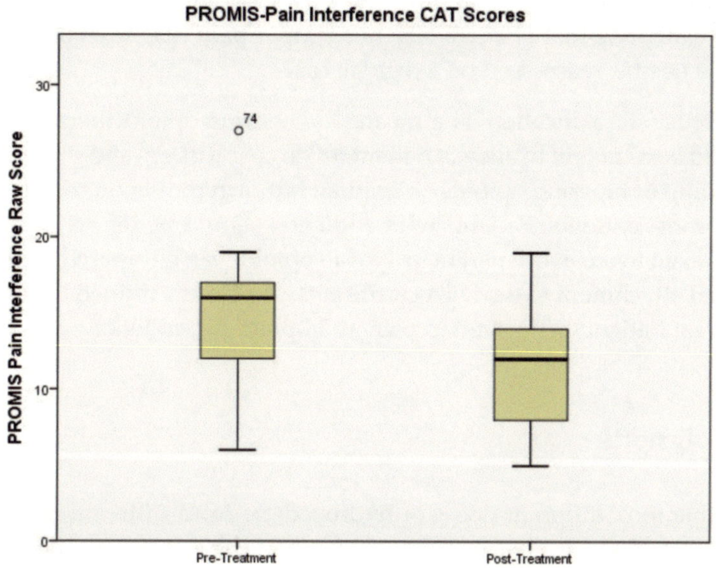

Figure 3. Pain interference scores

A significant group of patients did not pursue interdisciplinary treatment and no outcome data is available to compare with the patients who completed the program. However, the 45 patients who did reduce or eliminate opioids, their risk for overdose and diversion is probably significantly lower and their function is clearly improved, along with functional existence.

Perhaps patients who chose not to participate in interdisciplinary care have pain that was opioid responsive, and made the right decision. On the other hand, it is likely patients who did not participate would have benefitted if they had chosen to participate.

In any event, patients do need alternatives to continued chronic opioid therapy and interdisciplinary treatment is a viable option for at least some of the large number of patients who have been treated with opioids.

20.1. Tapering off

Many patients are prescribed opioid therapy by one doctor and then continue chronic opioid therapy with another doctor. Once patients have been exposed to opioids for a prolonged period of time, it becomes difficult to change the pain management approach and extinguish opioid-liking behaviors. However, continuing chronic opioid therapy that was initiated by another doctor is not addressed well in current guidelines. The single prescriber principle, interpreted literally, would mean that "taking over" opioid prescribing from another doctor would be prohibited. The reality is that patients change insurance, move, and choose to change doctors over the course of years for a number of valid reasons. Existing opioid therapy may not be an indication for continuing chronic opioid therapy, and primary care physicians, as well as specialists, need to be prepared to refer patients for detoxification if guidelines for opioid therapy cannot be met due to a lack of a proper pain diagnosis or red flags for abuse exist. Legitimate need is reassessed on a regular basis.

Patients may refuse detoxification as a means to continue opioid therapy. The prescribing physician should be reluctant to allow a patient to "go cold turkey" and should have some skill and understanding of tapering opioids. A gradual but firm reduction over a period of weeks is adequate for most patients. Patients with addiction should be referred for addictionology care and encouraged to receive expert help. Not all opioids can be tapered, such as Methadone, without a special attachment to the DEA certificates. Physicians trained in addictionology are best suited to treat patients who overlap pain and opioid dependence.

21. Clinical vignette

An elderly couple took different doses of hydrocodone from different doctors. They began sharing medication. Both needed to be tapered off and they refused and were discharged. Signed, written opioid agreements were in effect, which helped diffuse the situation.

Lesson learned-having opioid treatment agreements signed by the patient are helpful when patients need to be tapered of opioid and/or discharged for a medical practice. Patients who are terminated from a medical practice for cause should be sent a certified letter and followed for 30 days while alternative care is arranged.

Patients may be tapered off opioid over a period of days to weeks. Rapid Benzodiazepine withdrawal is associated with seizures and should proceed slowly in conjunction with psychiatric care if accessible. Clonidine patch 0.1 mg/day may be helpful managing symptoms of opioid withdrawal, as well as hydroxyzine as an anxiolytic.

22. REMS

Risk evaluation and mitigation strategies (REMS) training is required for long acting and sustained release opioid prescribing. These measures are varied depending on the specific opioid preparation. Standardization of REMS requirements will eventually assist to meet guidelines [84].

22.1. Alternatives to chronic opioids

Tamper resistant preparations, buprenorphine, tramadol and new agents may help reduce the diversion associated with chronic opioid therapy. Interdisciplinary evaluations including interventional pain evaluations, psychological and physical therapy evaluations invariably lead to alternatives to chronic opioid therapy. Many chronic pain patients may be managed without opioids, and adjunctive medications enhance sleep, diminish depression and anxiety observed as comorbidities.

22.2. Guidelines

Multiple guidelines have been promulgated for opioid treatment of chronic pain. Experts in the field have published guidelines but new information about the risks of opioids necessitates new guidelines at this time. The American Society of Interventional Pain Physicians (ASIPP) updates controlled substance guidelines every two years. This exhaustive effort is available for download on the internet at www.asipp.org [85].

22.3. Labeling

In 2013, The Food and Drug Administration in the United States required new labeling information for opioids that are long acting:

"TRADENAME is:

- A strong prescription pain medicine that contains an opioid (narcotic) that is used to manage pain severe enough to require daily around-the-clock, long-term treatment with an opioid, when other pain treatments such as non-opioid pain medicines or immediate-release opioid medicines do not treat your pain well enough or you cannot tolerate them.
- A long-acting (extended-release) opioid pain medicine that can put you at risk for overdose and death. Even if you take your dose correctly as prescribed you are at risk for opioid addiction, abuse, and misuse that can lead to death.
- Not for use to treat pain that is not around-the-clock."

The use of long acting drugs for acute post-operative pain should be limited to special circumstances such as opioid tolerance or burn pain.

Recently, the Federation of State Medical Boards issued a new model policy including the following statement: "Additionally, providers should not continue opioid treatment unless the patient has received a benefit, including demonstrated functional improvement." [86] Most studies of opioids for chronic pain have shown incremental improvements in pain but have failed to show functional improvement. Therefore, it seems as though chronic opioid therapy is unlikely to continue as an accepted treatment for most patients.

Washington State has developed new workers' compensation guidelines in response to an epidemic of overdoses. [87] These guidelines are an attempt to objectify treatment for subjective symptoms. The guidelines restrict the use of chronic opioid therapy to very few special cases. The guidelines reserve opioids for VAS >7 and limit the dose to 120mg/day of oral morphine equivalents. The duration of treatment is limited to weeks. Continuation of opioids must be associated with a 30% improvement on a 2-question instrument for pain and function. Interestingly, the guidelines allow for marijuana use even though marijuana use has been associated with the use of more dangerous illicit substances. Restrictive guidelines such as these are fraught with contradiction and the potential for limiting access to therapy.

New opioid prescribing guidelines with a "safe harbor" prescribing clause including doses and duration of intervals between follow –up visits for reevaluation and prescription refills. Most prescribing laws, rules and guidelines mandate a single prescriber and pharmacist yet a single decision maker model is a major factor in making an individual physician vulnerable to disciplinary action.

22.4. Clinical vignette

An elderly obese woman with intractable severe pain was bedridden and demanded more opioid. Her bedridden status was confirmed and no additional opioid was prescribed. She responded by saying "you want me to be in pain".

Lesson learned-in the current environment, increases in opioid doses need to be associated with increased function.

22.5. Cancer pain

The use of opioids for cancer pain is excluded from restrictions in most guidelines. However, many patients with cancer survive long-term and are really chronic pain patients. Cancer treatment may produce chemotherapy related neuropathy, radiation plexopathy, and chronic post-operative pain such as post mastectomy syndrome, post thoracotomy syndrome and phantom pain syndrome. Pathologic fractures, especially vertebral body fractures, respond to interventional procedures. Interventional options for vertebral fractures include vertebroplasty, facet injections, and lysis of adhesions, quadratus lumborum or psoas injections, or transforaminal catheter techniques for chronic pain.

Neuromodulation may be useful in patients with neuropathic pain resulting from successful cancer treatment. Patients need to be evaluated for myofascial pain, radiculopathy and other common pain syndromes with careful history taking and physical examination. Terminally ill patients do have options for treatment other than escalating opioid doses. Trigger point injections, lysis of adhesions and other interventional therapies are often very helpful managing patients with cancer who may or may not ultimately die from neoplasia.

CLINICAL VIGNETTE patient with pain in the groin, scrotum and sacral area following radiation left the patient unable to sleep in any position other than in a chair in a knees-to-chest position. The patient responded to sacral electrode stimulation bilaterally at S3. A year later, the patient had more pain and responded to stimulation at S2.

Lesson learned-Following aggressive cancer treatment, there are devastating pain conditions that are not terminal but do respond to interventional techniques but not to opioids.

Cancers of the cervix, rectum and other tissues produce pelvic pain syndromes that are often difficult to treat. Patients who have undergone abdominal-perineal resections have pain syndromes that may not respond well to opioids. This group of patients may have pain with sitting and tenderness to palpation over the ischial tuberosity (Racz's sign). Ricardo Plancarte describes the inferior hypogastric block may provide significant relief in some of these patients. [88]

A unilateral inferior hypogastric block is the preferred procedure for patients with unilateral pain and ischial tenderness. The inferior hypogastric plexus is more anatomically defined compared to the superior hypogastric plexus, which is more diffuse. A diagnostic block should be performed, preferably with a curved blunt needle, before a neurolytic block with phenol 6%, 4-5 ml. [89] Erdine reported a transdiscal approach that may be the most effective technique. [90]

"Morphinemia" (a lack of morphine) should not be considered as the primary problem in every patient with cancer related pain. Opioids are prescribed for patients who respond to them, but additional options are explored in order to respond to a patient in need of pain relief, who does not respond adequately to increasing doses of opioids.

Methylnaltrexone for opioid related constipation in palliative care patients may be used when laxatives and other measures are inadequate. Constipation can cause abdominal pain and treating this with more opioid continues the cycle. The dose of methylnaltrexone is 0.15 mg/kg.

Opioids also control rest pain, but not movement related pain. Opioids do reduce the likelihood of a patient becoming bedridden. Metastases usually do not invade vertebral pedicles early, and patients respond to lysis of adhesions enough to be able to walk. [91,92]

Clinical vignette-a patient with spinal metastasis responded for 3 months to lysis of adhesions. The patient became bedridden again and responded to a second procedure.

Lesson learned-some patients with terminal cancer may have improved quality of life with interventional techniques that otherwise would not be produced with opioids alone.

Patients with upper abdominal cancer pain may benefit from splanchnic radiofrequency ablation. Quality of life and pain control have been improved in studies using this technique. [93]

Patients with cancer related pain should be evaluated for interventional procedures that may improve their quality of life and suffering. Patients with terminal illness may become isolated from medical specialists and be treated by mid-level practitioners who are unfamiliar with options other than opioid escalation. Cancer pain treatment requires a team approach to afford optimal care.

Other conditions beyond cancer are legitimate palliative diagnosis for opioid use. Patients with end stage coronary artery disease and congestive heart failure are treated with morphine, not for chest pain, but for the venous dilatory effect, decrease cardiac preload, and reduction in shortness of breath. Patients who are bedridden with osteoporotic fractures are another example of patients with chronic pain at the end of life, and opioids are a compassionate treatment companion. Every drug used for pain has toxicity and side effects that sometimes precludes its use. Sometimes opioids are the least toxic option in the palliative care setting.

23. Conclusions

Patients who request relatively small doses of opioids for conditions such as arthritis pain often do well over a period of years. This experience reinforces a practitioner's belief in the efficacy of chronic opioid therapy. However, addictionologists and pain specialists often witness a very different side of pain treated with opioids.

The prescribing clinician strives to improve the ability to identify patients who will do poorly with opioids, but we also strive to identify patients who will do well with this option. Generally, lower doses, less potent drugs, and shorter durations of therapy are associated with improved outcome and reduced adverse events. Some have suggested that opioids are to be used intermittently, not on a daily basis, for "breakthrough pain" only, along with other drug classes for "basal" analgesia. Others believe long-acting pharmacokinetically smooth agents are best suited for chronic pain.

The public health problem of overdose deaths has overridden the notion that the individual patient and their physician are free to use opioids for chronic pain without fear of legal and regulatory action and physicians need to anticipate the substantial shift in policy of regulators who authorize the privilege of practicing medicine.

Physicians are encouraged to err on the side of less opioid, rather than more opioid, and improve their skills in providing patient satisfaction with other drugs for chronic pain known as adjuncts. Non-drug treatments for pain need to be maximized as well prior to initiating opioid therapy. Tramadol and low dose potent opioids with defined frequent follow-up visits for refills are a necessary part of the practice of standard care despite the lack of long term randomized controlled trials.

Although contradictory to the patient/physician relationship, physicians must improve their ability to say “no” to the patient who demands opioids. This is weighed against alienating patients who have legitimate pain, but co-morbidities that place them at risk for bad outcomes from chronic opioid therapy. [94] Pain research, public education, patient education and medical education need to improve so that pain can be treated more successfully and safely. Improved diagnosis and treatment should lead to more cost effective treatment.

Author details

Hans Hansen[1], Carl E. Noe[2] and Gabor B. Racz[3]

1 The Pain Relief Centers, Statesville, North Carolina, USA

2 University of Texas Southwestern Medical Center, Dallas, Texas , USA

3 Texas Tech University Health Science Center, Lubbock Texas, USA

References

[1] http://healthyamericans.org/reports/drugabuse2013/, 2013

[2] Sullivan, M.D., Ballantyne, J.C.: What are we learning with long term opioid therapy?Archives of Internal Medicine (2012) 172:433-434

[3] Braden, J.B., Young, A., Sullivan M.D., et.al.: Predictors of change in pain and physical functioning among post-menopausal women with recurrent pain conditions in the women's health initiative observational cohort. The Journal of Pain (2012) 13:64-72

[4] Laxmaiah Manchikanti, MD, et al. American Society of Interventional Pain Physicians (ASIPP) Guidelines for Responsible Opioid Prescribing and Chronic Non-Cancer Pain: Part 1 – Evidence Assessment. Pain Physician 2012; 15: S67-S116

[5] Report of the International Narcotics Control Board for 2004. New York, United Nations, 2005. www.incb.org/pdf/e/ar/2004/incb_report_2004_full.pdf

[6] Edlund MJ, Martin BC, Devries A, Fan MY, Braden JB, Sullivan MD. Trends in use of opioids for chronic noncancer pain among individuals with mental health and substance use disorders: the TROUP Study. Clin J Pain 2010; 26:1-8.

[7] Sullivan MD, Edlund MJ, Fan MY, Devries A, Brennan Braden J, Martin BC. Risks for possible and probable opioid misuse among recipients of chronic opioid therapy in commercial and Medicaid insurance plans: the TROUP Study. Pain 2010; 150:332-339.

[8] Fleming MF, Balousek SL, Klessig CL, Mundt MP, Brown DD. Substance use disorders in a primary care sample receiving daily opioid therapy. J Pain 2007; 8:573-582.

[9] Warner M, Chen LH, Makuc DM, Anderson RN, Miniño AM. Drug poisoning deaths in the United States, 1980-2008. NCHS data brief, no. 81. National Center for Health Statistics, Hyattsville, MD, 2011.

[10] Centers for Disease Control and Prevention. Vital signs: Overdoses of prescription opioid pain relievers – United States, 1999-2008. MMWR. Morb Mortal Wkly Rep 2011; 60:1487-1492.

[11] Pain Med. 2013 Oct;14(10):1534-47. doi: 10.1111/pme.12183. Epub 2013 Jul 10. The economic burden of opioid-related poisoning in the United States. Inocencio TJ1, Carroll NV, Read EJ, Holdford DA.

[12] Pain Physician. 2012 Jul;15(3 Suppl):ES9-38. Opioid epidemic in the United States. Manchikanti L1, Helm S 2nd, Fellows B, Janata JW, Pampati V, Grider JS, Boswell MV.

[13] Pain Physician. 2012 Jul;15(3 Suppl):ES9-38. Opioid epidemic in the United States. Manchikanti L1, Helm S 2nd, Fellows B, Janata JW, Pampati V, Grider JS, Boswell MV.

[14] Open Med. 2012 Apr 10;6(2):e41-7. Print 2012. Trends in prescriptions for oxycodone and other commonly used opioids in the United States, 2000-2010. Kenan K1, Mack K, Paulozzi L.

[15] Pain Physician. 2014 Mar-Apr;17(2):E119-28. Assessment of the trends in medical use and misuse of opioid analgesics from 2004 to 2011. Atluri S, Sudarshan G, Manchikanti L1.

[16] IMS Institute for Healthcare Informatics. The use of medicines in the United States: Review of 2011. April 2012. www.imshealth.com/ims/Global/Content/Insights/IMS%20Institute%20for%20Healthcare%20Informatics/IHII_Medicines_in_U.S_Report_2011.pdf

[17] Pain. 2013 Dec;154 Suppl 1:S94-100. doi: 10.1016/j.pain.2013.09.009. Epub 2013 Sep 11. Opioid therapy for chronic pain in the United States: promises and perils. Sullivan MD1, Howe CQ.

[18] Clin Perinatol. 1991 Mar;18(1):1-22. Animal models of opiate, cocaine, and cannabis use. Hutchings DE1, Dow-Edwards D.

[19] Chou R, Huffman L. Use of Chronic Opioid Therapy in Chronic Non-cancer Pain: Evidence Review. American Pain Society, Glenview, IL, 2009. www.ampainsoc.org/library/pdf/Opioid_Final_Evidence_Report.pdf

[20] Governale L. Outpatient prescription opioid utilization in the U.S., years 2000 – 2009. Drug Utilization Data Analysis Team Leader, Division of Epidemiology, Office of Surveillance and Epidemiology. Presentation for U.S. Food and Drug Administration, July 22, 2010. www.fda.gov/downloads/AdvisoryCommittees/CommitteesMeetingMaterials/Drugs/AnestheticAndLifeSupportDrugsAdvisoryCommittee/UCM220950.pdf

[21] Woolfe, SH. The Power of Prevention and What It Requires. JAMA 2008: 299; 2437-2439

[22] Time Magazine. Friday, May 2, 2008. Kathleen Kingsbury.

[23] Krueger, A. Lancet May 2003

[24] Greene, Carmen. 2005

[25] Donavan, MI. J of Pain Symptom Manage. 1999: 18; 38-48

[26] The Arthritis Foundation, "Pain in America: Highlights from a Gallop Survey.", 2000

[27] Smith, BH, et al. The Impact of Chronic Pain in the Community. Fam Pract 2001: 18 (3): 292-9

[28] Stewart, WF, et al. Loss Productive Time and Cost due to Common Pain Conditions in the U.S. Workforce. JAMA (2003) 290: 18, p. 2446

[29] Lawrence, RC, et al. Arthritis and Rheum. 1998: 41 (5): 778-799

[30] Makela, M, et al. Prevalence, Determinence, and Consequences of Chronic Neck Pain in Finland. AMJ Epidemiol 134: 1356-1357, 1991

[31] Kohlberg, L., LaCrosse, J., & Ricks, D. (1972). The predictability of adult mental health from childhood behavior. In B. Wolman (Ed.), Manual of child psychopathology (pp. 1217–1284). New York: McGraw-Hill.

[32] Merskey H, Bogduk N. Task Force on Taxonomy of the International Association for the Study of Pain. Classification of Chronic Pain: Descriptions of Chronic Pain Syndromes and Definition of Pain Terms. 2nd ed. IASP Press, Seattle, WA, 1994.

[33] Neuropsychopharmacology. 2014 Apr 1. doi: 10.1038/npp.2014.77. Persistent Pain Facilitates Response to Morphine Reward by Downregulation of Central Amygdala GABAergic Function. Zhang Z, Tao W, Hou YY, Wang W, Lu YG, Pan ZZ

[34] Institute of Medicine (IOM). Relieving Pain in America: A Blueprint for Transforming Prevention, Care, Education, and Research. The National Academies Press, Washington, DC, June 29, 2011.

[35] Pizzo PA, Clark NM. Alleviating suffering 101 – Pain relief in the United States. N Engl J Med 2012; 367:197-198.

[36] Martin BI, Turner JA, Mirza SK, Lee MJ, Comstock BA, Deyo RA. Trends in health care expenditures, utilization, and health status among US adults with spine problems, 1997-2006. Spine (Phila Pa 1976) 2009 34:2077-2084.

[37] Cicero TJ, Wong G, Tian Y, Lynskey M, Todorov A, Isenberg K. Co-morbidity and utilization of medical services by pain patients receiving opioid medications: Data from an insurance claims database. Pain 2009; 144:20-27.

[38] Sjøgren P, Grønbæk M, Peuckmann V, Ekholm O. A population-based cohort study on chronic pain: the role of opioids. Clin J Pain 2010; 26:763-769.

[39] Substance Abuse and Mental Health Services Administration. Results from the 2010 National Survey on Drug Use and Health: Summary of National Findings. NSDUH Series H-41, HHS Publication No. (SMA) 11-4658. Substance Abuse and Mental Health Services Administration, Rockville, MD, 2011. www.samhsa.gov/data/NSDUH/2k10NSDUH/2k10Results.pdf.

[40] Diabetes and Cardiovascular Disease Executive Summary Conference Proceeding for Healthcare Professionals From a Special Writing Group of the American Heart Association. Scott M. Grundy, MD, PhD; Barbara Howard, PhD; Sidney Smith Jr, MD; Robert Eckel, MD; Rita Redberg, MD; Robert O. Bonow, MD. http://circ.ahajournals.org/content/105/18/2231.full

[41] Pain. 1986 May;25(2):171-86. Chronic use of opioid analgesics in non-malignant pain: report of 38 cases. Portenoy RK, Foley KM.

[42] http://www.unodc.org/unodc/en/frontpage/the-1912-hague-international-opium-convention.html

[43] JAMA. 2011 Apr 6;305(13):1315-21. doi: 10.1001/jama.2011.370. Association between opioid prescribing patterns and opioid overdose-related deaths. Bohnert AS1, Valenstein M, Bair MJ, Ganoczy D, McCarthy JF, Ilgen MA, Blow FC.

[44] Manchikanti L, Whitfield E, Pallone F. Evolution of the National All Schedules Prescription Electronic Reporting Act (NASPER): A public law for balancing treatment of pain and drug abuse and diversion. Pain Physician 2005; 8:335-347.

[45] Centers for Disease Control and Prevention. CDC grand rounds: Prescription drug overdoses – a U.S. epidemic. MMWR Morb Mortal Wkly Rep 2012; 61:10-13.

[46] Centers for Disease Control and Prevention. Vital signs: Overdoses of prescription opioid pain relievers – United States, 1999-2008. MMWR. Morb Mortal Wkly Rep 2011; 60:1487-1492.

[47] Pain Physician. 2012 Jul;15(3 Suppl):ES9-38. Opioid epidemic in the United States. Manchikanti L1, Helm S 2nd, Fellows B, Janata JW, Pampati V, Grider JS, Boswell MV.

[48] Drug Alcohol Rev. 2014 Apr 16. doi: 10.1111/dar.12143. Opioid-related mortality and filled prescriptions for buprenorphine and methadone. Wikner BN1, Ohman I, Seldén T, Druid H, Brandt L, Kieler H.

[49] Pain Physician. 2003 Apr;6(2):173-8. Prevalence of illicit drug use in patients without controlled substance abuse in interventional pain management. Manchikanti L1, Pampati V, Damron KS, Beyer CD, Barnhill RC.

[50] Deyo RA, Smith DH, Johnson ES, Donovan M, Tillotson CJ, Yang X, Petrik AF, Dobscha SK. Opioids for back pain patients: Primary care prescribing patterns and use of services. J Am Board Fam Med 2011; 24:717-727.

[51] Manchikanti L, Abdi S, Atluri S, Balog CC, Benyamin RM, Boswell MV, Brown KR, Bruel BM, Bryce DA, Burks PA, Burton AW, Calodney AK, Caraway DL, Cash KA, Christo PJ, Colson J, Damron KS, Datta S, Deer TR, Diwan S, Eriator I, Falco FJE, Fellows B, Geffert S, Gharibo CG, Glaser SE, Grider JS, Hameed H, Hameed M, Hansen HC, Harned M, Hayek SM, Helm II S, Hirsch JA, Janata JW, Kaye AM, Kaye AD, Koyyalagunta D, Lee M, Manchikanti KN, McManus CD, Pampati V, Parr AT, Pasupuleti R, Patel V, Pope JE, Sehgal N, Silverman SM, Singh V, Smith HS, Solanki DR, Tracy DH, Vallejo R, Wargo BW. American Society of Interventional Pain Physicians (ASIPP) guidelines for responsible opioid prescribing in chronic non-cancer pain: Part 1 – Evidence assessment. Pain Physician 2012; 15:S1-S66

[52] Am J Ind Med. 2013 Dec;56(12):1452-62. doi: 10.1002/ajim.22266. Epub 2013 Oct 10. Opioid poisonings and opioid adverse effects in workers in Washington State. Ful-

ton-Kehoe D1, Garg RK, Turner JA, Bauer AM, Sullivan MD, Wickizer TM, Franklin GM.

[53] Richarz, U., Waechter, S., Sabatowski, R., Szczepanski, L., Binsfeld, H.: Sustained safety and efficacy of once –daily hydromorphone extended release compared to twice –daily oxycodone controlled release over 52 weeks in patients with moderate to severe chronic noncancer pain. Pain Practice 2013, 13:30-40.

[54] Afilalo, M., Etropolski, M.S., Kuperwasser, B., et.al: Efficacy and Safety of Tapentadol Extended Release Compared with Oxycodone Controlled Release for the Management of Moderate to Severe Chronic Pain Related to Osteoarthritis of the Knee. Clinical Drug Investigation 2010; 30:489-505.

[55] Lerner, D., Chang, H., Rogers, W.H., et.al.: Imputing at-work productivity loss using results of a randomized controlled trial comparing tapentadol extended release and oxycodone controlled release for osteoarthritis pain. Journal of Occupational and Environmental Medicine 54:933-938

[56] Steiner, D., Munera, C., Hale, M., Ripa, S., Landau, C.: Efficacy and safety of buprenorphine transdermal system for moderate to severe low back pain: a randomized, double blind study. Journal of Pain 12:1163-173

[57] Bohnert A.S., Valenstein, M., Bair, M.J., et.al.: Association between opioid prescribing patterns and opioid overdose –related deaths. JAMA (2011) 305:1315-1321.

[58] Miller, M., Sturmer, T., Azrael, D., Levin, R., Solomon, D.H.: Opioid analgesics and the risk of fractures in older adults with arthritis Journal of the American Geriatric Society (2011) 59:430-438

[59] Saunders, K.W., Dunn, K.M., Merrill, J.O., et.al.: Relationship of opioid use and dosage levels to fractures in older chronic pain patients Journal of General Internal Medicine 25(4):310-315

[60] Gomes, T., Redelmeier D.A., Juurlink D.N., et.al;.: opioid dose and risk of road trauma in Canada: a population-based study JAMA (2010) 173:196-201

[61] Seal, K.H., Shi, Y., Cohen, G., et.al.: Association of mental health disorders with prescription opioids and high –risk opioid use in US veterans of Iraq and Afghanistan JAMA (2012) 307:940-947

[62] Lee M, Silverman SM, Hansen H, Patel VB, Manchikanti L. A comprehensive review of opioid-induced hyperalgesia. Pain Physician 2011; 14:145-161.

[63] Braden J.B., Edlund, M.J., Martin, B,C., et.al.: Trends in use of opioids by noncancer pain type 2000-2005 among Arkansas Medicaid and healthcare enrollees: results from the TROUP study Journal of Pain (2008) 9:1026-1035

[64] Brede, E., Mayer, T.G., Gatchel, R.J.: Prediction of failure to retain work 1 year after interdisciplinary functional restoration in occupational injuries Archives of Physical Medicine and Rehabilitation (2012) 93:268-274

[65] Franklin G.M., Stover, B.D., Turner, J.A.,et.al: early opioid prescription and subsequent disability among workers with back injuries Spine (2008) 33:199-204

[66] Naliboff, B.D., Wu, S.M., Schieffer, B., et.al.: A randomized trial of 2 prescription strategies for opioid treatment of chronic nonmalignant pain Journal of Pain 12:288-296

[67] Peavy K.M., Banta-Green, C.J., Kingston, S., et.al.: "Hooked on " prescription-type opiates prior to using heroin: results from a survey of syringe exchange clients Journal of Psychoactive Drugs (2012) 44:259-265

[68] Manchikanti L, Whitfield E, Pallone F. Evolution of the National All Schedules Prescription Electronic Reporting Act (NASPER): A public law for balancing treatment of pain and drug abuse and diversion. Pain Physician 2005; 8:335-347.

[69] Wang J, Christo PJ. The influence of prescription monitoring programs on chronic pain management. Pain Physician 2009; 12:507-515

[70] Reifler LM, Droz D, Bailey JE, Schnoll SH, Fant R, Dart RC, Bucher Bartelson B. Do prescription monitoring programs impact state trends in opioid abuse/misuse? Pain Med 2012; 13:434-442.

[71] Yokell MA, Green TC, Rich JD. Prescription drug monitoring programs. JAMA 2012; 307:912; author reply 912-913.

[72] Paulozzi LJ, Kilbourne EM, Desai HA. Prescription drug monitoring programs and death rates from drug overdose. Pain Med 2011; 12:747-754.

[73] Gourlay DL, Heit HA, Almahrezi A. Universal precautions in pain medicine: A rational approach to the treatment of chronic pain. Pain Med 2005; 6:107-112.

[74] Lee M, Silverman SM, Hansen H, Patel VB, Manchikanti L. A comprehensive review of opioid-induced hyperalgesia. Pain Physician 2011; 14:145-161.

[75] Manchikanti L, Singh V, Caraway DL, Benyamin RM. Breakthrough pain in chronic non-cancer pain: Fact, fiction, or abuse. Pain Physician 2011; 14:E103-E117.

[76] https://archive.org/details/63310410R.nlm.nih.gov

[77] Soc Sci Med. 1984;18(6):515-23. Pain and the ethics of pain management. Edwards RB.

[78] http://www.cdc.gov/primarycare/materials/opoidabuse/docs/pda-phperspective-508.pdf

[79] Substance Abuse and Mental Health Services Administration. Results from the 2010 National Survey on Drug Use and Health: Summary of National Findings. NSDUH

Series H-41, HHS Publication No. (SMA) 11-4658. Substance Abuse and Mental Health Services Administration, Rockville, MD, 2011. www.samhsa.gov/data/NSDUH/2k10NSDUH/2k10Results.pdf.

[80] Substance Abuse and Mental Health Services Administration. Results from the 2010 National Survey on Drug Use and Health: Mental Health Findings. NSDUH Series H-42, HHS Publication No. (SMA) 11-4667. Rockville, MD: Substance Abuse and Mental Health Services Administration, 2012. www.samhsa.gov/data/NSDUH/2k10MH_Findings/2k10MHResults.pdf

[81] Smith, T.J., Coyne, P.J., Staats, P.S., et.al.: An implantable drug delivery system for refractory cancer pain provides sustained pain control, less drug-related toxicity, and possibly better survival compared with comprehensive medical management. Annals of Oncology 16:825-833, 2005

[82] Tao, W., Nguyen, A.P., Ogunnaike, B.O., Craig, M.G.: Use of a 23 gauge continuous spinal catheter for labor analgesia: a case series International Journal of Obstetrical Anesthesia 20(4):351-4

[83] Dominguez E, Sahinler B, Bassam D, Day M, Lou L, Racz GB, Raj PP: Predictive Value of intrathecal Narcotic Trials for Long-Term therapy with Implantable Drug Administration systems in Chronic Non-Cancer Pain Patients. Pain Practice 2(4)315-325, 2002

[84] Thompson CA. Long-awaited opioid REMS affects prescribers more than dispensers. Am J Health Syst Pharm 2011; 68:963-967.

[85] Manchikanti L, Abdi S, Atluri S, Balog CC, Benyamin RM, Boswell MV, Brown KR, Bruel BM, Bryce DA, Purks PA, Burton AW, Caraway DL, Christo PJ, Colson J, Damron KS, S, Deer TR, Diwan S, Eriator I, Falco FJE, Fellows B, Geffert S, Gharibo CG, Glaser SE, Grider JS, Hameed H, Hameed M, Hansen H, Harned M, Hayek SM, Helm II S, Hirsch JA, Janata JW, Jorden AE, Kaye AM, Kaye AD, Koyyalagunta D, Lee M, Manchikanti KN, McManus CD, Pampati V, Parr AT, Pasupuleti R, Patel V, Pope JE, Ruan X, Sehgal N, Silverman SM, Singh V, Smith HS, Solanki DR, Tracy DH, Vallejo R, Wargo BW, Trescot AM. American Society of Interventional Pain Physicians (ASIPP) guidelines for responsible opioid prescribing in chronic non-cancer pain: Part 2 – Guidance. Pain Physician 2012; 15:S67-S116.

[86] Federation of State Medical Boards Model Policy on the Use of Opioid Analgesics in the Treatment of Chronic Pain July 2013

[87] Franklin G.M., Mal, J., Turner, J., et.al.: Bending the prescription opioids dosing and mortality curves: impact of the Washington State opioid dosing guidelines American Journal of Industrial Medicine (2012) 55: 325-331

[88] Racz GB, O Arter, C Noe, JE Heavner: Diagnostic and neurolytic hypogastric plexus blockade for pelvic pain. Abs NYPGA, 293: 1989.

[89] Racz GB, Noe C Colvin J, Heavner JE: Sympathetic nerve block, pelvic, hypogastric plexus block. In Raj JJ (ed.): Practical Management of Pain, Second Edition., 813-817, 1992.

[90] Erdine, S., Yucel, A.: Transdiscal approach for hypogastric plexus block Regional anesthesia and pain medicine 28:304-308

[91] Arter OE, Racz GB: Pain Management of the Oncologic Patient. Seminars in Surgical Oncology 6:162-172, 1990

[92] Racz, G.B., Day, M.R., Heavner,J.E., Smith, J.P.: The Racz Procedure: Lysis of epidural adhesions (Percutaneous Neuroplasty) In: Comprehensive treatment of chronic pain by medical interventional and integrative approaches. American Academy of Pain Medicine Ed. T.R. Deer, et. al. p 521-534 Springer publisher

[93] Papadopoulos, D., Kostopanagiotou, G., Batistaki, C.: Bilateral Thoracic Splanchnic Nerve Radiofrequency Thermocoagulation for the Management of End-Stage Pancreatic Abdominal Cancer Pain Pain Physician 2013; 16:125-133

[94] Wang, E., Golden, A., Butterworth, P.J.: How to say no The Permanente Journal 6(4) http://xnet.kp.org/permanentejournal/fall02/sayno.html

Chapter 4

Multimodal Analgesia for the Management of Postoperative Pain

Borja Mugabure Bujedo, Silvia González Santos,
Amaia Uría Azpiazu, Anxo Rubín Noriega,
David García Salazar and Manuel Azkona Andueza

Additional information is available at the end of the chapter

http://dx.doi.org/10.5772/57401

1. Introduction

The US Congress declared the 10-year period between January 1st, 2001, and December 31st, 2010, the decade for the control and treatment of pain, while the IASP (International Association for the Study of Pain) declared the period ending in October 2011, the year dedicated to acute pain. In spite of this measure, we must recognize that this effort has been insufficient, and that pain is one of the main health problems in the 21st century [1]. There is no ideal analgesic regimen, as none encompasses the characteristics of a fast onset of action, good cost-effectiveness profile, absence of short and long-term adverse effects, nil interaction with other drugs and/or metabolites, and ease of administration, both for the patients and healthcare personnel. Furthermore, technical deficiencies in the drug-delivery systems have contributed to a worsening of this situation, which is why, over the past few years, new and more precise mechanisms have appeared to allow us to improve the overall quality of analgesic regimens, "making old drugs new", especially those in the opioids family [2].

In spite of advances in the knowledge of the neurobiology of nociception and the physiology of systemic and spinal analgesic drugs, postoperative pain remains undertreated. Hospitalized postoperative patients should have the best access to analgesia, nevertheless, more than 1/3 of these patients experience moderate to severe pain in the first 24 h after their procedure [2]. Further, around 60% of current surgery can be ambulatory, but in reality, almost 80% of patients complain about moderate postoperative pain. Inadequate treatment leads to an extension of the recovery time, an increase in the length of the hospitalization stay, of health-care costs, and greater patient dissatisfaction [3].

INTECH
open science | open minds

© 2015 The Author(s). Licensee InTech. This chapter is distributed under the terms of the Creative Commons Attribution License (http://creativecommons.org/licenses/by/3.0), which permits unrestricted use, distribution, and reproduction in any medium, provided the original work is properly cited.

The gap between the knowledge of the mechanism of pain production and the application of an effective treatment is great, and ever growing. Neither acute, nor chronic pain usually receives adequate treatment due to several reasons relating to culture, attitude, education, politics and logistics. The correct treatment of pain is considered a fundamental right of the patient; in fact, lawsuits have been launched due to the under-treatment of pain, as well as an indicator of good clinical practice and quality of care [4]. The ideal analgesic regimen must assess the risks against the benefits and consider the patient's preference, as well as the clinician's prior experience, and will be framed within a multimodal approach in order to facilitate postsurgical recovery. Effectiveness in the management of postoperative pain entails a multimodal approach involving several drugs with different mechanisms of action so as to achieve a synergistic effect and thus minimize the adverse effects of the different routes of administration [5].

The main objective of this review is to explain the multimodal approach to postoperative pain, defining the benefits and risks of the combination of the most common used analgesic drugs and techniques as well as the latest improvements in this field and experts' recommendations. For this purpose, a review on Ovid-Medline was carried out until December 2012, with the keywords: "postoperative pain", "postoperative convalescence", "multimodal analgesia", "non-steroidal anti-inflammatory drugs", "regional analgesia" and "opioids", focusing on systematic reviews with or without meta-analysis, randomized controlled trials and expert opinion articles concerning several controversial points.

2. Pathophysiology of postoperative pain

The study of the neurophysiology of pain [6] has produced important advances in the knowledge of the mechanism of the production of painful stimuli in the perioperative period, describing a dynamic system where multiple nociceptive afferent pathways, together with other downstream modulation mechanisms, are of relevance. Surgical incision triggers deep responses of an inflammatory nature and from the sympathetic system, which determines a first stage of peripheral sensitization that, if it is maintained over time, amplifies the transmission of the stimulus until it conditions a second stage of central sensitization. As a consequence, it leads to an increased release of catecholamines and increased oxygen consumption, with increased neuroendocrine activity, translating into hyperactivity in many organs and systems. This translates into cardiovascular, pulmonary, endocrine-metabolic, gastrointestinal, immunological and psychological complications.

There is a direct association between processes with a severe degree of postsurgical pain and the proportion of the appearance of *chronic pain,* such as with limb amputation (30-83%), thoracotomy (36-56%), gall bladder or breast surgery (11-57%), inguinal hernia (37%) and sternotomy (27%) or abdominal hysterectomy (3-25%) [7]. Chronic pain can be severe in about 2-10% of these patients representing a major largely unrecognized clinical problem. Iatrogenic neuropathic pain is probably the most important cause of long-term postsurgical pain and consequently surgical techniques that avoid nerve damage should be applied whenever possible. Also, early and aggressive pain therapy during the postoperative setting should be administered since the intensity of acute pain correlates with the risk of developing a persistent pain state. Finally, the role of genetic factors should be studied, since only a certain proportion of patients with intraoperative nerve damage develop chronic pain [8]. Many clinical trials have demonstrated the effectiveness of gabapentin and pregabalin administration in the perioperative period as an adjunct to reduce acute postoperative pain. However, very few clinical trials have examined their use in the prevention of chronic postsurgical pain (CPSP). Eight studies were included in a recent meta–analysis, the six of the gabapentin trials demonstrated a moderate–to–large reduction in the development of CPSP (pooled odds ratio [OR] 0.52; 95% confidence interval [CI], 0.27 to 0.98; P=0.04), and the two pregabalin trials found a very large reduction in the development of CPSP (pooled OR 0.09; 95% CI, 0.02 to 0.79; P=0.007). This review supports the view that the perioperative administration of gabapentin and pregabalin is effective in reducing the incidence of CPSP but better–designed clinical trials are needed to confirm these early findings [9].

We must hence carry out a thorough treatment of dynamic postoperative pain, as it is not enough to only treat pain at rest, and to avoid other predicting factors, such as pain more than one month prior to the intervention, aggressive or repeated surgery, associated nerve injury or prior psychopathological factors [10]. Moreover, factors predisposing patients to a greater postoperative pain are young age and the type of surgery, such as orthopaedic surgery (due to the involvement of periosteum, which has a very low pain sensitivity threshold) and thoraco-abdominal surgery (due to the large involvement of the functions of the corresponding organs) [10]. The concept of *pre-emptive analgesia* is based on the administration, prior to surgical incision, of an analgesic in order to mitigate or prevent central hypersensitivity phenomena, aiming to reduce analgesic consumption in the postoperative period and chronic pain. However, there is great controversy regarding its efficacy. In a meta-analysis [11], sixty-six studies with data from 3, 261 patients were analysed. Fixed-effect model combined data were used and the effect size index (ES) was used as the standardized mean difference. When the data from all three-outcome measures were combined, the ES was the most pronounced for the pre-emptive administration of epidural analgesia (ES, 0.38; 95% confidence interval [CI], 0.28-0.47), local anaesthetic wound infiltration (ES, 0.29; 95% CI, 0.17-0.40), and non-steroidal anti-inflammatory-drugs (NSAIDs) administration (ES, 0.39; 95% CI, 0.27-0.48). Whereas pre-emptive epidural analgesia resulted in consistent improvements in all three-outcome variables, pre-emptive local anaesthetic wound infiltration and NSAIDs administration improved analgesic consumption and time to first rescue analgesic request, but not postoperative pain scores. The least proof of efficacy was found for systemic NMDA antagonist (ES, 0.09; 95% CI, -0.03 to 0.22) and opioid (ES, -0.10; 95% CI, -0.26 to 0.07) administration, and the results remain equivocal. Epidural analgesia begun *prior* to the surgical stimulus and maintained for several days (2-4) in the postoperative period has previously shown to be effective in this setting, either for amputations or thoracotomy and laparotomy, focusing on the timing of the perioperative analgesia [12].

Hyperalgesia can occur after surgery either due to nervous system sensitization caused by surgical nociception (nociception-induced hyperalgesia) or as an effect of anaesthetic drugs, particularly opioids (opioid-induced hyperalgesia - OIH). Both are potentially undesirable and can share similar underlying mechanisms such as the involvement of excitatory amino acids via the N-methyl-D-aspartate (NMDA) receptors [13]. Hyperalgesia is characterized by a deviation down and to the left of the curve that associates the intensity of the stimulus to the degree of pain observed, so that a usually painful stimulus is perceived as a pain of greater intensity, and likewise, another stimulus that is not painful is perceived as painful (allodynia). This effect may be seen both in the peripheral and central nervous systems. *Primary hyperalgesia* is a consequence of the sensitization of peripheral nociceptors during the inflammatory phase which is sustained by the local ischemia and acidosis caused by thermal or mechanical stimuli in areas close to the surgical incision. *Secondary hyperalgesia* is, in turn, due to central sensitization by a painful afferent stimulus sustained over time that triggers a spontaneous increase in the neuronal activity of the posterior horn of the spinal cord, only manifesting when faced with mechanical stimuli in tissues far from the lesion [14].

The clinical importance of hyperalgesia lies, on the one hand, in the increased intensity of the pain, in the consumption of analgesics, in the morbidity and in the discomfort in the postoperative period, and also, in the greater presence of chronic pain, and a greater probability of developing a complex regional pain syndrome that has even been suggested [15]. Furthermore, the greatest inconvenience lies in how hard it is to quantify; this should be done against electrical stimuli on the region of the skin, as it is not usually reflected in traditional subjective pain assessment scales (visual or numeric analogic scales), and objective neuroplasticity assessment tests (Von Frey filaments) that provide complementary information for a correct adjustment of the treatment. This should be based on neuromodulator drugs like gabapentinoids (gabapentin or pregabalin), ketamine, or NSAIDs. Finally, effective perioperative blocking of nociceptive inputs from the wound with regional analgesia as well as the use of antihyperalgesic and analgesic drugs in a multimodal combination, seem to be the best way to prevent central sensitization [14, 15].

3. Systemic analgesia

3.1. Non-steroidal-anti-inflammatory-drugs: NSAIDS

The acceptance of the concept of multimodal analgesia and the appearance of parenteral preparations has increased the popularity of NSAIDs in the management of postoperative pain [16]. The potential beneficial effects are summarized in Table I.

The mechanism of action involves the peripheral and central inhibition of cyclooxygenase (COX) and to the reduced production of prostaglandins from arachidonic acid. Two isoenzymes have been described [17], *COX-1: Constitutive*, responsible for platelet aggregation, haemostasis and the protection of the gastric mucosa, but it also increases by 2-4 times in the initial inflammatory process and in the synovial fluid of chronic processes such as rheumatoid arthritis and *COX-2: Induced*, causing pain (by increasing by 20-80 times in the inflammation), fever and carcinogenesis (by facilitating tumour invasion, angiogenesis and metastasis). However, both forms are constitutive in the dorsal root ganglion and in the grey matter of the

IMPROVEMENT OF ANALGESIA:
• Reduced activation and sensitization of peripheral nociceptors • Attenuation of the inflammatory response. • Coverage of some types of pain better than opioids (osseous pain, pain during movement and when coughing). • Effectiveness in its use as part of a multimodal analgesia. • Synergistic effect with opioids (reduction of opioid dose by 20% to 50%). • Preventive analgesia (due to a reduction of neuronal desensitization and of production of medullary prostaglandins).
LESS ADVERSE EFFECTS THAN OPIOIDS:
• Lower individual dose variability than with opioids. • Long duration of action half-life. • No generation of dependence or addiction. • No respiratory depression • Lower incidence of paralytic ileus, nausea and vomiting than with opioids. • No production of central alterations (either cognitive or pupillary). • *COX-2:* Lower incidence of GI adverse effects and a no anti-platelet activity.

Table 1. Beneficial actions attributed to NSAIDs in the appropriate management of postoperative pain [16, 17]

spinal cord. Therefore, although the spinal administration of COX-1 inhibitors has not shown to be effective, COX-2 inhibitors (Coxib) may play an important role in central sensitization and in the anti-hyperalgesic effect by blocking the constitutive form at the medullary level and by reducing the central production of prostaglandin E-2. Although Coxib drugs present with a lower risk of gastrointestinal haemorrhage and a nil effect on platelet function, they have not been demonstrated to reduce renal complications (hypertension, oedema, nephrotoxicity) and the effects on osteogenesis, compared to non-selective NSAIDs are still controversial [16, 17, 18]. It has been proposed that COX-2 is a cardioprotective enzyme and that the cardiovascular risk associated with its inhibition is due to an alteration in the balance between prostacyclin I-2 (endothelial) and thromboxane A-2 (platelet) in favour of the latter which leads to platelet aggregation, vasoconstriction and vascular proliferation. Coxib drugs improve the side effect profile and maintain a similar analgesic power; however, the duration of the treatment with these drugs in at-risk patients, their adverse effects, cost/effectiveness and efficacy compared to that of conventional NSAIDs associated with gastric protectors and their reliability in patients who usually take anti-aggregate drugs have not yet been defined [17, 18]. On the basis of many human studies, one may conclude that perioperative COX-2 inhibitors, in standard doses, decrease opioid consumption, but it is not clear whether they decrease adverse events related to the opioids. Future investigations with different multimodal techniques may help elucidate and clarify the true benefits of perioperative COX-2 inhibitors in acute pain management strategies [18].

Celecoxib is a sulphonamide with a large volume of distribution (400 litres/200 mg), large tissue penetration, degradation through the cytochrome P450 2C9/3A4 system, and a half-life of 11 h, with inactive metabolites. *Rofecoxib* is a sulphone with a volume of distribution of 86-litres/

25 mg, it is metabolized by cytosolic reduction, without interacting with the cytochrome system, and its half-life is of 17 h, with active metabolites. The equipotent dose for the treatment of acute pain is 400 mg of celecoxib/50 mg of rofecoxib. This would explain the differences between COX-2/COX-1 selectivity, and the differences found in the incidence of cardiovascular adverse effects, which are greater for rofecoxib [19, 20]. The decision to withdraw this drug from the US market in September 2004 was based on a three year controlled clinical trial on the prevention of adenomatous polyposis, in which an increased relative risk of cardiovascular effects such as ischemia or myocardial infarction was found in patients who were on treatment for more than 18 months. The risk of myocardial infarction varies with individual NSAIDs. An increased risk was observed for diclofenac and rofecoxib, the latter having a clear dose-response trend. There was a suggestion of a small increased risk with ibuprofen. Data also suggest a small-reduced risk for naproxen present only in non-users of aspirin, mainly people free of clinically apparent vascular disease [20].

Etoricoxib is a selective cyclo-oxygenase-2 (COX-2) inhibitor licensed for the relief of chronic pain in osteoarthritis and rheumatoid arthritis, and acute pain in some jurisdictions. This class of drugs is believed to be associated with fewer upper gastrointestinal adverse effects than conventional non-steroidal anti-inflammatory drugs (NSAIDs). Single dose oral etoricoxib produces high levels of good quality pain relief after surgery and the incidence of adverse events did not differ from the placebo. The 120 mg dose is as effective as, or better than, other commonly used analgesics [21].

Parecoxib is a pro-drug used in Europe for parenteral administration in the treatment of moderate-to-severe postoperative pain. The IV administration of 40 mg produces analgesia at 14 min. and as it is rapidly hydrolysed in the liver into valdecoxib, it is not detected in urine. Its analgesic peak is detected after 2 h and its duration varies from between 5-22 h. Its usefulness in reducing pain after dental, gynaecological, abdominal, orthopaedic and cardiac surgery has been proven. The analgesic efficacy of 40 mg IV is similar to that of ketorolac 30 mg IV. The maximum daily dose recommended is of 80 mg [22]. Parecoxib is contraindicated in patients with ischaemic heart disease or established cerebrovascular disease, in patients with congestive heart failure (NYHA classes II-IV), as well as in the treatment of postoperative pain after coronary by-pass surgery.

The efficacy of *paracetamol or acetaminophen* [23] has been proven in the treatment of moderate postoperative pain and in many other types of acute pain. It appears it could act by blocking the COX-3 detected in the cerebral cortex, thus reducing pain and fever. This third isoenzyme, which is similar to the mRNA of COX-1, has a retained intron-1 that alters its genetic expression in humans, and it may lead to questions as to whether this is the pathway for its therapeutic action, which, centrally, could be favoured for its lower presence of endoperoxides in nerve cells. The main analgesic mechanism appears to be due to a modulation of the serotonergic system, and it is possible that it increases noradrenalin concentrations in the CNS and peripheral β-endorphins. Thus, even if the mechanism of action is not clearly understood, there is now evidence that paracetamol acts within the CNS, by inhibiting the prostaglandin synthesis, whereas it has very weak antiplatelet and anti-inflammatory effects at recommended dosages. It manifests with a potentiating effect on NSAIDs and opioids and at therapeutic doses it does not present with relevant adverse effects. It presents with a very favourable efficacy/tolerability ratio, which is why it has been turned into the first-line of treatment in postoperative multimodal analgesia regimens. Its peak effect in the CSF is achieved at 1-2 h and its concentration in this compartment remains above that of plasma after repeated doses. It has been suggested that better analgesia could be obtained with a 2 g starting dose instead of with the recommended dose of 1 g. Its maximum daily dose is 4 g, but 3 g per day should not be exceeded in alcohol abusers or patients with a coexisting disease causing glutathione depletion. The usual scheme of administration (1 g every 6 hours) has a less than 10 mg sparing effect on 24 hour morphine consumption and consequently does not significantly reduce morphine side effects [24]. In a meta-analysis, seven prospective randomized controlled trials, involving 265 patients in the group with PCA (patient-controlled-analgesia) morphine plus acetaminophen and 226 patients in the group with PCA morphine alone, were selected. Acetaminophen administration was not associated with a decrease in the incidence of morphine-related adverse effects or an increase in patient satisfaction. Adding acetaminophen to PCA was associated with a morphine-sparing effect of 20% (mean, -9 mg; CI -15 to -3 mg; P=0.003) over the first postoperative 24 h [24]. In a recent systematic review, it has been verified how the association of paracetamol with other NSAIDs (diclofenac, ibuprofen, ketoprofen, ketorolac, tenoxicam, rofecoxib and aspirin) improved the efficacy of paracetamol administered alone (85% of the studies), as well as that of anti-inflammatories (64% of the studies) [25]. The antinociception induced by the intraperitoneal co-administration of combinations of paracetamol with the NSAIDs; diclofenac, ibuprofen, ketoprofen, meloxicam, metamizole, naproxen, nimesulide, parecoxib and piroxicam was studied by isobolographic analysis in the acetic acid abdominal constriction test in mice (writhing test). As shown by isobolographic analysis, all the combinations were synergistic, the experimental ED50s being significantly smaller than the theoretically calculated ED50s. The results of this study demonstrate potent interactions between paracetamol and NSAIDs and validate the clinical use of combinations of these drugs in the treatment of pain conditions [26].

Metamizole or dipyrone is another powerful analgesic and antipyretic agent, with limited anti-inflammatory power, that is broadly used in Spain, Russia, South America and Africa, but that is not marketed in the US or the United Kingdom due to the possible risk of agranulocytosis and aplastic anaemia. Other inconveniences of metamizole include the possibility of episodes of severe allergic reactions and of hypotension after its administration via IV [16]. It presents with a spasmolytic action and an efficacy that is superior to that of salicylates, which is why it is indicated in moderate to severe postoperative pain and in colic-type pain. In a systematic review [27], over 70% of participants experienced at least 50% pain relief over 4 to 6 hours with 500 mg of oral dipyrone compared to 30% with a placebo in five studies (288 participants). Fewer participants needed rescue medication with dipyrone (7%) than with the placebo (34%; four studies, 248 participants). There was no difference in participants experiencing at least 50% pain relief with 2.5 g intravenous dipyrone and 100 mg intravenous tramadol (70% versus 65%; two studies, 200 participants). No serious adverse events were reported.

Diclofenac is an anti-inflammatory with a great analgesic capacity, especially after orthopaedic and traumatological surgery, due to its great penetration into inflamed tissues and synovial fluid. It is also of use in pains of a colic nature, such as renal pain. The maximum daily dose is of 150 mg, distributed in 2 doses, and it is important to remember that some countries only approve it for deep intramuscular use [28]. Its greatest contraindication is kidney failure and gastrointestinal bleeding disorders. A new formulation of the non-selective NSAID diclofenac sodium suitable for intravenous bolus injection has been developed using hydroxypropyl beta-cyclodextrin as a solubility enhancer (HPbetaCD diclofenac). HPbetaCD diclofenac intravenous bolus injection was shown to be bioequivalent to the existing parenteral formulation of diclofenac containing propylene glycol and benzyl alcohol as solubilizers (PG-BA diclofenac), which is relatively insoluble and requires slow intravenous infusion over 30 minutes. For patients with acute moderate and severe pain after abdominal or pelvic surgery, repeated 18.75 mg and 37.5 mg doses of HPβCD diclofenac provided significant analgesic efficacy, as compared to a placebo. Significant analgesic efficacy was also provided by the active comparator ketorolac. Both HPβCD diclofenac and ketorolac significantly reduced the need for opioids [29].

Dexketoprofen trometamol is one of the most potent "in vitro" inhibitors of prostaglandin synthesis; it is a soluble salt of the (S)-(+) right-handed enantiomer of ketoprofen. It is administered at doses of 12.5-25 mg orally, with a fast absorption with an empty stomach, and recently has been administered at 50 mg IV with a maximum daily dose of 150 mg for only 48 h, binding strongly to albumin, and with a renal excretion of inactive metabolites after glucuronidation. Ketoprofen at doses of 25 mg to 100 mg is an effective analgesic in moderate to severe acute postoperative pain with an NNT for at least 50% pain relief of 3.3 with a 50 mg dose. This is similar to that of commonly used NSAIDs such as ibuprofen (NNT 2.5 for a 400 mg dose) and diclofenac (NNT 2.7 at a 50 mg dose). The duration of action is about five hours. Dexketoprofen is also effective with NNTs of 3.2 to 3.6 in the dose range 10 mg to 25 mg. Both drugs were well tolerated in single doses and its main indication is acute postoperative pain and nephritic colic [30].

Ketorolac is an anti-inflammatory with a great analgesic power, equitable to that of meperidine and even morphine, but with a roof therapeutic effect. It is absorbed orally, by IM, IV and topically through the eye, as it is well tolerated by all human tissues. It binds to plasma proteins to a degree of 99%, and it´s eliminated by the renal pathway as an active drug and metabolites. It is very useful in postoperative pain, of the renal colic and spastic bladder-type. It has also been used successfully in IV regional anaesthesia together with lidocaine [31]. The recommended doses are 10 mg orally or 30 mg parentally, with a maximum duration of five and two days, respectively. Its main adverse effects are dyspepsia and nausea, although it must be used cautiously in patients with a history of gastrointestinal bleeding. A European multicentre study that compared ketorolac with ketoprofen and naproxen used postoperatively (≤ 5 days) evaluated the risk of death (0.17%), surgical bleeding (1.04%), gastrointestinal bleeding (0.04%), acute kidney failure (0.09%) and allergic reactions (0.12%) on 11, 245 patients, and found no significant differences among them [32].

It is a proven fact that NSAIDs are effective in the postoperative treatment of moderate to severe pain, but it is yet to be verified what systematic reviews suggest: *that they can be as effective as opioids* [5, 16, 33]. (See Table II, Oxford Listing about the efficacy of single-dose analgesics based on Systematic Reviews. *NOTE: The lower the NNT, the greater the potency*)

NSAIDS	**NSAIDS + OPIOIDS**	**OPIOIDS**
Etoricoxib PO 60 mg NNT 2.2 (1.7-3.2) 80 mg NNT 1.6 (1.5-1.8) 180-240 mg NNT 1.5 (1.3-1.7) *Valdecoxib PO* 40 mg NNT 1.6 (1.4-1.8) 20 mg NNT 1.7 (1.4-2.0) *Parecoxib IV* 40 mg NNT 1.7 (1.3-2.4) 20 mg NNT 2.5 (2.0-4.8) *Celecoxib PO* 200 mg NNT 3.5 (2.9-4.4) 400 mg NNT 2.1 (1.8-2.1) *Rofecoxib PO* 50 mg NNT 2.2 (1.9-2.4)	*Paracetamol 1 g + Codeine 60 mg PO* NNT 2.2 (1.7-2.9) *Paracetamol 500 mg + Oxycodone IR 5 mg* NNT 2.2 (1.7-3.2) *Paracetamol 500 mg + Oxycodone IR 10 mg* NNT 2.6 (2.0-3.5) *Paracetamol 650 mg + Tramadol 75 mg PO* NNT 2.6 (2.0-3.0) *Paracetamol 1000 mg + Oxycodone IR 10 mg PO* NNT 2.7 (1.7-5.6) *Paracetamol 650 mg + Tramadol 112 mg PO* NNT 2.8 (2.1-4.4)	*Oxycodone PO 15 mg* NNT 2.4 (1.5-4.9)
Diclofenac PO, IM 100 mg NNT 1.8 (1.5-2.1) 50 mg NNT 2.3 (2.0-2.7) 25 mg NNT 2.8 (2.1-4.3) *Ketoprofen PO* 50 mg 3.3 (1.6-4.5) Dexketoprofen 10 mg PO NNT 3.2 (2.8-3.4) 25 mg PO NNT 3.6 (2.6-4.2) 50 mg IV similar to diclofenac IM	*Paracetamol 1000 mg + Oxycodone IR 5 mg PO* NNT 3.8 (2.1-20.0)	*Morphine IM 10 mg* NNT 2.9 (2.6-3.6) *Meperidine IM 100 mg* NNT 2.9 (2.3-3.9)
Ibuprofen PO 400 mg + Paracetamol 1 g NNT 1.5 (1.4-1.7) 200 mg + Paracetamol 500 mg NNT 1.6 (1, 5-1.8) 600 mg NNT 2.4 (1.9-3.3) 400 mg NNT 2.7 (2.5-3.0) 200 mg NNT 3.3 (2.8-4.0) *Flurbiprofen PO* 100 mg NNT 2.5 (2.0-3.1) 50 mg NNT 2.7 (2.3-3.3) *Metamizole PO, IV* 500 mg NNT 2.4 (1.9-3.2) 2 g IV similar to 100 mg tramadol	*Paracetamol 600/650 mg + Codeine 60 mgPO* NNT 4.2 (3.4-5.3) *Paracetamol 650 mg + Dextropropoxifen 65 mg PO* NNT 4.4 (3.5-5.6)	*Tapentadol PO:* - Bunionectomy pain (50, 75, 100 mg) NNT 3.6 -3.8 -2.5 - Dental pain (50, 75, 100, 200 mg) NNT 13, 5, 2, 3

NSAIDS	NSAIDS + OPIOIDS	OPIOIDS
Ketorolac PO 10 mg NNT 2.6 (2.3-3.1) *Ketorolac IM 30 mg* NNT 3.4 (2.5-4.9)	*Aspirin 650 mg + Codeine 60 mg PO* NNT 5.3 (4.1-7.4)	*Tramadol PO 100 mg* NNT 4.8 (3.4-8.2) *Tramadol PO 50 mg* NNT 7.1 (4.6-18)
Naproxen Na PO 550 mg NNT 2.6 (2.2-3.2) *Piroxicam 20 mg PO* NNT 2.7 (2.1-3.8)	*Paracetamol 325 mg + Oxycodone IR5 mg PO* NNT 5.5 (3.4-14.0)	*Dextropropoxifen PO 65 mg* NNT 7.7 (4.6-22)
Paracetamol PO 1 g NNT 3.8 (3.4-4.4) 650 mg NNT 5.3 (4.1-7.2) *Aspirin PO* 1200 mg NNT 2.4 (1.9-3.2) 1 g NNT 4.0 (3.2-5.4) 650 mg NNT 4.4 (4.0-4.9)	*Paracetamol 300 mg + Codeine 30 mg PO* NNT 5.7 (4.0-9.8)	*Dihydrocodeine PO 30 mg* NNT 8.1 (4.1-540) *Codeine PO 60 mg* NNT 9.1 (6.0-23.4)

PO: Per Os (orally)

IM: Intramuscularly

IV: Intravenously

IR: Immediate release

(Between brackets after NNT: 95% confidence interval)

Table 2. Relative efficacy of several analgesics according to the nnt in acute pain [5, 16, 33] (NNT: Number of patients necessary to treat in order to achieve a 50% relief of moderate to severe postoperative pain after a single dose)

3.2. Opioids

Opioids are the drugs with the greatest known analgesic efficacy. This is because their action is the result of a combined interaction on four types of receptors in turn divided into several subtypes (μ_{1-3}, δ_{1-2}, κ_{1-3}, ORL-1) that are located at different levels of the nerve axis, from the cerebral cortex to the spinal cord, and in some peripheral locations, and that intervene both in afferent and efferent mechanisms of nociceptive sensitivity. They are also a part of the endogenous neuromodulator system of pain, and are associated with the adrenergic, serotonergic and GABAergic system [16].

Opioids produce a high degree of analgesia, without a roof effect, but are limited by the appearance of side effects such as respiratory depression, nausea and itching. Their parenteral use in moderate to severe pain achieves a good analgesic effect in a short period of time; the intravenous route being preferable to the intramuscular route due to their greater bioavailability. The oral route with sustained-release drugs is also showing its usefulness in this setting [34, 35]. The features of the main parenteral opioids are summarized in table III.

OPIOIDS	Onset of action (min)	Peak effect (min)	Duration of the clinical effect (h)	Potency compared to morphine	IV-PCA bolus dose	Time of closure of IV-PCA (min)	Continuous IV infusion *
Morphine **	2-4	15-20	2	1	1-2 mg	6-10	0-2 mg h-1
Hydromorphone	2-3	10-15	2	5	0.2-0.4mg	6-10	0-0.4 mg h-1
Meperidine ***	10	30	3-4	1/10	10-20 mg	6-10	0-20 mg h-1
Fentanyl	1-2	5	1-2	100	20-50 µg	5-10	0-60 µg h-1
Sufentanil	1	5	1	1000	4-6 µg	5-10	0-8 µg h-1
Tramadol	10	35	4-6	1/10	10-20 mg	6-10	0-20 mg h-1
Methadone	2-3	5-6	6-12	1	0.5 mg	10-15	0-0.5 mg h-1

* Not recommended for initial programming except in patients undergoing chronic treatment with opioids or insufficient analgesia with PCA alone.

**Not recommended in patients with serum creatinine levels > 2 mg/dL, due to an accumulation of the active metabolite morphine-6-glucuronide.

*** Contraindicated in patients with kidney failure, convulsive disorders (due to their neurotoxic metabolite normeperidine), or patients who take MAOIs due to the risk of malignant hyperthermia syndrome. Only recommended in patients with intolerance to all other opioids.

Table 3. Recommended dosage for most common IV opioids [5, 16, 34, 35]

3.3. Opioids with special characteristics

Tramadol [36] is a synthetic opioid with a weak affinity for receptor μ (6, 000 times lower than morphine) and also for receptors κ and σ; it presents with a *non-opioid mechanism*, as it inhibits the central reuptake of serotonin and adrenaline, and has mild properties as a local peripheral anaesthetic. It produces a smaller number of side effects, such as nausea, due to a lower potency compared to morphine (1/5-1/10 depending on whether its administration is oral or parenteral) and it has an active metabolite [M1 (mono-O-desmethyltramadol)] with a greater affinity for opioid receptors than the original compound, which is why it contributes to the overall analgesic effect. It has shown its usefulness in a large variety of processes with moderate pain, with a dose of 100 mg /8 h IV recommended in the postoperative period. The efficacy of tramadol for the management of moderate to severe postoperative pain has been demonstrated in both inpatients and day surgery patients. Most importantly, unlike other opioids, tramadol has no clinically relevant effects on respiratory or cardiovascular parameters. It may prove particularly useful in patients with poor cardiopulmonary function, including the elderly, the obese and smokers, in patients with impaired hepatic or renal function, and in patients in whom NSAIDs drugs are not recommended or need to be used with caution. Parenteral or oral tramadol has proved to be an effective and well-tolerated analgesic agent in the perioperative setting.

Oxycodone [37] is a semisynthetic pure agonist derived from the natural opioid alkaloid thebaine, which is becoming the most used opioid in North America for the treatment of moderate to severe pain, as its pharmacodynamics are similar to those of morphine. Because its chemical structure only varies in a CH3 group in position 3, and an oxygen in position 6, it has certain pharmacokinetic advantages over morphine. Its administration, aside from analgesia, produces anxiolysis, euphoria, a sensation of relaxation, and inhibits coughing. It is available as immediate-release and sustained-release oral tablets, releasing 38% during the first two hours and the rest during the following 6-12 h, which is why they must be swallowed without chewing, to avoid an overdose. It differs from morphine in terms of its greater oral bioavailability (60-87% in the retarded form, and almost 100% in the immediate-release form), a slightly greater half-life (3-5 h) and in its liver metabolism, which occurs by means of the cytochrome P-450 (CPY2D6) rather than by glucuronidation, which is why it can interact with sertraline and fluoxetine, potent inhibitors of said enzyme. It reaches a plasma steady state after 24-36 h of treatment. It is metabolized mainly into noroxycodone, which has a relative analgesic potency of 0.6 and to a lesser extent, in oxymorphone which has a high analgesic power, both of which are eliminated by the kidney. The plasma clearance for adults is of 0.8 L/min, and about 40% binds to proteins. Its administration must not be adjusted with respect to age, although it is reduced by 20-50% in patients with liver or kidney failure and concomitant treatment with other CNS depressants, such as benzodiazepines. A better risk/benefit ratio in the postoperative period appears to be associated with the use of ibuprofen or paracetamol and it has a neuropathic pain efficacy due to its "*κ-agonist*" action. As a treatment guide, 10 mg of oxycodone are equal to 20 mg of oral morphine. Oxycodone is highly effective and well tolerated in different types of surgical procedures and patient groups, from preterm to aged patients. In the future, the use of trans mucosal administration and enteral oxycodone-naloxone controlled-release tablets is likely to increase, and an appropriate concurrent use of different enteral drug formulations will decrease the need for more complex administration techniques, such as intravenous patient-controlled analgesia [38].

Tapentadol [39] is a new mixed analgesic of dual central action, μ-opioid agonist and noradrenalin reuptake inhibitor. It is 2-3 times less potent than morphine, but it is in turn, twice as potent as tramadol. It was approved in November 2008 by the FDA for the treatment of moderate to severe pain in adult patients. It is available in immediate-release (IR) tablets of 50, 75, 100, 150 mg, with a half-life of 4-6 h and a maximum daily dose of 600 mg. A 12-h sustained-release presentation has recently been marketed for the management of chronic pain. It has a better safety profile for nausea and/or vomiting and constipation compared to oxycodone IR and also has a significantly lower rate of treatment discontinuation. It has been successfully tested after otorhinolaryngological and dental surgery, in chronic osteoarticular pain, both of the rachis and is associated with knee and hip arthrosis. The observed efficacy across different pain models and favourable gastrointestinal tolerability profile associated with tapentadol IR indicate that this novel analgesic is an attractive treatment option for the relief of moderate-to-severe acute pain [40].

3.4. Non-opioid analgesic coadjutants

Good pain control after surgery is important in preventing negative outcomes such as tachycardia, hypertension, myocardial ischemia, decrease in alveolar ventilation and poor wound healing. Exacerbations of acute pain can lead to neural sensitization and the release of mediators both peripherally and centrally. Clinical wind up occurs as a consequence of the processes of N-Methyl D-Aspartate (NMDA) activation, wind up central sensitization, the long-term potentiation of pain and transcription-dependent sensitization. Advances in the knowledge of molecular mechanisms have led to the development of multimodal analgesia and new pharmaceutical products to treat postoperative pain. They include extended-release epidural morphine and analgesic adjuvants such as capsaicin, ketamine, gabapentin, pregabalin, dexmedetomidine and tapentadol. Newer postoperative patient-controlled analgesia (PCA) in modes such as intranasal, regional, transdermal, and pulmonary presents another interesting avenue of development [41].

NMDA-antagonist drugs are used as modulators of pain, hyperalgesia and allodynia after surgical trauma. *Ketamine* is involved in opioid, cholinergic and monoaminergic systems; it may act on sodium channels, although the optimal dose and route of administration are yet to be defined. It has been tested as an analgesic potentiation drug, and in a systematic review on 2, 240 patients [42], it was verified that, in the treatment of acute postoperative pain at sub anaesthetic doses (0.1-0.25 mg/kg), either IV, IM or epidural (0.5-1 mg/kg), it is effective in reducing morphine consumption during the first 24 h after surgery, and reducing nausea and vomiting with a low incidence of side effects. Further, intravenous ketamine is an effective adjunct for postoperative analgesia. Particular benefit was observed in painful procedures, including upper abdominal, thoracic and major orthopaedic surgeries. The analgesic effect of ketamine was independent of the type of intraoperative opioid administered, the timing of ketamine administration, and the ketamine dose [43]. Despite using less opioid, 25 out of 32 treatment groups (78%) experienced less pain than the placebo groups at some point postoperatively when ketamine was efficacious. This finding implies an improved quality of pain control in addition to decreased opioid consumption. Hallucinations and nightmares were more common with ketamine but sedation was not. When ketamine was efficacious for pain, postoperative nausea and vomiting were less frequent in the ketamine group. The dose-dependent role of ketamine analgesia could not be determined. *Dextromethorphan* (40-120 mg IM) and *amantadine* (200 mg IV) are other drugs of this group that have been used with varying efficacy [16].

Agonists of α_2–adrenergic receptors, such as *clonidine* (2-8 μg/kg IV) and *dexmedetomidine* (2.5 μg/kg IM) enhance the analgesic and sedative effects of opioids centrally, at the level of the *locus coeruleus* and of the posterior medullary horn, respectively, but its side effects such as hypotension and bradycardia limit their routine use intravenously or through the medulla. A very recent systematic review and meta-analysis [44], looked at 30 relevant studies (1, 792 patients, 933 received clonidine or dexmedetomidine). There was evidence of postoperative morphine sparing at 24 h; the weighted mean difference was -4.1 mg (95% confidence interval, -6.0 to -2.2) with clonidine and -14.5 mg (-22.1 to -6.8) with dexmedetomidine. There was also evidence of a decrease in pain intensity at 24 h; the weighted mean difference was -0.7 cm (-1.2 to -0.1) on a 10 cm visual analogic scale with clonidine and -0.6 cm (-0.9 to -0.2) with dexmedetomidine. The incidence of early nausea was decreased with both (number needed to treat, approximately nine). Clonidine increased the risk of intraoperative (number needed to harm, approximately nine) and postoperative hypotension (number needed to harm, 20). Dexmedetomidine increased the risk of postoperative bradycardia (number needed to harm, three). Recovery times were not prolonged. No trial reported on chronic pain or hyperalgesia.

Gabapentin and *pregabalin,* structural analogues of γ–amino butyric acid, are the first-line treatment for neuropathic pain, and their usefulness in postoperative pain is due to their action on the $\alpha_2\delta$-1 subunit of voltage-dependent calcium channels of the posterior medullary horn. Their oral administration, and their central adverse effects, such as dizziness and somnolence, limit their use. Which is why their effective dose and treatment duration are yet to be defined. Their greatest usefulness lies in their ability to reduce the consumption of opioids in the postoperative period, as well as to reduce pain in movement and quality of sleep, which is why it is being used successfully in orthopaedic surgery, improving rehabilitation [45]. They are also useful in patients who are used to opioids by reducing their consumption in the postoperative period. They have also recently shown their usefulness in the prevention of postsurgical chronic pain [9]. In a recent meta-analysis [46], pregabalin administration reduced the amount of postoperative analgesic drugs (30.8% of non-overlapping values - odds ratio=0.43). There was no effect with 150, and 300 or 600 mg/day provided identical results. Pregabalin increased the risk of dizziness or light-headedness and of visual disturbances, and decreased the occurrence of postoperative nausea and vomiting (PONV) in patients who did not receive anti-PONV prophylaxis. The authors concluded that the administration of pregabalin during a short perioperative period provides additional analgesia in the short term, but at the cost of additional adverse effects. The lowest effective dose was calculated as 225-300 mg/day.

Postoperative nausea and vomiting are the most common complications after anaesthesia and surgery, and both female sex and laparoscopic technique are risk factors. It is certainly of a remarkably high incidence after laparoscopic gynaecological surgery, which is reported as being at nearly 70% within the first postoperative 24 hours. *Corticoids* have analgesic and anti-inflammatory properties due to the joint inhibition of cyclooxygenase and lipoxygenase, and it has been shown that the preoperative use of dexamethasone (4-8 mg IV) also prevents the appearance of postoperative vomiting and nausea, especially after laparoscopy. In a recent meta-analysis [47], prophylactic dexamethasone administration decreased the incidence of nausea and vomiting after laparoscopic gynaecological operations in post-anaesthesia care units and within the first postoperative 24 hours. In a review of the current mechanisms for reducing postoperative pain, nausea and vomiting, epidural anaesthesia did not reduce the length of a hospital stay or the incidence of PONV despite reducing pain intensity and ileus. NSAIDs are more effective than paracetamol in reducing postoperative opioid consumption and PONV, while dexamethasone and 5-HT3 antagonists are both effective in reducing PONV [48]. *Dehydrobenzperidol* is also used as a first-line agent in the treatment of postoperative vomiting and in a quantitative systematic review of randomized controlled trials of 2, 957 patient´s doses below 1mg was determined as the optimal IV dose. Two patients receiving 0.625mg of droperidol had extrapyramidal symptoms. Cardiac toxicity data were not reported. The authors concluded that because adverse drug reactions are likely to be dose-dependent, there is an argument to stop using doses of more than 1mg [49].

In a meta-analysis of 1, 754 patients, it has been verified that the *perioperative infusion of lidocaine* [50] reduced the intensity of pain and the consumption of opioids postoperatively, the incidence of paralytic ileus and of nausea and vomiting, as well as the length of hospital stay. The efficacy was greater in patients who underwent abdominal surgery. Considering that in some cases, toxic levels were detected, and that adverse effects were not collected systematically in all the studies, we must establish a safety range before recommending their systematic use. In another recent systematic review of 764 patients, having open and laparoscopic abdominal surgery, as well as ambulatory surgery patients [51], intravenous perioperative infusion of lidocaine resulted in significant reductions in postoperative pain intensity and opioid consumption. Pain scores were reduced at rest and with coughing or movement for up to 48 hours postoperatively. Opioid consumption was reduced by up to 85% in lidocaine-treated patients when compared with controls. The infusion of lidocaine also resulted in earlier return of bowel function, allowing for earlier rehabilitation and a shorter duration of hospital stay. First flatus occurred up to 23 hours earlier, while first bowel movement occurred up to 28 hours earlier in the patients treated with lidocaine. The duration of the hospital stay was reduced by an average of 1.1 days in the patients treated with lidocaine. The administration of an intravenous lidocaine infusion did not result in toxicity or clinically significant adverse events. Lidocaine had no impact on postoperative analgesia in patients undergoing tonsillectomy, total hip arthroplasty or coronary artery bypass surgery. Systemic lidocaine also improves the postoperative quality of recovery in patients undergoing outpatient laparoscopy. In a recent study [52], patients who received lidocaine had less opioid consumption, which was translated to a better quality of recovery. The authors concluded that lidocaine is a safe, inexpensive and effective strategy for improving the quality of recovery after ambulatory surgery.

IV Magnesium has been reported to improve postoperative pain, however, the evidence is inconsistent. The objective of a very recent quantitative systematic review was to evaluate whether or not the perioperative administration of IV magnesium can reduce postoperative pain. Twenty-five trials comparing magnesium with a placebo were identified. Apart from the mode of administration (bolus or continuous infusion), perioperative magnesium reduced cumulative IV morphine consumption by 24.4% (mean difference: 7.6 mg, 95% CI -9.5 to -5.8 mg; $p < 0.00001$) at 24 h postoperatively. Numeric pain scores at rest and on movement at 24 h postoperatively clearly improved and both were reduced by 4.2 (95% CI -6.3 to -2.1; $p < 0.0001$) and 9.2 (95% CI -16.1 to -2.3; $p = 0.009$) out of 100, respectively. The authors concluded that perioperative IV magnesium reduces opioid consumption and, to a lesser extent, pain scores, in the first 24 h postoperatively, without any reported serious adverse effects [53].

Non-pharmacological techniques, such as transcutaneous electrical nerve stimulation (TENS), which works by activating the opioid receptors and thick Aβ fibres, auricular acupuncture, music therapy or psychotherapy, may also be useful in the postoperative period, but more studies are needed to verify their efficacy as coadjutant to pharmacological therapy [54].

4. Patient-controlled analgesia

4.1. IV-PCA

Relief of acute pain during the immediate postoperative period is an important task for anaesthesiologists. Morphine is widely used to control moderate-to-severe postoperative pain and the use of small IV boluses of morphine in the post-anaesthesia care unit (PACU) allows for a rapid titration of the dose needed for adequate pain relief. The essential principle of a titration regimen must be to adapt the morphine dose to the pain level. Although morphine would not appear to be the most appropriate choice for achieving rapid pain relief, this is the only opioid assessed in many studies of immediate postoperative pain management using titration. More than 90% of the patients achieve pain relief using a protocol of morphine titration (2-3 mg/ 5 min.) and the mean dose required to obtain pain relief is 12 mg, after a median of four boluses. Sedation is frequent during IV morphine titration and should be considered as a morphine-related adverse event and not evidence of pain relief. The incidence of respiratory depression is very low when the criteria for limiting the dose of IV morphine are enforced. Morphine titration can be used with caution in elderly patients, in children, or in obese patients. In real practice, morphine titration allows the physician to meet the needs of individual patients rapidly and limits the risk of overdose making this method the first step in postoperative pain management [55].

The introduction of patient-controlled analgesia (PCA) has provided us a very useful tool in the adjustment of opioid doses within a broad range of postoperative needs, in turn minimizing adverse effects. Patients can self-administer a rescue dose, with or without a background regimen, thus maintaining plasma therapeutic levels. The basis of the treatment consists of a period of closure after the administered bolus in which a new administration is not allowed, thus avoiding the appearance of side effects, such as excessive sedation or respiratory depression [35].

In a practical sense [35], it is advised to administer 2-4 mg of morphine IV every 5-10 min. in the post anaesthetic recovery unit until the pain is controlled, and then start with 1 mg every 6-8 min, without a baseline infusion. If the patient does not achieve an adequate analgesia, the dose of the bolus will be increased to 1.5-2 mg and, as a last resort, a continuous infusion of 1-2 mg/h will be implemented, as long as it does not constitute > 50% of the total administered dose (see fig. nº1). In case of patients with chronic opioid treatment, this opioid infusion could be of up to 80%. The total dose to be scheduled may be calculated according to the rule mg/day/morphine = 100 - age. The systematic review showed a better analgesic quality, together with a lesser morbidity, compared to other analgesic IV regimens without PCA, but there were no differences in the total consumption of opioids, side effects or days of hospital stay. The incidence of adverse effects, such as respiratory depression (< 0.5%) does not seem to differ from other routes of opioids administration, such as the parenteral or neuraxial routes, and it is lower in the pure form of IV PCA.

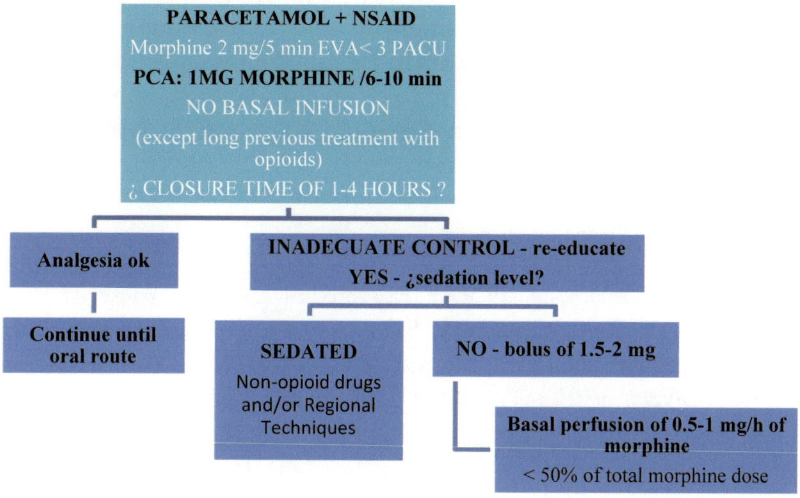

Figure 1. Titration of IV morphine in bolus or PCA in the PACU [35, 55]

4.2. Transdermal PCA

Transdermal Iontophoresis [56] is a drug delivery system by which a molecule with an electrical charge penetrates through the skin in the presence of an electric field. There is a need for an active infusion system, either local or systemic, that delivers lipophilic drugs, composed of small, positively charged particles. It has been tested with transdermal fentanyl in a system similar to a credit card, with an autonomous battery, and a button for the administration of boluses, placed on the arm or on the chest. The administered dose is prefixed at 40 μg, with a closure of 10 min, and with a limit of 80 doses a day and/or 24 h of treatment, whichever occurs first. The on-demand dosing and pharmacokinetics of this system differentiate it from the passive transdermal formulation of fentanyl designed for the management of chronic pain. Its results appear to be comparable to morphine in IV PCA in the treatment of acute postoperative pain, with a good-excellent overall satisfaction of 74-80%, and with a similar incidence of adverse effects, being nausea the most frequent in almost 40% of the patients The use of this system may serve as an alternative modality for the management of acute pain without increasing such adverse effects as bleeding, intravenous catheter infiltration, or manual pump malfunction.

4.3. Intranasal PCA

There is also the possibility of carrying out a *patient controlled intranasal analgesia* (*PCINA*) [57] with a rapid absorption of opioids. Intranasal drug administration is an easy, well-tolerated, non-invasive trans mucosal route that avoids first-pass metabolism in the liver. The nasal mucosa provides an extensive, highly vascularized surface of pseudo stratified ciliated epithelium. It secretes mucus that is subjected to mucociliary movement that can affect the duration of the contact between the drug and the surface. Absorption is influenced by anatomical and physiological factors as well as by properties of the drug and the delivery system. The drug most used is fentanyl at similar doses to intravenous route, but other opioids have been used to treat acute pain like meperidine, diamorphine and butorphanol. The adverse systemic effects are similar to those described for intravenous administration, the most common being drowsiness, nausea and vomiting. Local effects reported are a burning sensation with meperidine and a bad taste.

4.4. Patient-controlled regional analgesia

Patient-controlled regional analgesia (PCRA) [58] encompasses a variety of techniques that provide effective postoperative pain relief without systemic exposure to opioids. Using PCRA, patients control the application of pre-programmed doses of local anaesthetics, most frequently ropivacaine or bupivacaine (occasionally in combination with an opioid), via an indwelling catheter, which can be placed in different regions of the body depending on the type of surgery. Infusions are controlled either by a staff-programmed electronic pump (similar to that used for IV PCA) or a disposable elastomeric pump. An elastomeric pump is a device that has a distensible bulb inside a protective bulb with a built-in filling port, delivery tube and bacterial filter. Analgesia can be delivered directly into a surgical incision (incisional PCRA), intra-articular (IA), tissue (IA PCRA), or perineural site (perineural PCRA).

In recent years, continuous peripheral nerve blockade has gained increasing acceptance as a safe and effective technique that provides better analgesia than opioids. A meta-analysis [59] that compared systemic opioids with regional peripheral techniques confirms a superior analgesia in the latter; regardless of whether they are used in the form of a single bolus or in a continuous infusion. In this review, perineural analgesia provided better postoperative analgesia compared with opioids ($P<0.001$). This effect was seen for all time periods measured for both mean visual analogic scale (VAS) and maximum VAS at 24 h ($P < 0.001$), 48 h ($P < 0.001$), and 72 h (mean VAS only) ($P < 0.001$) postoperatively. Perineural catheters provided superior analgesia to opioids for all catheter locations and time periods ($P < 0.05$). Nausea/ vomiting, sedation and pruritus all occurred more commonly with opioid analgesia ($P<0.001$). A reduction in opioid use was noted with perineural analgesia ($P < 0.001$). In spite of this, the overall benefit to the prognosis of postoperative patients has not been statistically proven.

4.5. Patient-controlled epidural analgesia

Patient-controlled epidural analgesia (PCEA) allows for an individualized postoperative regimen that reduces pharmacological requirements, improves the degree of satisfaction and provides a higher analgesic quality. In series of more than 1, 000 patients, 90% were satisfied, with a VAS score of 1 at bed rest to 4 in motion. The presence of side effects was similar to the continuous epidural technique, standing out: itching (16.7%), nausea (14.8%), sedation (13.2%), hypotension (6.8%), motor block (2%) and respiratory depression (0.3%). The specific site of action of LAs is located at the level of the sheath of spinal nerve roots, the ganglion of the dorsal root and through the meninges in the spinal cord itself. The LAs most used are *bupivacaine* (≤ 0.125%), *ropivacaine* (≤ 0.20%), and *levobupivacaine* (≤ 0.125%), together with fentanyl (2-5 μg/mL) or sufentanil (0.5-1 μg/mL) which enhance their analgesic action and allow for a reducing of their total dose [60]. This route of administration has proven to be superior to the IV PCA formula with opioids. Continuous epidural techniques include the benefits of the metameric localized delivery of analgesic drugs with extended delivery in infusion and the capability to adjust the optimal degree of quality and depth in each patient, producing a sensitive postoperative block, with a minimal compromise to movement [61]. The combined use of regional-general anaesthesia improves the immediate recovery after surgery, and allows for an analgesic control of a higher quality than that offered by systemic opioids [62]. The location of the epidural catheter must be, whenever technically possible, *metameric to the surgical zone*, as it has been demonstrated that a thoracic catheter for thoraco-abdominal surgery reduces cardiorespiratory morbidity and mortality, improves analgesic quality and reduces the incidence of adverse effects such as urine retention and motor block [63].

A broad meta-analysis of data from 141 randomized controlled trials, which studied a total of 9, 559 patients, showed that the use of epidural or spinal anaesthesia was associated with a 30% decrease in 30 day mortality, in addition to other beneficial effects such as a 55% decrease in the incidence of pulmonary embolism, a 39% decrease in pneumonia, a 50% decrease in transfusion requirements, and a 44% decrease in deep venous thrombosis. There was also evidence of further benefits such as a decrease in the risk of respiratory depression, myocardial infarction and renal failure [64]. However, data from more recent studies in patients undergoing major surgery failed to show any decrease in mortality with perioperative epidural analgesia when compared with a combination of general anaesthesia and the use of systemic opioids [65]. Further, an Australian multicentre study (*The Master Trial*), on epidural anaesthesia in abdominal surgery in high-risk patients, on 888 cases collected over six years (1995-2001) did not show such beneficial effects. There was no reduction in the morbidity in the group receiving epidural administration compared to the control group with opioids and parenteral administration, and the mortality at 30 days was similar (4.3% in the control versus 5.1% in the group with epidural administration). Only acute respiratory failure (ARF) was less frequent in the epidural group (23% in epidural versus 30% in the control, $p = 0.02$). An NNT of 15 patients was calculated to achieve the prevention of an ARF episode. The pain score was lower and statistically significant in the epidural group, although the VAS was only reduced by 1 cm in the scale 0-10 cm [66].

For catheter placement, the loss of resistance using saline has become the most widely used method. Patient positioning, the use of a midline or paramedian approach, and the method used for catheter fixation can all influence the success rate. When using equipotent doses, the difference in clinical effect between bupivacaine and the newer isoforms levobupivacaine and ropivacaine appears minimal. With continuous infusion, the dose is the primary determinant of epidural anaesthesia quality, with volume and concentration playing a lesser role. The addition of adjuvants, especially opioids and epinephrine, may substantially increase the success rate of epidural analgesia. The use of patient-controlled epidural analgesia (PCEA) with background infusion appears to be the best method for postoperative analgesia [67].

In spite of what was demonstrated above, the thoracic epidural with a local anaesthetic and opioid is the technique of choice for reducing the consumption of IV opioids in the postoperative period for high-risk patients, patients undergoing open vascular and major thoracoabdominal surgery [68], but some authors question the routine use of this mode of analgesia in the postoperative period for patients having abdominal surgery [69] or thoracic surgery in favour of a paravertebral blockade (PVB)[70]. There is also some evidence that the use of epidural analgesia may decrease the risk of cancer recurrence [71] and surgical site infection [72], although the published data supporting these effects is not yet convincing [73]. More controlled studies are needed to confirm these potentially exciting findings.

5. Paravertebral blockade (PVB)

Paravertabral blockades (PVB) have been used to achieve unilateral analgesia for surgical and traumatic processes in the chest and abdomen. Its analgesic capacity is compared to the gold standard for this setting, which is thoracic epidural analgesia, always at the expense of the administration of more volume and a greater concentration of LA although adverse effects such as hypotension, urinary retention and vomiting are much less. Its greatest inconvenience is the variable distribution of LA after the single injection technique, with a measure of four sensitive levels blocked after the initial recommended dose of 0.2-0.3 mL/kg of 0.5% bupivacaine with adrenaline, as well as the time to the peak onset of action, which is 40 min and therefore it cannot be used as a preventive analgesia [74]. The failure rate for this technique is lower than that of the thoracic epidural and it is estimated to be above 6-10%, although the use of a stimulator helps improve the success rate. A systematic review and meta-analysis [75] on 520 patients in which both techniques were compared reflected a similar anaesthetic quality with a better profile of adverse effects and pulmonary complications in favour of a paravertebral block. Moreover, it is advantageous in patients who receive anti-aggregation and are under general anaesthesia. Its advantages for use with video thoracoscopy have not been well demonstrated, but they have been demonstrated in breast surgery [76].

In a review by Scarci et al., [70] PVB was found to be of equal efficacy to epidural anaesthesia in patients undergoing thoracotomy surgery, but with a favourable side effect profile, and a lower complication rate. The reduced rate of complication was most marked for pulmonary complications and was accompanied by a quicker return to normal pulmonary function. The epidural block was associated with frequent side effects [urinary retention (42%), nausea (22%), itching (22%) and hypotension (3%) and, rarely, respiratory depression (0.07%)]. Additionally, it prolonged operative time and was associated with technical failure or displacement (8%). Epidurals were also related to a higher complication rate (atelectasis/pneumonia) compared to the PVB.

6. Epidural coadjutants

6.1. Opioids

The spinal administration of an opioid drug does not guarantee selective action and segmental analgesia in the spine. Evidence from experimental studies in animals indicates that bioavailability in the spinal cord biophase is negatively correlated with liposolubility, and is higher for hydrophilic opioids, such as morphine, than lipophilic opioids, such as fentanyl, sufentanil and alfentanil. All opioids administered produce part of their analgesic effect via spinal selectivity, although lipophilic opioids also rapidly reach higher centres of the brain due to their good vascular uptake and redistribution. Clinical trials have demonstrated that the administration of lipophilic opioids by continuous epidural infusion does not produce analgesia due to a spinal mechanism, nevertheless, by strengthening local anaesthesia they enable total doses to be reduced. This contrasts with single epidural injections of fentanyl, which with sufficiently high quantities of the drug can reach specific areas at the spinal level [77].

Morphine [78] is probably the opioid with the greatest medullary selective action after epidural (3-5 mg/day) or intradural administration. *Morphine* is the most used epidural opioid, and it could be considered the gold standard of spinal drugs (which does not imply it is the ideal one), because, due to its medullary selectivity, the epidural dose used is much lower than the parenteral dose (1/5-1/10), with a recommended daily maximum dose of 10 mg. It can be administered both in the form of boluses (30-100 μg/kg) and in a continuous infusion (0, 2-0, 4 mg /h), as the latter appears to induce a greater analgesic quality, and as a single drug or together with LAs, because these two drugs potentiate the global analgesic effect by means of a synergistic action, resulting in a postoperative analgesia of great quality and duration, but at the expense of a greater incidence of adverse effects. Despite epidural morphine being regarded as an effective drug via a route of administration that is just as effective, its use as a single dose is limited by its effective half-life of less than 24 h, a short duration compared with that of postoperative pain. Liposomes are spherical particles formed by an external phospholipid layer and an internal aqueous chamber, where the drug is located. This is why in 2004, the FDA approved extended release epidural morphine (EREM) liposome injections only for lumbar epidural use, with a half-life of 48 h after a single injection, delaying the peak concentration in the CSF by up to 3 h, without the problems associated with the catheter and with the expectation of improving the global failure rate by close to 30% of the continuous epidural technique. The basic points for its use include administration prior to surgery or after clamping the umbilical cord during a caesarean section and at least 15 min. after the epidural test dose of LA and that no more epidural drugs be given for 48 h, since the continuous infusion of LA increase the release of morphine. The formulation must not be injected through a filter as the particles may be disrupted [79]. As with all opioids, the chief hazard is respiratory depression especially in elderly and debilitated patients and in those with compromised respiratory function. In a meta-analysis on the risk of respiratory depression compared to intravenous morphine in patient-controlled analgesia (PCA), an odds ratio (OR) of 5.80 (95% CI 1.05 - 31.93; $p = 0.04$) was estimated for the use of EREM [80].

The continuous, solely epidural administration of *fentanyl and sufentanil [77]* offers very few advantages compared to its intravenous administration, which is why it is used with LAs to reduce its minimum effective analgesic concentration improving overall patient satisfaction. Lipophilic opioids such as fentanyl and sufentanil produce an analgesic effect mainly through systemic reuptake and their administration as a single drug does not offer any advantages compared to the parenteral route. However, their use with LAs enhances the analgesic effect, reducing the total dose of each of the drugs, as well as their adverse effects, such as hypotension and motor block. Fentanyl and sufentanil given epidurally or intradurally are the drugs of choice in obstetrics and ambulatory surgery, and are the coadjutants most commonly used together spinally with local anaesthetics in the perioperative period, improving analgesia without prolonging motor blockade. The spinal administration of *alfentanil* produces analgesia through systemic reuptake and redistribution to cerebral opioid receptors, as it has the greatest volume of distribution. Only fentanyl in bolus appears to present a specific medullary action in the group of lipophilic opioids in the epidural route at a concentration > 10 µg/ml. Finally, [78] epidural methadone and hydromorphone are suitable alternatives for analgesia in the postoperative period, given that they have intermediate pharmacokinetic characteristics with respect to the two aforementioned groups of opioids.

6.2. Other coadjutants

The components of an ideal epidural solution for the control of postoperative pain are yet to be defined, as none achieves a total relief of the baseline pain at rest and of the breakthrough pain of a dynamic nature, without adverse effects such as hypotension, motor block, nausea, itching or sedation. However, from the studies published to date (clinical, randomized, controlled trials), we may draw the following conclusions with a high level of clinical evidence associated with the use of epidural *adrenalin* [81]:

- The combination of adrenalin with a mixture of low doses of bupivacaine (0.1 %) and fentanyl (2 µg/ml) has proven to be very effective in continuous infusion after major thoracoabdominal surgery, reducing the consumption of two other epidural drugs, as well as reducing their vascular absorption from the epidural space and improving the overall analgesic quality, efficacy and safety.
- The minimum analgesic concentration of adrenalin has been estimated to be 1.5 µg/ml.
- Ropivacaine has proven to be equipotent to bupivacaine in the same epidural mix.
- The location of the epidural catheter must be metameric at the level of the thorax, as there is not enough scientific evidence to recommend the use of adrenalin in continuous infusion at the lumbar level.

Clonidine (5-20 µg/h) enhances the analgesic effect of the epidural mix, but the appearance of side effects such as hypotension, bradycardia or sedation limits its routine use. *Neostigmine*, a cholinesterase inhibitor, has been described as a strong analgesic coadjutant when using this route, at doses of 1-10 µg/kg after orthopaedic surgery to the knee, abdominal and gynaecological surgery, although it is limited by adverse effects such as sedation and nausea [82].

The objectives of a very recent quantitative systematic review were to assess both the analgesic efficacy and the safety of neuraxial magnesium. Eighteen published trials, comparing magnesium with placebos, have examined the use of neuraxial *magnesium* in its use as a perioperative adjunctive analgesic since 2002, with encouraging results. However, concurrent animal studies have reported clinical and histological evidence of neurological complications with similar weight-adjusted doses. The time to first analgesic request increased by 11.1% after intrathecal magnesium administration (mean difference: 39.6 min; 95% CI 16.3-63.0 min; $p = 0.0009$), and by 72.2% after epidural administration (mean difference: 109.5 min; 95% CI 19.6-199.3 min; $p = 0.02$) with doses of between 50 and 100mg. Four trials were monitored for neurological complications: of the 140 patients included, only a 4-day persistent headache was recorded. The authors concluded that despite promising perioperative analgesic effects, the risk of neurological complications resulting from neuraxial magnesium has not yet been adequately defined [83].

7. Intradural opioid analgesia

Intrathecal opioid administration can provide an excellent method of controlling acute postoperative pain and is an attractive analgesic technique since the drug is injected directly into the CSF, close to the structures of the central nervous system where the opioid acts. The procedure is simple, quick and has a relatively low risk of technical complications or failure. It is ever more frequent to associate opioids of different characteristics in the intradural route, a lipophilic opioid, such as fentanyl (20-40 µg), and/or a hydrophilic opioid such as morphine (100-300 µg), in the form of a bolus prior to surgery, together with LA, in order to guarantee coverage both during the immediate (2-4 h) and the late (12-24 h) postoperative period. Thus, associating a lipophilic opioid with bupivacaine or lidocaine leads to a shortening of the onset of the block and to an improvement of intraoperative analgesia as well as during the first hours of the postoperative period without prolonging the motor block or lengthening the time to discharge making it a good choice for ambulatory surgery [84].

In an excellent review by Rathmell JP et al. [85] on the use of intrathecal drugs in the treatment of acute pain, a maximum effective dose of morphine was advised, the negative effects of which seem to surpass the beneficial effects; after doses > 300 µg, nausea and itching usually appear, as well as severe urinary retention, and in studies on healthy volunteers, all of them presented with respiratory depression when the doses went beyond 600 µg.

In a meta-analysis [86] of 27 studies (15 concerning cardiothoracic, nine abdominal, and three spinal surgery) on a total of 645 patients who received doses between 100 and 4000 μg, it was demonstrated that among those given intrathecal morphine VAS at rest, on a scale of 10cm, was 2cm lower at 4 h and 1cm lower at 12 and 24 h, and this effect was more pronounced with movement, the relative improvement being more than 2cm throughout the period of monitoring. This lower score on a VAS was significantly better than the outcome with other analgesic techniques such as the administration of IV ketamine at low doses (scores fell by 0.4cm), a regimen of postoperative NSAID (scores fell by 1cm), and even the continuous epidural infusion technique (scores fell by 1cm), as assessed by the same authors previously [87]. The doses of opioids required intra- and postoperatively up to 48 h were lower among those given intrathecal morphine and the use of morphine up to 24 h was significantly lower in the abdominal surgery group (−24.2mg, CI: −29.5 to −19) than the cardiothoracic surgery group (−9.7mg, CI: −17.6 to −1.80). This more marginal benefit in the latter group makes the use of intrathecal morphine in thoracic surgery questionable, as a similar reduction in the amount of morphine required intravenously can be achieved using other strategies, such as the use of intraoperative ketamine (−16 mg/24 h) or postoperative NSAID (−10 to 20 mg/24 h) and even 4mg of IV paracetamol may be able to avoid using up to 8mg of morphine in the first day after surgery [88]. The adverse effects were indeed more common in the group given intrathecal morphine with an odds ratio of 7.8, 3.8 and 2.3 for respiratory depression, pruritus and urine retention, respectively, although interestingly there was not a higher rate of nausea or vomiting. Further, a recent meta-analysis has demonstrated that the addition of clonidine to intrathecal morphine extends the time to the first rescue analgesia in a postoperative setting by more than 75min. compared with morphine alone and it also reduces the amount of postoperative morphine by a mean of 4.45mg (95% CI: 1.40-7.49). However, as the effects are small, and the results are heavily influenced by a study in which intrathecal fentanyl was also given, the authors concluded that this must be balanced with the increased frequency of hypotension [89].

Attempts have been made to define the optimal doses and drugs for a series of surgical procedures with the following recommendations [84-86]:

- *Sufentanil* 5-12.5 μg, or *fentanyl* 10-25 μg for orthopaedic, ambulatory surgery and caesarean section, and *fentanyl* 5 μg and *sufentanil* 2.5-5 μg for pain in labour, as sufentanil doses > 7.5 μg are associated with foetal bradycardia.
- *Morphine:* 50-500 μg (Summarized in Figure nº2)

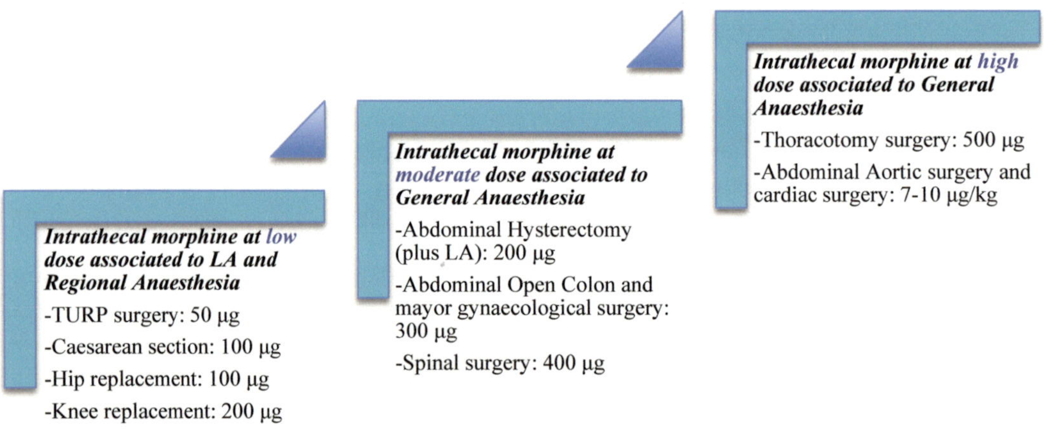

Figure 2. Recommended intrathecal morphine dosage for various surgical procedures in adults [84-86]

Key points for choosing the correct dose of intradural opioids [84-89]:

- Correct patient selection and minimum effective dose for each surgical procedure.

- Do not use morphine for ambulatory patients. Lyophilic opioids such as fentanyl and sufentanil are a better choice.

- Morphine DOSES ≥ 300 μg → have an elevated *risk of late respiratory depression 6-12 h.*

- Morphine DOSES < 300 μg have a similar risk to the parenteral administration of opioids.

- Monitored surveillance is recommended in the recovery or waking room or a mínimum monitoring for respiratory rate, oxygen levels (pulse oxymetry, if necessary) and above all, to monitor the level of consciousness for 12-24 h after intradural morphine and 4-6 h after fentanyl or sufentanil.

8. Peri-incisional analgesia

Peri-incisional analgesia is experiencing a great increase due to its ease of placement by the surgeon and its low profile of complications in the hospitalization ward (rate of infections < 0.7%, without the systemic toxicity risk of LA). It is carried out using a multi-perforated catheter of a similar length to the surgical wound, with an infusion of a long action LA without a vasoconstrictor, in a variable location in the literature, but predominantly in a subcutaneous or subfascial location. It has advantages in a large variety of processes with incisions of 7 to 15cm in length, with a lower VAS score, both at rest and in motion, as well as a lower consumption of opioids and a greater satisfaction for the patients, without affecting the hospital stay [16]. A systematic review, including 16 RCTs of patients undergoing major orthopaedic surgery and 15 RCTs undergoing cardiothoracic surgery, showed that postoperative pain management by wound catheter infusion was associated with decreased pain scores at rest and activity, opioid rescue dose, incidence of PONV and increased pain satisfaction [90]. However, a more recent meta-analysis was far less positive [91]. A total of 753 studies primarily fitted the search criteria and 163 were initially extracted. Of these, 32 studies were included in the meta-analysis. Wound catheters provided no significant analgesia at rest or during activity, except in patients undergoing gynaecological and obstetric surgery at 48 h (P=0.03). The overall morphine consumption was lower (≈13 mg) during 0-24 h (P<0.001) in these patients. No significant differences in side effects were found, except for a lower risk of wound breakdown (P=0.048) and a shorter length of hospital stay (P=0.04) in patients receiving LA. Some authors disagree about these results arguing that these conclusions were due to the exclusion of orthopaedic patients and patients in whom catheters were not actually placed in the surgical wound [92].

A recent study has evaluated the efficacy of the preperitoneal continuous wound infusion (CWI) of ropivacaine for postoperative analgesia after open colorectal surgery in a multicentre randomized controlled trial. Over the 72-hour period after the end of surgery, CWI analgesia was not inferior to continuous epidural analgesia (CEA). The difference of the mean VAS score between CEI and CWI patients was 1.89 (97.5% confidence interval = -0.42, 4.19) at rest and 2.76 (97.5% confidence interval = -2.28, 7.80) after coughing. Secondary end points, morphine consumption and rescue analgesia, did not differ between groups. Time to first flatus was 3.06 ± 0.77 days in the CWI group and 3.61 ± 1.41 days in the CEI group (P = 0.002). Time to first stool was shorter in the CWI than the CEI group (4.49 ± 0.99 versus 5.29 ± 1.62 days; P = 0.001). The mean time to hospital discharge was shorter in the CWI group than in the CEI group (7.4

± 0.41 and 8.0 ± 0.38 days, respectively). More patients in the CWI group reported an excellent quality of postoperative pain control (45.3% versus 7.6%). The quality of night sleep was better with CWI analgesia, particularly at the postoperative 72-hour evaluation (P = 0.009). Postoperative nausea and vomiting were significantly less frequent with CWI analgesia at the 24 hours (P = 0.02), 48 hours (P = 0.01), and 72 hours (P = 0.007) after surgery evaluations [93].

Appropriate catheter positioning is important, as it seems that preperitoneal placing is associated with better analgesia in patients undergoing open colorectal surgery, whilst subfascial placing provides good analgesia after caesarean section. The evidence-based PROSPECT recommendations include wound infiltration for inguinal herniotomy, laparoscopic cholecystectomy, hysterectomy, open colon surgery (preperitoneal infusion), total knee arthoplasty and haemorrhoidectomy [94]. This technique is also recommended by the ASA (*American Society of Anesthesiology*) practice guidelines as a part of a multimodal analgesia strategy for the management of postoperative pain [95].

9. Evidenced-based clinical recommendations

Due to the large variability of surgical interventions and the multiplicity of factors involved in postoperative pain, two initiatives have been put forward for drafting a practical guideline based on clinical evidence, specific for each process, and both are available on the Internet. One of them comes from the Veterans Health Administration of the US, in collaboration with the Defence Department and the University of Iowa (www.oqp.med.va.gov/cpg/cpg.htm), and the other from a working group of European anaesthesiologists and surgeons, the Prospect Working Group (www.postoppain.org). In the latter, the level of recommendation for each drug or medical acts for all of the perioperative periods are defined, and it currently contains 10 surgical procedures [94]. The Prospect Group helps physicians choose the most adequate drugs and technique combinations based on the published medical evidence and they are specialized in providing evidence-based and procedure-specific recommendations and clinical decision support for the management of postoperative pain. These are some examples for postoperative pain management:

This is the *modus operandi* of the Prospect Group:

1. Procedure-specific recommendations take into consideration the differences in character, location and severity of pain associated with different surgical procedures.

2. Evidence from a systematic review is supplemented with transferable evidence and expert knowledge from a Working Group of surgeons and anaesthesiologists.

3. Consensus recommendations are formulated by the Prospect Working Group, using established methods for group decision-making (Delphi method, Nominal Group Process).

4. Recommendations are graded to indicate the strength of recommendations (A–D).

5. Recommendations are provided with an explanation of the evidence on which they are based, including the level (LoE 1–4) and source of evidence (procedure-specific or transferable).

6. All evidence from systematic reviews, as well as transferable evidence, is summarized and abstracts of all references are provided.

7. Studies included in the reviews are assessed and assigned a level of evidence: study design, quality, consistency and directness are taken into consideration.

8. Procedure-specific evidence, transferable evidence and clinical practice information (expert opinion) are clearly separated.

9. Benefits and harms of different interventions are indicated with a system of ticks and crosses, and the balance of benefits and harms is considered in formulating the recommendations.

10. Evidence and recommendations are freely accessible on the Internet at www.postop-pain.org (Consult the original website for clarification of each level of recommendation)

- *Recommendations for colonic surgery*:

    - Continuous thoracic epidural anaesthesia and analgesia at a level appropriate to the site of incision are recommended for routine use, based on superior postoperative analgesic and safety benefits compared with systemic techniques, if there is no contraindication for epidural administration. (Grade A)

    - Where epidural techniques are used, it is recommended that a combination of strong opioid and LA must be used because of the increased analgesic efficacy compared with a strong opioid alone and to reduce the dose of opioids and their associated side effects. (Grade A)

    - Preoperative administration of a single-shot epidural analgesia produces a similar postoperative analgesic efficacy to postoperative administration

    - Continuous epidural anaesthesia and postoperative analgesia are recommended for routine use in colonic resection (Grade A), based on their benefits for reducing postoperative pain, systemic opioid use and improving bowel recovery time [(Level of evidence 1 (LoE 1)]

    - A combination of epidural local anaesthetic (LA) and strong opioid is recommended for epidural analgesia (Grade A), based on procedure-specific evidence of their combined efficacy, in reducing postoperative pain and systemic opioid use, compared with LA alone (LoE 1). However, the addition of opioid to epidural LA results in an increase in time to the first bowel movement. (LoE 1)

    - Where epidural techniques are used, it is recommended that the epidural catheter be inserted preoperatively because this is the most practical timing for insertion. (Grade D, LoE 4)

- COX-2-selective inhibitors (Grade B) (only for patients who do not receive epidural analgesia)
- Continuous administration of pre/intraoperative IV lidocaine if continued during the immediate postoperative period (Grade B), when epidural analgesia is not feasible or contra-indicated.
- Spinal analgesia is not recommended in combination with epidural anaesthesia (Grade B), based on the lack of benefit in reducing postoperative pain in colonic resection (LoE 2). Moreover, it introduces a greater level of complexity. (LoE 4)
- The decision concerning the type of operative technique or incision to use for colonic resection should be primarily based on factors other than the management of postoperative pain, e.g., malignancy versus benign disease operative risk factors of the patient, risk of wound infection, and availability of surgical expertise (Grade D)
- Laparoscopic colonic resection is recommended over open colon surgery for reducing postoperative pain, if the conditions outlined above allow (Grade A)
- A horizontal/curved (transverse) incision is recommended over a vertical incision for analgesic and other benefits if the operative conditions allow (Grade B). In addition, the horizontal/curved incision is preferred for its cosmetic benefits (Grade D)
- Diathermy is recommended over the scalpel (Grade C)
- Maintenance of normothermia is recommended for improved clinical outcomes, but it is not helpful for reducing postoperative pain (Grade A)
- Postoperative Recommended Systemic Analgesia:
- COX-2-selective inhibitors (Grade B) (only for patients who are not receiving epidural analgesia or upon the cessation of epidural analgesia)
- Conventional NSAIDs (Grade A) (only for patients who are not receiving epidural analgesia or upon the cessation of epidural analgesia)
- IV lidocaine (Grade B) (when epidural is not feasible or contra-indicated)
- Strong opioids (Grade B) (for high-intensity pain)
- Weak opioids (Grade B) in association with other non-opioid analgesics (for moderate- or low-intensity pain), or if non-opioid analgesia is insufficient or contra-indicated
- Paracetamol (Grade B) for moderate- or low-intensity pain (only for patients who do not receive epidural analgesia, or after the cessation of epidural analgesia)

* *Recommendations for post-thoracotomy pain*:
  - Pre- and intraoperative thoracic epidural or Paravertebral Blockade (PVB) are recommended based on the reduction in pain compared with postoperative administration alone. (Grade A)

- PVB LA or thoracic epidural LA plus a strong opioid is recommended as a preoperative bolus followed by an infusion continued for 2–3 days postoperatively, based on a reduction in pain compared with systemic analgesia. (Grade A)
- There are not enough data to recommend one specific combination of LA over another, or a specific concentration or volume.
- There are not enough data to recommend lipophilic opioids in preference to hydrophilic opioids or vice versa, in combination with LA.
- Thoracic epidural LA plus an opioid is recommended in preference to a spinal strong opioid based on evidence that the analgesic effect of thoracic epidural analgesia has a longer duration than 24 h. (Grade A)
- A preoperative single bolus of a spinal strong opioid is recommended as part of a multi-analgesic regimen (Grade A), when epidural analgesia or paravertebral blocks are not possible for any reason (Grade D). Repeated perioperative doses via the spinal route are not recommended because they are not considered to be safe or practical. (Grade D)
- Spinal opioids are recommended in preference to intravenous PCA opioids, based on a greater reduction in pain for up to 24 hours, with no difference in respiratory function. (Grade A)
- Lumbar epidural strong opioid is not recommended as the first choice based on evidence that the thoracic epidural route is more effective for pain relief (Grade A). However, there is procedure specific evidence that lumbar hydrophilic strong opioid reduces pain compared with systemic analgesia.
- Epidural epinephrine is recommended if a low dose of epidural LA and/or opioid is used (Grade B).
- Intercostal nerve block with LA (bolus at the end of surgery, followed by continuous infusion), if thoracic epidural analgesia and paravertebral blocks are not possible (Grade D)
- Postoperative Recommended Systemic analgesia:
- Conventional NSAIDs, if regional analgesia is inadequate (Grade A)
- COX-2-selective inhibitors, if regional analgesia is inadequate (Grade B)
- Intravenous PCA strong opioid, if regional analgesic techniques fail or are not possible (Grade D)
- Weak opioids for moderate- (VAS>30<50 mm) or low- (VAS<30 mm) intensity pain in the late postoperative period, only if conventional NSAIDs/COX-2-selective inhibitors plus paracetamol are insufficient or contra-indicated (Grade D)
- Paracetamol, if regional analgesia is inadequate, as part of a multianalgesic regimen (Grade D)

- *Recommendations for Abdominal Hysterectomy*:
  - General anaesthesia, or single dose spinal anaesthesia with or without light general anaesthesia in low-risk patients (grade D)
  - Epidural anaesthesia combined with light general anaesthesia or combined spinal-epidural anaesthesia, in high-risk patients (grade A)
  - Strong opioids administered in time to secure sufficient analgesia when the patient wakes up (grade A)
  - Wound infiltration before closure (grade A)
  - LAVH or VH rather than abdominal hysterectomy, only if allowed by the surgical requirements (based on technical feasibility, patient indication for hysterectomy and risk factors) (grade A)
  - Pfannenstiel incision, only if allowed by the surgical requirements (based on technical feasibility, patient indication for hysterectomy and risk factors) (grade B)
  - Diathermy incision (grade B)
  - Active patient warming in high-risk patients (grade A)
  - Intraoperative music (grade A)
  - Postoperative Recommended Systemic Analgesia:
  - COX-2 selective inhibitors or conventional NSAIDs, in combination with strong opioids for high-intensity pain (VAS>50mm) or with weak opioids for moderate- (VAS<50>30) or low-intensity pain (VAS<30 mm) (grade A)
  - Strong opioids via IV PCA or via fixed IV dosing titrated to pain intensity (grade A)
  - Paracetamol for moderate- (VAS>30<50) or low-intensity (VAS<30 mm) pain, in combination with COX-2 inhibitors or conventional NSAIDs (grade A)
- *Recommendations for total hip arthroplasty*:
  - COX-2-selective inhibitors or conventional NSAIDs (grade A) in combination with paracetamol and/or strong opioids for high-intensity pain (grade A) or with paracetamol and/or weak opioids for moderate- or low-intensity pain (grade D)
  - Strong opioids in combination with non-opioid analgesia to manage high-intensity pain (grade A), in time to provide analgesia in the early postoperative recovery period, administered by IV patient-controlled analgesia (grade A) or IV titrated for pain intensity (grade D)
  - Weak opioids for moderate- or low-intensity pain if conventional NSAIDs or COX-2-selective inhibitors are insufficient or are contra-indicated (grade D)
  - Paracetamol (grade A) in combination with conventional NSAIDs or COX-2-selective inhibitors, with or without rescue opioids (grade B)

  - Epidural infusion with local anaesthetic plus opioid for cardiopulmonary risk patients (grade B), in time to provide analgesia in the early postoperative recovery period (grade D)

  - Posterior lumbar plexus block (psoas sheath blocks) (grade A) or femoral nerve block (grade B) or single-bolus spinal morphine as a part of spinal anaesthesia (grade B), depending on the balance of efficacy and risks for the individual patient

  - Intraoperative, high-volume, low-concentration wound infiltration (LIA) (grade A)

- *Recommendations for total knee arthroplasty*:

  - Pre or postoperative Femoral nerve block is recommended (Grade A) based on evidence of a reduction in pain scores and supplemental analgesia (procedure-specific evidence, LoE 1)

  - No recommendation can be made concerning continuous femoral infusion techniques versus a single bolus because of the heterogeneity in the study design and the inconsistency of procedure-specific data (LoE 4).

  - Spinal LA + opioid is recommended (Grade A, LoE 1), but not as the first choice of analgesic technique because of a greater potential for adverse events compared with femoral nerve block (transferable evidence, LoE 3)

  - Morphine is recommended as the opioid in the spinal LA + opioid combination (Grade A) based on evidence for a longer duration of analgesic effect than other opioids (procedure-specific evidence, LoE 1)

  - Preoperative epidural analgesia (LA and/or opioid) is not recommended as the first choice but it can be used if a femoral blockade is not possible (Grade B).

There is also overall scientific evidence published on the treatment of APP, which is summarized in figure nº3 [97]. In the case of *ambulatory surgery,* [98] multimodal or balanced regimens of analgesia based on non-opioid drugs have been imposed in order to reduce adverse effects such as nausea and/or vomiting. Moreover, preventive analgesia has been promoted which aims to achieve better control of postoperative pain, as it is one of the most important factors for readmission. It has been proven that a combined regimen of dexamethasone at a single preoperative dose, incision LA (at the beginning or at the end of the surgery) and a postoperative regimen of 3-5 days of NSAIDs (COXIB or non-selective NSAIDs) achieved the best results in the control of pain and in the reduction of the time of convalescence. The association of paracetamol, gabapentinoids and the continuous infusion of peri-incisional LA in an ambulatory setting have also achieved a beneficial effect in patients. In the case of a poor control of pain, opioid rescue medication, such as tramadol or oral oxycodone could be necessary.

(Ia) meta-analysis, including at least one controlled and randomized study with a large number of cases, (Ib) the same, but with fewer cases, (II) well designed cohort or case-control studies, (III) well designed descriptive, non-experimental studies (IV) studies based on expert opinions or committees, (V) insufficient evidence to reach an opinion.

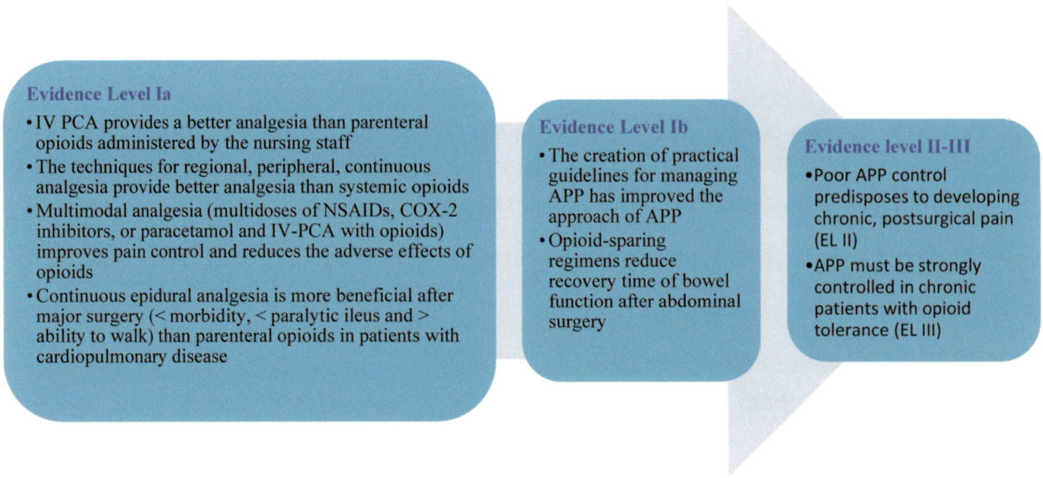

Figure 3. Analgesic strategies with the Evidence Level (EL) in APP [97]:

10. Combination of drugs and rehabilitation programme in surgical patients

It is normal daily practice to combine analgesics in order to improve the overall quality and patient satisfaction, but this does not mean we always meet our goal. Based on the studies that included controlled clinical trials or systematic reviews, that compare one drug with a combination of the same drug with one or more additional drugs via the same route of administration, Curatolo M et al. obtained the conclusions summarized in table IV [96].

The data currently available show that a *multimodal programme of postoperative physical therapy and rehabilitation* [99] can reduce the length of hospital stay, improve the control of dynamic pain and reduce the morbidity and mortality associated with the surgical procedure. We must begin with postoperative care that includes pain as the fifth vital sign, the use of regional analgesia to decrease opioid consumption, a responsible fluid therapy, maintaining normal body temperature, early mobilization, shortening the return to oral intake, avoiding motion-restriction factors such as drains, as well as improving postoperative sleep and stress, as they play a key role in reducing convalescence. This has led to the creation of ambulatory surgery units requiring coordination between all the healthcare specialists involved. Acute postoperative pain units are the key starting point for setting these programmes into motion.

Among the variety of surgical procedures, the recovery programme for colorectal surgery is one of the most studied and evaluated in the last decade. A recent meta-analysis concluded that the implementation of four or more elements of the Enhance Recovery After Surgery (ERAS) pathway leads to a reduction in the length of hospital stay by more than two days and an almost 50% reduction in complication rates in patients undergoing major colonic/colorectal surgery [100]. However, on the other hand, a Cochrane review of fast track surgery versus conventional recovery strategies for colorectal surgery concluded that the quality of the trials and the lack of other sufficient outcomes parameters do not justify the implementation of fast-track surgery as the standard for care [101].

Drug Combination	Efficacy in Acute Postoperative Pain (APP)
Adding NSAIDs to opioids	Improved analgesia and less side effects
Adding paracetamol to opioids	Improved analgesia and less side effects
Associating paracetamol + opioids	Better than each one separately
Adding a weak opioid to paracetamol	Questionable usefulness in minor surgery
Adding a weak opioid to an NSAID	Questionable usefulness in minor surgery
Adding IV ketamine to an opioid	Probable usefulness→ Monitor the narrow therapeutic range
Adding an epidural opioid to the LA	Useful
Adding clonidine to the epidural mix	There is no clear benefit
Adding adrenalin to the epidural mix	Useful in thoracic epidural analgesia

Table 4. Efficacy of pharmacological combination in acute postoperative pain (APP) [96]

11. Discussion

In 2007, a review was published on the clinical evidence of the effect of postoperative analgesia on the major postoperative complications with the following conclusions [102]: the positive effects of epidural analgesia on cardiovascular events or on lung function are limited to high-risk patients or to major vascular surgery, which, in some cases, is irrelevant when using an endovascular technique, and those that are beneficial in the presence of paralytic ileus can be minimized by laparoscopic techniques and fast-track programmes. Moreover, they found no evidence that the perineural or peri-incisional administration of LA, the administration of opioids by PCA, or the programmes of postoperative multimodal analgesia had any positive beneficial effects on postoperative complications, although they do improve overall patient satisfaction.

Indeed, many authors have questioned the use of epidural analgesia as the first choice of technique in the recovery protocols after mayor surgery. Rawal N. [103] thinks that epidural analgesia is a well-established technique that has commonly been regarded as the gold standard in postoperative pain management. However, newer, evidence-based outcome data show that the benefits of epidural analgesia are not as significant as previously believed, and that there are some benefits by decreasing the incidence of cardiovascular and pulmonary complications, but these benefits are probably limited to high-risk patients undergoing major abdominal or thoracic surgery who receive thoracic epidural analgesia with local anaesthetic drugs only. In the review, it was demonstrated that there is increasing evidence that less invasive regional analgesic techniques are as effective as epidural analgesia. These include paravertebral block for thoracotomy, femoral block for total hip and knee arthroplasty, wound catheter infusions for caesarean delivery and colon surgery, and local infiltration analgesia techniques for lower limb joint arthroplasty. Wound infiltration techniques and their modifications are simple and safe alternatives for a variety of other surgical procedures. The author also argues that although pain relief associated with epidural analgesia can be outstanding, clinicians expect more from this invasive, high-cost, labour-intensive technique and that the number of indications for the use of epidural analgesia seems to be decreasing for a variety of reasons. The main conclusion is that the decision about whether to continue using epidural techniques should be guided by regular institutional audits and careful risk-benefit assessment rather than by tradition.

Finally, practice guidelines for acute postoperative pain management have been recently published. The experts recommend anaesthesiologists who manage perioperative pain to use therapeutic options such as epidural or intrathecal opioids, systemic opioid PCA, and regional techniques after thoughtfully considering the risks and benefits for the individual patient. These modalities should be used in preference to IM opioids ordered "as needed". Consultants and ASA members also strongly agree that the therapy selected should reflect the individual anaesthesiologist's expertise, as well as the capacity for the safe application of the modality in each practiced setting. Special caution should be taken when continuous infusion modalities are used, as drug accumulation may contribute to adverse events. [95]

12. Conclusions

Although great work is being carried out in the area of postoperative pain, there is still a long way to go. It is necessary to apply a *multimodal approach to pain* that includes the routine use of regional techniques, a combination of analgesics such as paracetamol, non-specific or COX-2 NSAIDs and opioids by different routes, making a responsible choice for the type of patient, the surgical management and the predicted adverse effects. The true role of coadjutant drugs and non-pharmacological therapies is yet to be seen, and in the future, it will be essential to have a *practical guide based on clinical evidence* for each process, that includes postsurgical rehabilitation.

We must delve into the pathophysiology of pain, and in the direct application of this knowledge to new drugs and new systems for drugs delivery that achieve a lower number of postoperative complications, as well as a better overall recovery and general well-being of the patients. Healthcare professionals must be trained in the field of pain and their work must be coordinated within an acute postoperative pain unit, the structure of which must be stable and multidisciplinary, so as to arrive at agreed analgesic regimens with surgical and nursing departments. In the future, the goal must be to also cover the late postoperative period with the creation of postsurgical acute and chronic pain units.

Author details

Borja Mugabure Bujedo, Silvia González Santos, Amaia Uría Azpiazu, Anxo Rubín Noriega, David García Salazar and Manuel Azkona Andueza

Department of Anaesthesiology, Critical Care and Pain Medicine, Donostia University Hospital, San Sebastian, Spain

References

[1] Boswell MB, Giordano J. Reflection, analysis and change: the decade of pain control and research and its lessons for the future of pain management. Pain Physician 2009; 12(6) 923-928.

[2] Heitz JW, Witkowski T, Viscusi ER. New and emerging analgesics and analgesic technologies for acute pain management. Current Opinion in Anesthesiology 2009; 22(5): 608-617

[3] Shang AB, Gan TJ. Optimizing postoperative pain management in the ambulatory patient. Drugs 2003; 63(9) 855-867

[4] Cousins MJ, Brennan F, Car DB. Pain relief: a universal human right. Pain 2004; 112(1-2) 1-4

[5] Brown AK, Christo PJ, Wu CL. Strategies for postoperative pain management. Best Practice & Research Clinical Anesthesiology 2004; 18(4) 703-717

[6] Joshi GP, Ogunnaike BO. Consequences of inadequate postoperative pain relief and chronic persistent postoperative pain. Anesthesiology Clinics of North America 2005; 23(1) 21-36

[7] Perkins FM, Kehlet H. Chronic pain as an outcome of surgery. A review of predictive factors. Anesthesiology 2004; 93(4) 1123-1133

[8] Kehet H, Jensen TS, Woolf CJ. Persistent postsurgical pain: risk factors and prevention. Lancet 2006; 13; 367(9522) 1618-1625

[9] Clarke H, Bonin RP, Orser BA, Englesakis M, Wijeysundera DN, Katz J. The Prevention of Chronic Postsurgical Pain Using Gabapentin and Pregabalin: A Combined Systematic Review and Meta-Analysis. Anesthesia & Analgesia 2012; 115(2) 428-442

[10] Ip HY, Abrishami A, Peng PW, Wong J, Chung F. Predictors of postoperative pain and analgesic consumption: a qualitative systematic review. Anesthesiology 2009; 111(3) 657-677

[11] Ong CK, Lirk P, Seymour RA, Jenkins BJ. The efficacy of preemptive analgesia for acute postoperative pain management: a meta-analysis. Anesthesia & Analgesia 2005; 100(3) 757-73,

[12] Moiniche S, Kehlet H, Dahl JB. A qualitative and quantitative systematic review of preemptive analgesia for postoperative pain relief: the role of timing of analgesia. Anesthesiology 2002; 96(3) 725-41.

[13] Koppert W, Schmelz M. The impact of opioid induced hyperalgesia for postoperative pain. Best Practice & Research Clinical Anesthesiology 2007; 21(1) 65-83

[14] Wilder-Smith OH, Arendt-Nielsen L. Postoperative Hyperalgesia: its clinical importance and relevance. Anesthesiology 2006; 104(3) 601-607

[15] Lavand'homme P. Perioperative pain. Current Opinion in Anaesthesiology 2006; 19(5) 556-561

[16] Mugabure Bujedo B, Tranque Bizueta I, González Santos S, Adrián Garde R. Multimodal approaches to postoperative pain management and convalescence. Revista de la Sociedad Española de Anestesiología 2007; 54(1) 29-40

[17] Gajraj NM, Joshi GP. Role of cyclooxygenase-2 inhibitors in postoperative pain management. Anesthesiology Clinics of North America 2005; 23(1) 49-72

[18] Kaye AD, Baluch A, Kaye AJ, Ralf G, Lubarsky D. Pharmacology of cyclooxygenase-2 inhibitors and preemptive analgesia in acute pain management. Current Opinion in Anesthesiology 2008; 21(4) 439-445

[19] Caldwell B, Aldington S, Weartherall M, Schirtcliffe P, Beasley R. Risk of cardiovascular events and celecoxib: a systematic review and meta-analysis. Journal of the Royal Society of Medicine 2006; 99(3) 132-140

[20] Hernández-Díaz S, Varas-Lorenzo C, García Rodríguez LA. Non-steroidal anti-inflammatory drugs and the risk of acute myocardial infarction. Basic & Clinical Pharmacology & Toxicology 2006; 98(3) 266-274

[21] Clarke R, Derry S, Moore RA.. Single dose oral etoricoxib for acute postoperative pain in adults. The Cochrane Database of Systematic Reviews 2012; 18(4) CD004309

[22] Kranke P, Morin AM, Roewer N, Eberhart LH. Patients' global evaluation of analgesia and safety of injected parecoxib for postoperative pain: a quantitative systematic review. Anesthesia & Analgesia 2004; 99(3) 797-806,

[23] Remy C, Marret E, Bonnet F. State of the art of paracetamol in acute pain therapy. Current Opinion in Anesthesiology 2006; 19(5) 562-565

[24] Remy C, Marret E, Bonnet F. Effects of acetaminophen on morphine side effects and consumption after major surgery: meta-analysis of randomized controlled trials. British Journal of Anaesthesia 2005; 94(4) 505-513

[25] Ong KS, Seymour RA, Lirk P, Merry AF. Combining paracetamol with NSAIDs: A qualitative systematic review of analgesic efficacy for acute postoperative pain. Anesthesia & Analgesia 2010; 110(4) 1170-1179

[26] Miranda HF, Puig MM, Prieto JC, Pinardi G. Synergism between paracetamol and nonsteroidal anti-inflammatory drugs in experimental acute pain. Drugs 2006; 121(1-2) 22-28

[27] Edwards J, Meseguer F, Faura C, Moore RA, McQuay HJ, Derry S. Single dose dipyrone for acute postoperative pain. Cochrane Database of Systematic Reviews 2010; 8(9) CD003227

[28] Derry P, Derry S, Moore RA, McQuay HJ. Single dose oral diclofenac for acute postoperative pain in adults. Cochrane Database of Systematic Reviews 2009; 15(2) CD004768

[29] Gan TJ, Daniels SE, Singla N, Hamilton DA, Carr DB. A Novel Injectable Formulation of Diclofenac Compared with Intravenous Ketorolac or Placebo for Acute Moderate-to-Severe Pain After Abdominal or Pelvic Surgery: A Multicenter, Double Blind, Randomized, Multiple-Dose Study. Anesthesia & Analgesia 2012; 115(5) 1212-1220

[30] Barden J, Derry S, Moore RA, McQuay HJ. Single dose oral ketoprofen and dexketoprofen for acute postoperative pain in adults. Cochrane Database of Systematic Reviews 2009; 7(4) CD007355

[31] Smith LA, Carroll D, Edwards JE, Moore RA, McQuay HJ. Single doses ketorolac and pethidine in acute postoperative pain: systematic review with meta-analysis. British Journal of Anaesthesia 2000; 84(1) 48-58

[32] Forrest JB, Camu F, Greer IA, H Kehlet, Abdalla M, Bonnet F, et al. Ketorolac, diclofenac and ketoprofen are equally safe for pain relief after major surgery. British Journal of Anaesthesia 2002; 88(2) 227-233,

[33] Moore RA, Derry S, McQuay HJ, Wiffen PJ. Single dose analgesics for acute postoperative pain in adults. Cochrane Database of Systematic Reviews 2011; 7(9) CD008659

[34] Guindon J, Walczak JS, Beaulieu P. Recent advances in the pharmacological management of pain. Drugs 2007; 67(15) 2121-2133

[35] Grass JA. Patient-controlled analgesia. Anesthesia & Analgesia 2005; 101(5 Suppl) 44-61

[36] Scott LJ, Perry CM. Tramadol: a review of its use in perioperative pain. Drugs 2000; 60(1) 139-176

[37] Lugo RA, Kern SE. The pharmacokinetics of oxycodone. Journal of Pain & Palliative Care Pharmacotherapy 2004; 18(4) 17-30

[38] Kokki H, Kokki M, Sjövall S. Oxycodone for the treatment of postoperative pain. Expert Opinion on Pharmacotherapy 2012; 13(7) 1044-1058

[39] Nossaman VE, Ramadhyani U, Kadowitz PJ, Nossaman BD. Advances in perioperative pain management: use of medications with dual analgesic mechanisms, tramadol & tapentadol. Anesthesiology Clinics 2010; 28(4) 647-666

[40] C.T. Hartrick. Tapentadol immediate release for the relief of moderate to severe acute pain. Expert Opinion on Pharmacotherapy 2009; 10(16) 2687-2696

[41] Vadivelu N, Mitra S, Narayan D. Recent advances in postoperative pain management. The Yale Journal of Biology and Medicine 2010; 83(1) 11-25

[42] Bell RF, Dahl JB, Moore RA, Kalso A. Perioperative ketamine for acute postoperative pain. Cochrane Database of Systematic Reviews 2006; 25(1) CD004603

[43] Laskowski K, Stirling A, McKay WP, Lim HJ. A systematic review of intravenous ketamine for postoperative analgesia. Canadian Journal of Anaesthesia 2011; 58(10) 911-923

[44] Blaudszun G, Lysakowski C, Elia N, Tramer MR. Effect of perioperative systemic α-2 agonists on postoperative morphine consumption and pain intensity: systematic review and meta-analysis of randomized controlled trials. Anesthesiology 2012; 116(6) 1312-1322

[45] Dauri M, Faria S, Gatti A, Celedonio L, Carpenedo R, Sabato AF. Gapapentin and pregabalin for the acute postoperative pain management. A systematic-narrative review of the recent clinical evidences. Current Drugs Targets 2009; 10(8) 716-733

[46] Engelman E, Cateloy F. Efficacy and safety of perioperative pregabalin for postoperative pain: a meta-analysis of randomized-controlled trials. Acta Anaesthesiologica Scandinavica 2011; 55(8) 927-943

[47] Wang B, He KH, Jiang MB, Liu C, Min S. Effect of prophylactic dexamethasone on nausea and vomiting after laparoscopic gynecological operation: meta-analysis. Middle East Journal of Anesthesiology 2011; 21(3) 397-402

[48] Rawlinson A, Kitchingham N, Hart C, McMahon G, Ong SL, Khanna A. Mechanism of reducing postoperative pain, nausea and vomiting: a systematic review of current techniques. Evidence-Based Medicine 2012; 17(3) 75-80

[49] Schaub I, Lysakowski C, Elia N, Tramér MR. Low-dose droperidol (≤ 1mg or ≤ 15 µg/kg-1) for the prevention of postoperative nausea and vomiting in adults: quantitative systematic review of randomized controlled trials. European Journal of Anaesthesiology 2012; 29(6) 286-294

[50] Vigneault L, Turgeon AF, Coté D, Lauzier F, Zarychanski R, Moore L, et al. Perioperative intravenous lidocaine for postoperative pain control: a meta-analysis of randomized controlled trials. Canadian Journal of Anesthesia 2010; 58(1) 22-37

[51] McCarthy CG, Megalla SA, Habib AS. Impact of intravenous lidocaine infusion on postoperative analgesia and recovery from surgery: a systematic review of randomized controlled trials. Drugs 2010; 70(9) 1149-1163

[52] De Oliveira GS Jr, Fitzgerald P, Streicher LF, Marcus RJ, McCarthy RJ. Systemic lidocaine to improve postoperative quality of recovery after ambulatory laparoscopic surgery. Anesthesia & Analgesia 2012; 115(2) 262-267

[53] Albrecht E, Kirkham KR, Liu SS, Brull R. Peri-operative intravenous administration of magnesium sulphate and postoperative pain: a meta-analysis. Anaesthesia 2013; 68(1) 79-90

[54] White PF. The changing role of non-opioid analgesic techniques in the management of postoperative pain. Anesthesia & Analgesia 2005; 101(5 Suppl) 5-22

[55] Aubrun F, Mazoit JX, Riou B. Postoperative intravenous morphine titration. British Journal of Anaesthesia 2012; 108(2) 193-201

[56] Mayes S, Ferrone M. Fentanyl HCI patient-controlled iontophoretic transdermal system for the management of acute postoperative pain. The Annals of Pharmacotherapy 2006; 40(12) 2178-2186

[57] Añez Simón C, Rull Bartomeu M, Rodríguez Pérez A, Fuentes Baena A. Intranasal opioids for acute pain. Revista de la Sociedad Española de Anestesiología 2006; 53(10) 643-652

[58] Viscusi ER. Patient-controlled drug delivery for acute postoperative pain management: a review of current and emergency technologies. Regional Anesthesia and Pain Medicine 2008; 33(2) 146-158

[59] Richman JM, Liu SS, Courpas G, Wong R, Rowlingson AJ, McGready J et al. Does continuous peripheral nerve block provide superior pain control to opioids? A Meta-analysis. Anesthesia & Analgesia 2006; 102(1) 248-257

[60] Handley GH, Silbert BS, Mooney PH, Schweitzer SA, Allen NB. Combined general and epidural anaesthesia versus general anaesthesia for major abdominal surgery: post anesthesia recovery characteristics. Regional Anesthesia and Pain Medicine 1997; 22(5) 435-441

[61] Wheatley RG, Schug SA, Watson D. Safety and efficacy of postoperative epidural analgesia. British Journal of Anaesthesia 2001; 87(1) 47-61

[62] Wigfull J, Welchew E. Survey of 1057 patients receiving postoperative patient-controlled epidural analgesia. Anaesthesia 2001; 56(1) 70-75

[63] Block BM, Liu SS, Rowlingston AJ, Cowan AR, Cowan JA Jr, Wu CL. Efficacy of postoperative epidural analgesia: A meta-analysis. The Journal of the American Medical Association 2003; 290(18) 2455-2463

[64] Rodgers A, Walker N, Schug S, McKee A, Kehlet H, Van Zundet A, et al. Reduction of postoperative mortality and mobility with epidural or spinal anaesthesia: results from overview of randomized trial. British Medical Association 2000; 321(7275) 1493-1496

[65] Peyton PJ, Myles PS, Silbert BS, Rigg JA, Jamrozik K, Parsons R. Perioperative epidural analgesia and outcome after major abdominal surgery in high-risk patients. Anesthesia & Analgesia 2003; 96(2) 548-554

[66] Rigg JR, Jamrozik K, Myles PS, Silbert BS, Peyton PJ, Parsons R, Collins KS., MASTER Anaesthesia Trial Study Group: Epidural Anaesthesia and analgesia and outcome of major surgery: a randomized trial. Lancet 2002; 359(9314) 1276-1282

[67] Hermanides J, Hollmann MW, Stevens MF, Lirk P. Failed epidural: causes and management. British Journal of Anaesthesia 2012; 109(2) 144-154

[68] Kehlet H. Procedure-specific postoperative pain management. Anesthesiology Clinics of North America 2005; 23(1) 203-210

[69] Low J, Jonhnston N, Morris C. Epidural analgesia: First do no harm. Anaesthesia 2008; 63(1) 1-3

[70] Scarci M, Joshi A, Attia R. In patients undergoing thoracic surgery is paravertebral as effective as epidural analgesia for pain management? Interactive Cardiovascular Thoracic Surgery 2010; 10(1) 92-96

[71] Yeager MP, Rosenkranz KM. Cancer recurrence after surgery: A role for regional anaesthesia. Regional Anesthesia and Pain Medicine 2010; 35(6) 483-484

[72] Chang CC, Lin HC, HW Lin, Lin HC. Anesthetic management and surgical site infections in total hip and knee replacement: A population-based study. Anesthesiology 2010; 113(2) 279-284

[73] Tsui BCH, Green JS. Type of anaesthesia during cancer surgery and cancer recurrence. British Medical Journal 2011; 342: d1605

[74] Cheema S, Richardson J, McGurgan P. Factors affecting the spread of bupivacaine in the adult thoracic paravertebral space. Anaesthesia 2003; 58(7) 684-687.

[75] Davies RG, Myles PS, Graham JM. A comparison of the analgesic efficacy and side effects of paravertebral vs. epidural blockade for thoracotomy: A systematic review and meta-analysis of randomized trials. British Journal of Anaesthesia 2006; 96(4) 418-26

[76] Schnabel A, Reichl SU, Kranke P, Pogatzki-Zahn EM, Zahn PK. Efficacy and safety of paravertebral blocks in breast-surgery: a meta-analysis of randomized trials. British Journal of Anaesthesia 2010; 105(6) 842-852

[77] Bernards CM. Recent insights into the pharmacokinetics of spinal opioids and the relevance to opioid selection. Current Opinion in Anaesthesiology 2004; 17(5) 441-447

[78] Bujedo BM, Santos SG, Azpiazu AU. A review of epidural and intrathecal opioids used in the management of postoperative pain. Journal of Opioid Management 2012; 8(3) 177-192

[79] Hartrick CT, Hartrick KA. Extended-released epidural morphine (Depodur™): review and safety analysis. Expert Review of Neurotherapeutics 2008; 8(11) 1641-1648,

[80] Sumida S, Lesley MR, Hanna MN, Murphy JD, Kumar K, Wu CL. Meta-analysis of the effect of extended-release epidural morphine versus intravenous patient-controlled analgesia on respiratory depression. Journal of Opioid Management 2009; 5(5) 301-305

[81] Niemi G. Advantages and disadvantages of adrenaline in regional anaesthesia. Best Practice & Research Clinical Anaesthesiology 2005; 19(2) 229-245

[82] Congedo E, Sgreccia M, De Cosmo G. New Drugs for epidural analgesia. Current Drug Targets 2009; 10(8) 696-706

[83] Albrecht E, Kirkham KR, Liu SS, Brull R. The analgesic efficacy and safety of neuraxial magnesium sulphate: a quantitative review. Anaesthesia 2013; 68(2): 190-202.

[84] Mugabure Bujedo B. A clinical approach to neuraxial morphine for the treatment of postoperative pain. Pain Research and Treatment 2012; 2012:612145

[85] Rathmell JP, Lair TR, Nauman B. The role of intrathecal drugs in the treatment of acute pain. Anesthesia & Analgesia 2005; 101(5 Suppl), S30-S43

[86] Meylan N, Elia, Lysakowski, Tramèr MR. Benefit and risk of intrathecal morphine without local anaesthetic in patients undergoing major surgery: meta-analysis of randomized trials. British Journal of Anaesthesia 2009; 102(2) 156-67

[87] Elia N, Lysakowski C, Tramèr MR. Does multimodal analgesia with acetaminophen, no steroidal anti-inflammatory drugs, or selective cyclooxygenase-2 inhibitors and patient-controlled analgesia morphine offer advantages over morphine alone? Meta-analyses of randomized trials. Anesthesiology 2005; 103(6) 1296–1304

[88] Remy C, Marret E, Bonnet F. Effects of acetaminophen on morphine side effects and consumption after major surgery: meta-analysis of randomized controlled trials. British Journal of Anaesthesia 2005; 94(4) 505–513

[89] Engelman E, Marsala C. Efficacy of adding clonidine to intrathecal morphine in acute postoperative pain: a meta-analysis. British Journal of Anaesthesia 2013; 110(1) 21-7

[90] Liu SS, Richman JM, Thyrby RC, Wu CL. Efficacy of continuous wound catheters delivering local anesthetic for postoperative analgesia: a quantitative and qualitative systematic review of randomized controlled trials. Journal of the American College of Surgeons 2006; 203(6) 914-932

[91] Gupta A, Favaios S, Perniola A, Magnuson A, Berggren L. A meta-analysis of the efficacy of wound catheters for postoperative pain management. Acta Anaesthesiologica Scandinavica 2011; 55(7) 785-796

[92] Rawal N, Borgeat A, Scott N. Wound catheters for postoperative pain: overture or finale? Acta Anaesthesiologica Scandinavica 2012; 56(3) 395-396

[93] Bertoglio S, Fabiani F, Negri PD, Corcione A, Merlo DF, Cafiero F, et al. The Postoperative Analgesic Efficacy of Preperitoneal Continuous Wound Infusion Compared to Epidural Continuous Infusion with Local Anesthetics after Colorectal Cancer Surgery: A Randomized Controlled Multicenter Study. Anesthesia & Analgesia 2012; 115(6) 1442-50

[94] Procedure-Specific Postoperative Pain Management (PROSPECT). Available at: www.postoppain.org. Accessed July 18, 2013

[95] Practice guidelines for acute pain management in the perioperative setting. An updated report by the American Society of Anesthesiologists Task Force on Acute Pain Management. Anesthesiology 2012; 116(2) 248-273

[96] Curatolo M, Sveticic G. Drug combinations in pain treatment: a review of the published evidence and a method for finding the optimal combination. Best Practice & Research Clinical Anaesthesiology 2002; 16(4) 507-519

[97] Santeularia MT, Catalá E, Genové M, Revuelta M, Moral MV. New trends in the treatment of postoperative pain in general and gastrointestinal surgery. Cirugía Española 2009; 86(2) 63-71

[98] White PF, Ofelia L. The role of multimodal analgesia in pain management after ambulatory surgery. Current Opinion in Anaesthesiology 2010; 23(6) 697-703.

[99] Joshi GP. Multimodal analgesia techniques and postoperative rehabilitation. Anesthesiology Clinics of North America 2005; 23(1) 185-202

[100] Varadhan KK, Neal KR, Dejong CHC, Fearon CH, Ljungqvist O, Lobo DN. The enhanced recovery after surgery (ERAS) pathway for patients undergoing major elective open colorectal surgery: a meta-analysis of randomized trials. Clinical Nutrition 2010; 29(4) 434-440

[101] Spanjersberg WR, Reurings J, Keus F, van Laarhoven CJ. Fast track surgery versus conventional recovery strategies for colorectal surgery. Cochrane Database of Systematic Reviews 2011; 2: CD007635

[102] Liu SS, Wu CL. Effect of postoperative analgesia on major postoperative complications: a systematic update of the evidence. Anesthesia & Analgesia 2007; 104(3) 689-702

[103] Rawal N. Epidural technique for postoperative pain: gold standard no more? Regional Anesthesia and Pain Medicine 2012; 37(3) 310-7.

Chapter 5

Noninvasive Neuromodulation Methods in the Treatment of Chronic Pain

Richard Rokyta and Jitka Fricova

Additional information is available at the end of the chapter

http://dx.doi.org/10.5772/57449

1. Introduction

Non-invasive neurostimulation is recommended for patients with chronic neuropathic pain lasting more than six months.

Neurostimulation methods represent a firm place in the treatment of chronic pain. In this article, the respective mechanisms of action and efficacy of TENS(transcutaneous electrical nerve stimulation), rTMS (repetitive transcranial magnetic stimulation), tDCS (transcranial direct current stimulation) are described. In addition to the positive effects, side effects and complications are mentioned and discussed in detail. In conclusion, neuromodulatory (neurostimulatory) techniques are highly recommended for the treatment of different types of pharmacoresistant pain.

2. Neurostimulation methods

Neurostimulation, as a treatment of pain method, has been shown to be beneficial for patients suffering from pharmacoresistant chronic pain. Currently, neurostimulation methods are indicated only after exhaustion of all other therapies; however, it is expected that, in the near future, neurostimulation methods will become a first line treatment. Chronic pain is thought to occur in up to 30% of the adult population, although some authors suggest that it is less than 10%; others researchers, particularly in developed countries, put the prevalence as high as 50%. Neurostimulation methods are mainly used for chronic intractable pain, in which long-term treatment had been ineffective. Invasive or non-invasive neurostimulation is often recommended for patients with chronic neuropathic pain lasting more than six months, which was

INTECH
open science | open minds

© 2015 The Author(s). Licensee InTech. This chapter is distributed under the terms of the Creative Commons Attribution License (http://creativecommons.org/licenses/by/3.0), which permits unrestricted use, distribution, and reproduction in any medium, provided the original work is properly cited.

refractory to well-established first and second-line analgesic therapy or in which first and second-line analgesic therapy produced unacceptable side effects. Most neurostimulation pain treatments are classified based on invasivity; they are classified as either invasive or non-invasive [29-32].

3. Invasive neurostimulation methods

- PNS - peripheral nerve stimulation SCS (spinal cord stimulation) - stimulation of the anterolateral and dorsal spinal cord tracts
- DBS - Deep brain stimulation
- MCS -Motor cortex stimulation [29]
- Stimulation of vagus nerve [37]
- Occipital nerve stimulation [22,23]

4. Non-invasive stimulation methods

- TENS (transcutaneous electrical nerve stimulation)
- rTMS (repetitive transcranial magnetic stimulation) [10]
- tDCS (transcranial direct current stimulation)

5. Transcutaneous electrical nerve stimulation (TENS)

TENS is a simple and relatively little used method with several probable mechanisms of pain relief [10]. These techniques are rather inexpensive and non-invasive, but the evidence for their effectiveness is overall of low quality [26]. The restrictive definition of TENS is the administration by surface electrodes of electric current produced by a device to stimulate cutaneous sensory nerves to reduce pain, both acute and chronic. TENS treatment targets painful regions instead of specific nerves. Based on the stimulation frequency, TENS can be subdivided in low frequency (frequency < 10 Hz) or high frequency (frequency > 10 Hz). As the biological basis of analgesia by TENS remains speculative, the 'gate control theory' of pain was the most tenable explanation but now release of endogenous opioids is the most acceptable explanation. [11]

Transcutaneous electrical nerve stimulation is known to work via multiple pathways and to have multiple indications and uses:

- TENS stimulates sensory nerves, activates the endogenous opioid system, stimulates the release of enkephalins and endorphins and increases blood flow in the stimulated areas.

- TENS produces pain relief at both low and high frequencies.
- TENS is mediated via release of μ and δ opioids in the CNS and by a reduction in substance P.
- TENS affects the cardiovascular system: it increases heart rate and lowers blood pressure [18,24].
- TENS has been successfully used for the treatment of pelvic pain when applied to the dam and its dermatomes [37]
- TENS is used in geriatrics as valuable alternative treatment method for pharmacothera-py. [1].
- TENS can be used to treat muscle spasms and pains in specific areas such as surgical scars or post-herpetic neuralgia.
- TENS is simple to cooperate with patients and they can use it at home for self-analgesia.
- TENS can be used as electroanalgesia, for the treatment of pain during labor; it is used along the projections of Th10, Th 11, Th 12 and L1.
- TENS can be used as a complement of rehabilitation methods; threshold stimulation affects spinal mechanisms and supra-threshold stimulation affects supraspinal modulating mechanisms.
- TENS is also effective for neuropathic pain (including diabetic neuropathic pain [34], stump and phantom pain, post-herpetic neuralgia, spinal cord injury [27,5] and fibromyalgia [4]; it has also started to be used for cancer pain [19].
- TENS is contraindicated for use in the patients with implanted pacemakers

A number of complementary therapies have been found to have some efficacy among the older population, including acupuncture, TENS and massage. Such approaches can affect pain and anxiety and are worth further investigation.

Difference scores for movement-evoked pain during the Timed "Up & Go" Test (TUG) which is used in ipsilateral and contralateral knees during transcutaneous electrical nerve stimulation (TENS). Significant decreases were observed ipsilaterally for all 3 groups (placebo TENS [P], low-frequency TENS [LF], and high-frequency TENS [HF]). Data are expressed as the mean and standard error of the mean. *=significantly different from baseline [33]

Difference scores for pain at rest in ipsilateral and contralateral knees during transcutaneous electrical nerve stimulation (TENS). Significant decreases were observed ipsilaterally for all 3 groups (placebo TENS [P], low-frequency TENS [LF], and high-frequency TENS [HF]). Data are expressed as the mean and standard error of the mean. *=significantly different from baseline [33]

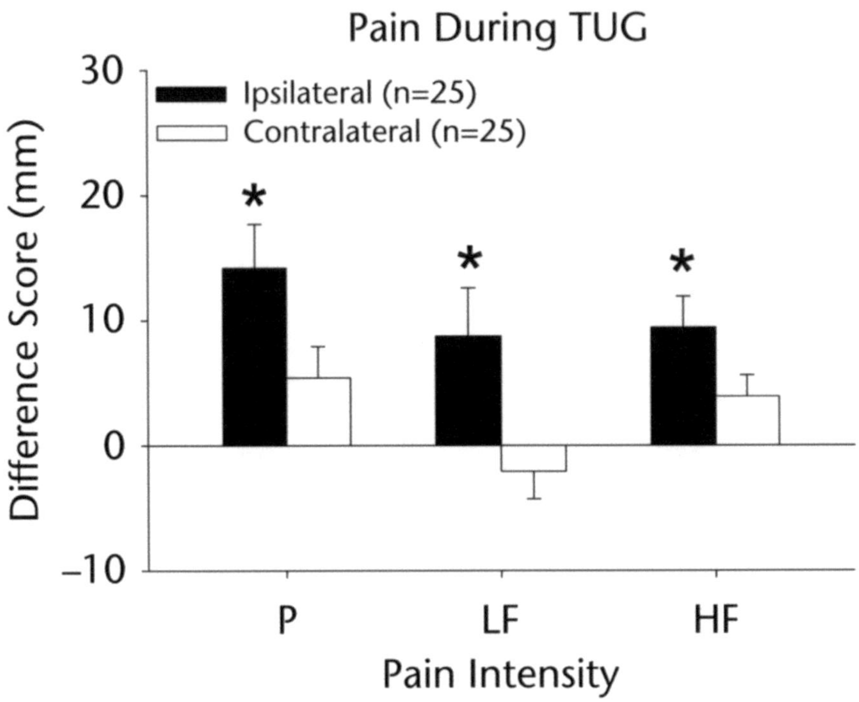
Pain During TUG
Ipsilateral (n=25)
Contralateral (n=25)
Difference Score (mm)
30
20
10
0
–10
*
*
*
P
LF
HF
Pain Intensity

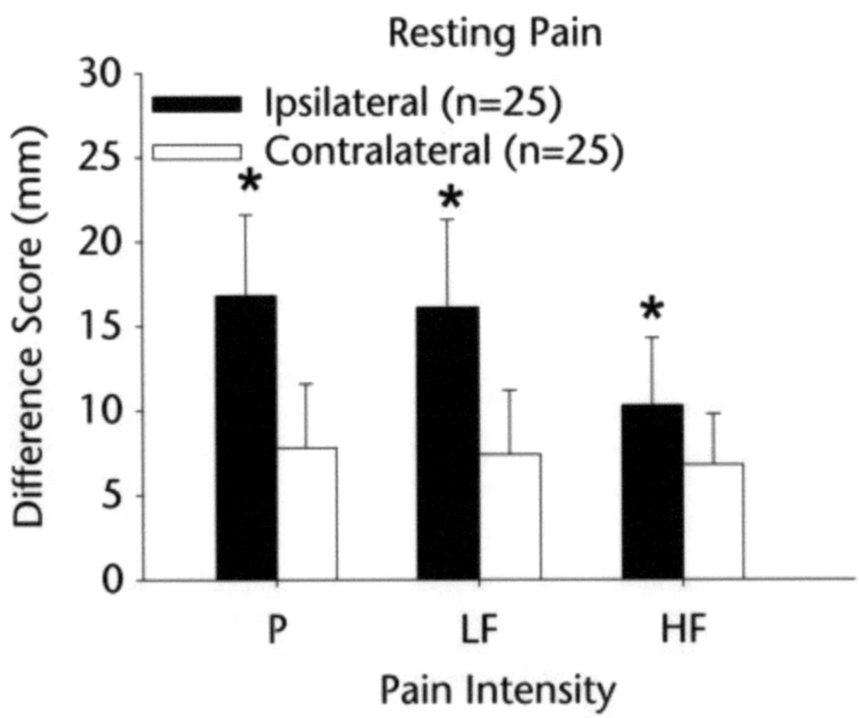
Resting Pain
Ipsilateral (n=25)
Contralateral (n=25)
Difference Score (mm)
30
25
20
15
10
5
0
*
*
*
P
LF
HF
Pain Intensity

In this study, participants were able to correctly identify active TENS 92% of the time. We previously reported similar responses to active TENS in healthy controls. Despite participants knowing that they received active TENS, there was no difference between active TENS and placebo TENS in subjective pain rating. Blinding of an electrical modality such as TENS has always been difficult, and few studies have reported blinding of active TENS.[33]

In summary, the present randomized clinical trial examined the effects of single treatments of HF-TENS and LF-TENS on knee OA pain and function. The use of various outcome measures, different frequencies, and an improved placebo provided insight for the management of knee OA pain with TENS. The pilot study tested a series of outcome measures designed to parallel and validate animal models of TENS and to test the effects of TENS in a true double-blind manner. Using PPT as an objective measure of pain sensitivity, showed that both HF-TENS and LF-TENS reduced primary hyperalgesia and that only HF-TENS reduced secondary hyperalgesia in people with OA. Quantitative sensory testing with cutaneous mechanical and heat pain measures was not affected by HF-TENS, LF-TENS, or placebo TENS, suggesting that TENS has no effect on cutaneous hyperalgesia. Alternatively, it is possible that the participants with OA did not have cutaneous mechanical and heat hyperalgesia. All treatments had similar but minimal effects on subjective pain measures, suggesting a placebo component of the effect of TENS. [33]

Side effects of TENS therapy:

High frequency TENS delivered at low intensities is associated with paraesthesia over the area of stimulation, and low frequency TENS delivered at high intensities is associated with a sharp flicking sensation or even muscle contractions. These sensations hamper proper blinding in controlled trials.[21]

TENS is completely contraindicated for use in patients with an implanted pacemaker.

6. Repetitive transcranial magnetic stimulation (rTMS)

Repetitive transcranial magnetic stimulation (rTMS) has been used for more than 20 years as treatment for various neurological disorders, including the treatment of chronic pain conditions.

rTMS is a noninvasive method that rarely has any side effects.

In 2008, rTMS of the left dorsolateral prefrontal cortex was approved for treatment of depression in the USA.

TMS can be used with a single pulse (single-pulse TMS), with a pair of applied pulses with a variable interval (paired-pulse TMS) or with repeating pulses (repetitive) rTMS.

rTMS is distinguished according to the selected frequency; it can be fast, i.e. high-frequency rTMS, which operate at frequencies of more than 1 Hz, or slow, i.e. low-frequency rTMS, which operate at frequencies of 1 Hz or less.

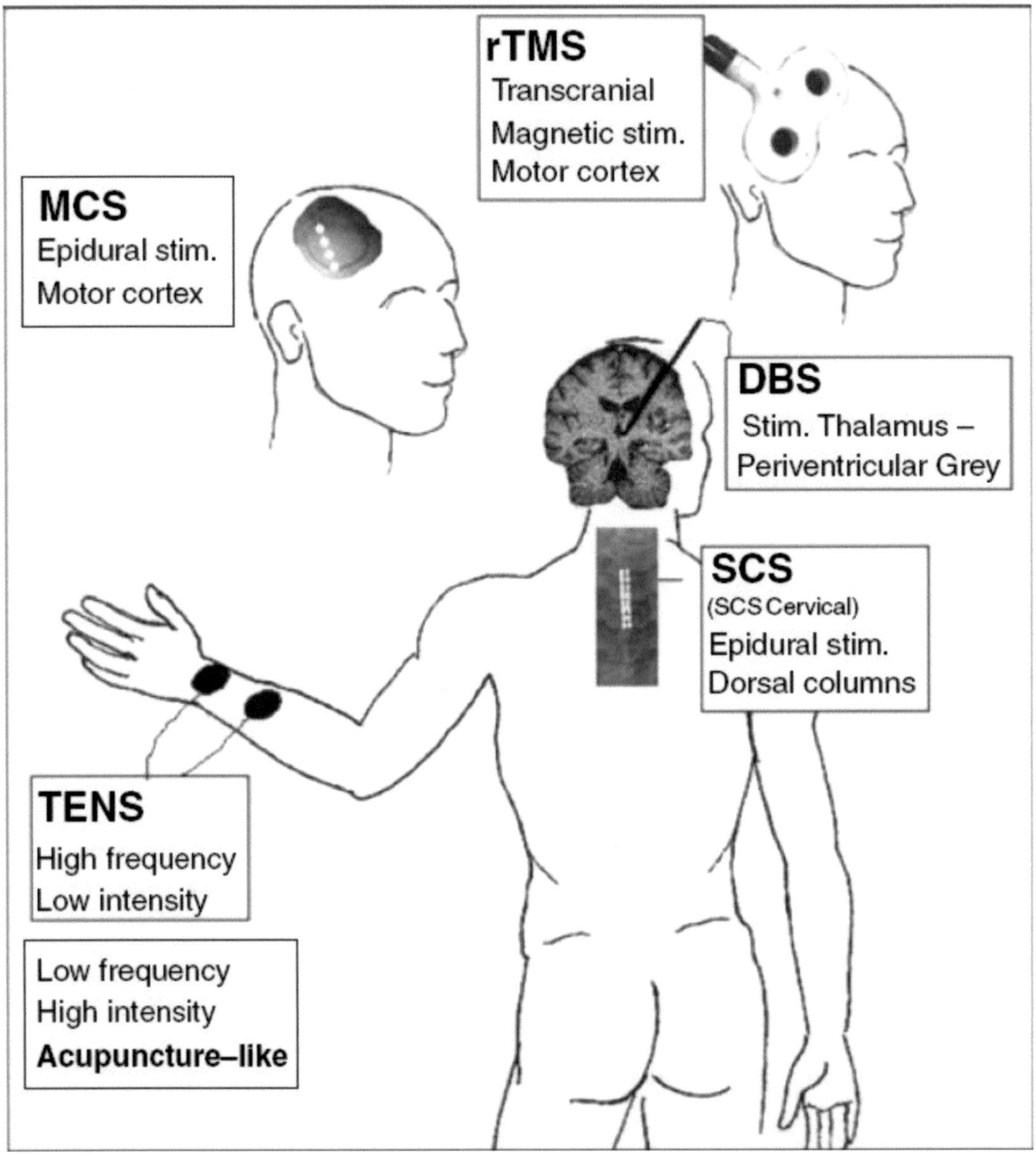

Figure 1. Guidelines of European Federation of Neurological Societes for the Neurostimulation Therapy in Neuropathic Pain [6].

This classification is based on a variety of physiological effects and degrees of risk associated with low and high frequency stimulation.

The effects of rTMS involved in a variety of mechanisms, including changes resembling experimental synaptic long term depression (LTD) and long-potentiating (LTP) mechanisms, activation of feedback loops, as well as changes in neuronal excitability. The treatment of pain using rTMS began mainly as a test to demonstrate the efficiency of cortical stimulation. The pioneers of this method were Lefaucheur et al. from Paris (2004, 2008) [11-13] and Leung et al. (2009) [17], which when using rTMS on healthy volunteers observed a decrease in sensory pain threshold.

Later it was shown that this effect was also present in patients suffering from various types of chronic pain. Studies using imaging techniques have shown that rTMS causes not only electrochemical changes in the brain, but also leads to a reorganization (changing the structure) of the cerebral cortex and other areas of the brain associated with chronic pain.

The TMS principle involves a magnetic field, with an intensity of 1-2 T, which generates an electric field that acts on the cell membrane of neurons and leads to changes in the electrochemical membrane potential.

Mechanism of action of rTMS pain treatment: The exact mechanism behind rTMS pain relief remains unknown. Stimulation of the motor cortex has been associated with pain relief in various pharmacoresistant pain syndromes. Stimulation of the motor cortex using rTMS alters the sensory threshold in healthy individuals and inhibits transmission of sensory information in the spinothalamic tract; depending on stimulation duration of each treatment, rTMS has been shown to induce a long-term increase in synaptic transmission.

Measurements of stimulation effects: In our research [10] we tested rTMS effects by making before and after rTMS using a VAS (visual analogue scale) and QST (quantitative sensory testing). QST consisted of thermal stimulation, which measured the thermal sensation threshold and tactile sensation testing using von Frey hairs. Testing must be individualized by establishing individual motor thresholds.

Contralateral motor stimulation provoked an immediate response and was associated with stimulation levels that produced relief from pain. Immediately after stimulation there is a temporary increase in pain, the changes in thermal threshold and tactile sensation. The benefits of rTMS, in the form of pain relief, are usually seen 2 to 4 days after treatment. rTMS outcomes depends on the origin and location of the treated pain and the degree of sensory deficit.

rTMS can also be used, in addition to its own analgesic effects, to determine if cortical brain stimulation would be effective in a particular patient.

6.1. Types of pain suitable for rTMS stimulation

Intractable chronic pain: neuropathic pain (postherpetic neuralgia), pain after stroke, deafferentation pain (very often after brachial plexus avulsion), trigeminal neuralgia, and thalamic pain. Other analgesic indications are atypical orofacial pain) [10], spinal stenosis, low back pain, phantom pain, stump pain, KRBS, fibromyalgia, and migraines.Best practices, for neurostimulation have been standardized and are available in the European Federation of Neurological Societies for neurostimulation therapy for neuropathic pain (G. Cruccu TZ Aziz, L. Garcia-Larrea, d, P. Hansson, TS Jensen; J.-P. Lefaucheur, BA Simpson and RS Taylor, European Journal of Neurology 2007).

rTMS, used in accordance with the guidelines, is considered to be a safe and non-invasive method of neuromodulation pain therapy. It offers an important next step in the treatment of chronic intractable pain. Our research has confirmed the benefits of rTMS stimulation in patients with trigeminal and orofacial pain. For most of patients, we observed a change in the nature and a reduction in the frequency of painful episodes. Two patients in our research group became pain-free and 1 patient was indicated for cortical stimulation two years after stimulation [8-10].

The use of rTMS in the treatment of chronic intractable pain is reserved for pain that does not respond to analgesics and for pain in which the cause is difficult to remove. If it can be demonstrated to have an analgesic effect, then rTMS could be considered for inclusion in the current methods of pain treatment [30]. The advantage of magnetic stimulation is that it is a non-invasive procedure that is not time-consuming. Before rTMS can be routinely used in the treatment of chronic pain, it is necessary to accurately determine the amount and duration for each stimulation session, thereby ensuring the optimal duration of effect. From our results it is possible to conclude that the more effective rTMS was obtained with 20 Hz stimulation if compared wit our results with 10 Hz stimulation [9]. These results were measured with subjective evaluation of the pain, VAS, and with objective measurement using QTS. In objective evaluation the tactile measurement proved to be more important, while the results from measurement of thermal thresholds were not significant.The two treatment groups (active vs. sham) were comparable with respect to baseline demographic and clinical characteristics. rTMS was well tolerated, and no serious adverse effects were reported. In our study we combined both, sham or real stimulation. Another advantage over other neuromodulatory methods is the price of the equipment.

rTMS has also been tested on healthy subjects and was found to cause facilitation of motor evoked potentials, leading to an alternative interpretation of the effects of rTMS, which involves the activation of plasticity in the cerebral cortex [37]. Another possible pathophysiological explanation is that low-frequency stimulation (1 Hz) reduces the activity of excitatory circuits in the human motor cortex. Our results did not completely confirm this hypothesis.rTMS has also been investigated in depression, Parkinson's disease, spinocerebellar degeneration, epilepsy, urinary incontinence, movement disorders, chronic pain, migraines and chronic tinnitus The method did very well in comparison with epidural motor cortex stimulation and transcranial direct current electrical stimulation both in terms of effect and having a favorable cost / effectiveness ratio rTMS has also been tested in monkeys Effectiveness of rTMS also depends on the type of neuropathic pain [16,17].

Application of rTMS induces not only subjective pain relief [16,17] but also objective changes in Quantitative Sensory Testing (QST), namely changes in thermal threshold [14,15]and the threshold for tactile sensation [14,15]. Changes in the threshold of tactile sensation can be easily and reliably accessed with techniques using von Frey monofilaments and a Peltier thermal generator can be used to determine changes in thermal threshold [14,17].

Information regarding the prevalence of orofacial pain varies considerably from study to study and depends on the source of pain, however, it appears to affect between 10 to 50% of the adult population. The most common cause of facial pain is pain of dental origin, which begins after dental reparation or dental surgeries. Very often it is an intractable pain and pharmacological treatment is unsuccessful. Recent studies have suggested the involvement of the peripheral and central nervous system in the pathophysiology of atypical odontalgia.

Today rTMS is used with short-term success in the treatment of pain, mostly neuropathic pain. Previous studies have confirmed the ability of high (> 1 Hz) rTMS to stimulate the M1 in the treatment of facial pain. They have shown that the application of rTMS to the M1 changes the thermal pain threshold in this and related areas. Also of interest is the DLPFC (dorsolateral prefrontal cortex) coil position, which seems to have a substantial influence on neuronal circuits involved in the processing of cognitive and emotional aspects of pain.

6.2. Other effects of rTMS on pain

1 Hz (low frequency) rTMS reduces acute pain induced by capsaicin temporarily improves phantom pain and reduces pain in fibromyalgia High-frequency rTMS has been shown to produce changes in the pain threshold in people with chronic pain. Higher frequency rTMS (5-10 Hz) also reduces deafferentation intractable pain in spinal cord injury and in peripheral nerves. We enlarged these indications of high frequency stimulation by using 20 Hz stimulation, which was found to be very suitable for treatment of orofacial pain.

rTMS suppresses the perception of painful CRPS (Complex Regional Pain Syndrome)and suppresses neuropathic pain, in particular pain with a central origin rTMS is also effective in treating migraines with or without aura Low-frequency vertex rTMS (1 Hz) has been shown to have a prophylactic effect on migraines.

Our study confirmed that rTMS at a frequency of 20 Hz, functionally localized to the area of the motor cortex contralateral to the position corresponding to the somatotopic location of the pain source is effective in the treatment of chronic orofacial pain. Subjective evaluation of intra- and inter-group VAS scores, compared with the control group, showed both immediate and delayed treatment effects in subsequent measurements. The results of the VAS ratings are consistent with results of previous studies.Changes in thermal sensation were not statistically different between groups. Intragroup comparison confirmed the reduction of thermal threshold for hot air stimulation after repeated rTMS application. Some studies have confirmed the influence of rTMS to reduce the threshold for thermal stimulation of both cold air and hot air [14,15] Other studies however, have shown an increased thermal threshold for hot air stimulation after rTMS Inter-group comparisons of tactile sensations showed acute effects after repeated stimulation (days 2, 4 and 5) but not when measured using a longer interval (day 21). Confirmation of the influence of rTMS on QST, specifically its ability to reduce the threshold for tactile (mechanical) sensation, supports the hypothesis that modulation of tactile and thermal perception in the painful zone interacts with the analgesic effect of cortical stimulation [15,16]

Our data are consistent with previous studies which reported that the use of a higher frequency increased number of pulses during an rTMS application and an increased number of applications [17] led to increased efficacy of the method in the treatment of pain. The best frequency of stimulation for the most effective pain treatment has not yet been resolved. Our results support the effect of 20 Hz rTMS. rTMS appears to be a safe and potentially effective tool for treatment of chronic migraine patients who showed resistance to pharmacological treatments [20]. Further studies are needed to assess factors underlying therapeutic effects (change in cortical excitability, better antinociceptive control).It's also to seek for optimal stimulation parameters (intensity,frequency, number and duration of stimulation sessions). Another important point may be the best cortical areas to be modulated for pain control in migraine, and the most efficacy side of stimulation, though the left side has been more frequently employed in studies on pain control.

6.3. Complications of rTMS

Low frequency rTMS stimulation can cause nausea, probably via stimulation of the posterior cranial fossa. rTMS of the premotor cortex reduces painful axial spasms in generalized secondary dystonia. [14-17] rTMS can also have side effects and randomly caused convulsions in control patients, one patient was reported to suffer from depression and parietal epilepsy.Side effects include induction of epileptic seizures (less than 1% of patients), which is more likely in high-frequency rTMS and rarely occurs in low-frequency rTMS. A more common problem is the formation of transient pain, which is precisely located and depends on the site of stimulation.

7. Transcranial direct current stimulation (tDCS)

Another non-invasive and simple neurostimulation technique is tDCS (transcranial direct current stimulation), which uses a cathode and anode, and is applied to the head using a low intensity direct current (0.029 to 0.08 mA/cm2) to stimulate the surface of the skull. tDCS is a noninvasive stimulation technique that is affordable and easy to use compared to other neuromodulation techniques [9].tDCS methods: anode stimulation increases cortical excitability, while cathodic stimulation decreases it. tDCS is a promising method for the treatment of chronic pain, as well as for patients with neuropsychiatric diseases and other neurological disorders.

7.1. Mechanisms of action tDCS

tDCS affects the brain's motor cortex excitability, which in humans is in area M1 (gyrus precentralis). Stimulation with the anode increases excitability of cortical brain cells by affecting the GABAergic system through depolarization. Anode stimulation reduces GABA concentrations in the cerebral cortex. Cathode stimulation reduces excitability of cortical brain cells via hyperpolarization of the glutamate system. Cathode stimulation produces a homeostatic effect. Low electric current rapidly increases the electrical conductivity of biological membranes by increasing permeability to ions and both small and large molecules. tDCS increases intracellular calcium. Neuroplasticity modulates the motor cortex through changes in opioid activity [7] glutamatergic, GABAergic, dopaminergic (D1 and D2 receptors), serotonergic and cholinergic system [25].Nicotine reduces inhibitory plastic changes after

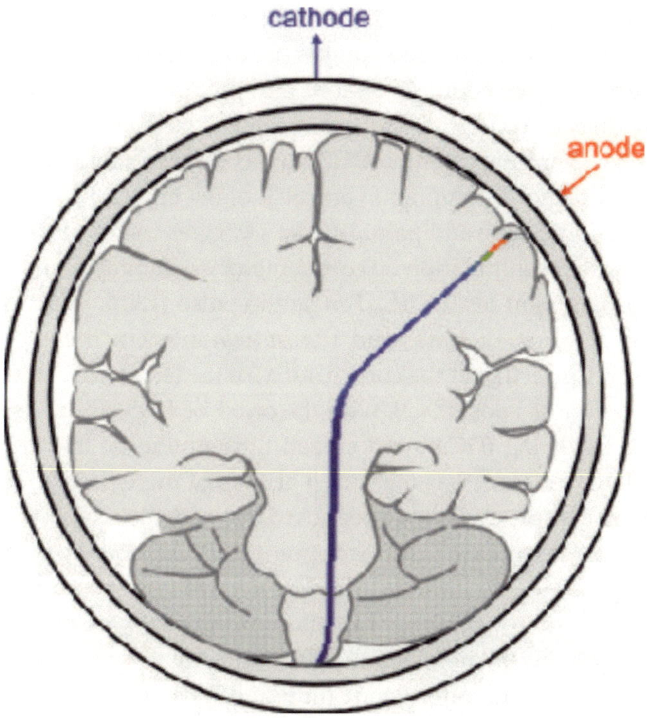

Figure 2. The placement of cathode and anode transcranial direct current stimulation tCDS

cathode stimulation and facilitatory plasticity after anode stimulation. tDCS has also been shown to stimulate glial cells; tDCS not only impacts neuroplasticity; tDCS is also neuroprotective.

7.2. Therapeutic indication tDCS

Therapeutic indication include chronic neuropathic pain [13] including refractory orofacial pain and pain after ERCP (endoscopic retrograde cholangiopancreatography), trigeminal pain, fibromyalgia [35], phantom pain [3] and back pain[28].

Therapeutic indications for psychiatric disorders include: depression (including severe depression), bipolar disorder, schizophrenia, Alzheimer's disease (here mainly it acts through GABAergic pathways during anode stimulation) and modulation of associative learning. Therapeutic indications in neurological diseases include: Parkinson's disease, postictal problems after stroke and tinnitus.

7.3. tDCS perspectives

In particular it is useful for stimulation of the prefrontal dorsolateral cortex and other spreading localization of tDCS stimulation. [27]. In recent Study [12] they using a randomized, cross-over design; each participant was exposed to 13 minutes of sham, unilateral-anodal or bilateral tDCS applied at 1.0 mA.In all tDCS conditions, the anode was placed over the "hot spot" of the non-dominant extensor carpi radialis longus (ECRL) muscle as determined by TMS. The order of these conditions were counterbalanced and randomized across participants, with a one week rest between each condition. This was achieved as the tDCS machine used, allowed for the use of a code to determine whether tDCS was active or inactive (sham). Within the sham condition, 50% of the unilateral stimulation and 50% of the bilateral stimulation was randomized for sham stimulation. Single and paired-pulse TMS was used to assess the after-effects of unilateral, bilateral or sham stimulation on corticomotor excitability of the right M1 and motor function of the non-dominant left ECRL. Ten single-pulse (130% of active motor threshold [AMT]), 10 paired-pulse (70% of AMT) and 10 test (test-intensity set to produce MEPs of ~1 mV) TMS stimuli were applied over the cortical area for the left ECRL at baseline, immediately following, 30 and 60 minutes post tDCS, with the order of TMS stimuli (single, paired-pulse or test) prior to and following tDCS, randomized throughout the trials (30 trials in total for each time point). Motor function was measured at each of these time points in all conditions by having participants complete a Purdue pegboard test with their left hand only. Importantly, all electrophysiological measures for each time point were measured prior to the performance of the pegboard, as post MEP facilitation and the effectiveness of SICI has been shown to be modulated immediately following the completion of the pegboard test. They examined the effects of a single-session of unilateral stimulation, bilateral and sham stimulation on modulating motor function of the non-dominant limb and indices of corticomotor plasticity. In healthy adults, the extent of motor function improvement and corticomotor plasticity were similar between unilateral and bilateral tDCS. Therefore, the physiological mechanisms regulating motor function were not different. Nevertheless, the present data indicate that tDCS induces behavioral changes in the non-dominant hand as a consequence of mechanisms associated with use-dependent cortical plasticity and is not influenced by the tDCS electrode arrangement. [12]

At a cellular level, direct current stimulation (DCS) may enhance plasticity in a given synaptic pathway while stimulated at a preferential frequency 0.1 Hz or consolidate a specific pattern of activity presented during DCS. DCS may preferentially modulate the level of potentiation in the activated pathway. DCS may facilitate long-term potentiation through membrane polarization and removal of Mg^{+} block but only those pathways activated during DCS (by a task or experimental stimulation) would benefit from this facilitation. DCS may be too weak and/or unspecific in isolation to enhance synaptic efficacy, but may boost ongoing (e.g., Hebbian) plasticity activated by task performance (i.e., modulation of input specific plasticity along an activated synaptic pathway while sparing quiescent synapses). In humans, transcranial electrical stimulation may also preferentially modulate networks with heightened oscillatory activity or preferentially change the progression of an active network during memory consolidation or synaptic downscaling [20]Anatomical specificity and functional specificity, through either ongoing activity-selectivity or input-selectivity, are not exclusive and may potentially be leveraged together in the development of rational tDCS protocols. In general, we propose that understanding the basis for tDCS selectivity is essential. Although we have focused our discussion to tDCS, the approaches described here would apply to other brain stimulation techniques including DBS, VNS, TMS, tRNS, and tACS as well as ultrasound and light based approaches [2

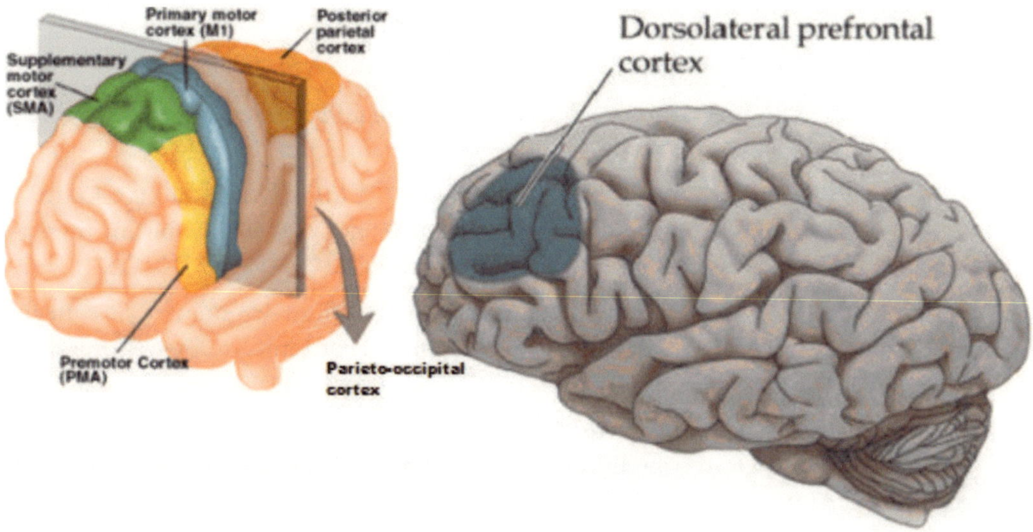

Figure 3. Localisation of dorsolateral prefrontal cortex which is very perspective for tDCS treatment

Acknowledgements

This work was supported by the grant of Charles University in Prague PRVOUK P 34.

Author details

Richard Rokyta[1*] and Jitka Fricova[2]

*Address all correspondence to: richard.rokyta@lf3.cuni.cz

1 Charles University in Prague, Third Faculty of Medicine, Department of Normal, Pathological and Clinical Physiology, Prague, Czech Republic

2 Charles University in Prague, First Faculty of Medicine and General Faculty Hospital, Department of Anaesthesiology, Resuscitation and Intensive Care, Pain Management Center, Prague, Czech Republic

References

[1] Abdulla A., Adams N., Bone M., Elliott AM., Gaffin J., Jones D., Knaggs R., Martin D., Sampson L., Schofield P. British Geriatric Guidance on the management of pain in older people. Age Ageing. 2013, 42 Suppl.

[2] Bikson M, Name A, Rahman A.. Origins of specificity during tDCS: anatomical, activity-selective, and input-bias mechanisms. Front Hum Neurosci. 2013, 21

[3] Bolognini N., Olgiati E., Maravita A,. Ferraro F., Fregni F. Motor and parietal cortex stimulation for phantom limb pain and sensations.Pain. 2013; 154(8):1274-80.

[4] Carbonario F., Matsutani LA., Yuan SL., Marques AP. Effectiveness of high-frequency transcutaneous electrical nerve stimulation at tender points as adjuvant therapy for patients with fibromyalgia.Eur J Phys Rehabil Med. 2013; 49(2):197-204.

[5] Celik EC., Erhan B., Gunduz B., Lakse E. The effect of low-frequency TENS in the treatment of neuropathic pain in patients with spinal cord injury. Spinal Cord. 2013; 51(4):334-7.

[6] Cruccu G., Aziz TZ., Garcia-Larrea L, Hansson P., Jensen TS., Lefaucheur JP., Simpson BA., Taylor RS. European EFNS guidelines on neurostimulation therapy for neuropathic pain. Eur. J. Neurol. 2007; 14 (9): 952-70.

[7] DosSantos MF., Love TM., Martikainen IK., Nascimento TD., Fregni F., Cummiford C., Deboer MD., Zubieta JK., Dasilva AF. Immediate effects of tDCS on the μ-opioid system of a chronic pain patient.Front Psychiatry. 2012;3:93.

[8] Fricová J., Klírová M., Novák T., Rokyta R.: Repetitive transcranial stimulation in chronic orofacial neurogenic pain treatment. International Neuromodulation Society – 10th World Congress, 21.5. – 27.5.2011, London, Great Britain.

[9] Fricová J., Klírová M., Šóš P., Tišlerová B., Masopust V., Haeckel M., Rokyta R. Repetitive transcranial stimulation in chronic neurogenic pain. 5th World Congress Institute of Pain, New York, USA, Pain Practice 2009; 9 (Suppl. 3):38.

[10] Fricová J., Klírová M., Masopust V., Novák T,Vérebová K,Rokyta R. Repetitive Transcranial Magnetic Stimulation in the treatment of chronic orofacial pain. Physiol. Res. 2013; 62 (Suppl. 1)

[11] Han JS., Chen XH., Sun SL., Xu XJ., Yuan Y., Yan SC., Hao JX., Terenius L. Effect of low- and high-frequency TENS on Met-enkephalin-Arg-Phe and dynorphin A immunoreactivity in human lumbar CSF. Pain 1991, 47:295–8

[12] Kidgell DJ., Goodwill AM., Frazer AK., Daly RM. Induction of cortical plasticity and improved motor performance following unilateral and bilateral transcranial direct current stimulation of the primary motor cortex. BMC Neurosci. 2013; 1;14(1):64.

[13] Knotkova H., Portenoy RK., Cruciani RA. Transcranial Direct Current Stimulation (tDCS) Relieved Itching in a Patient with Chronic Neuropathic Pain. Clin J Pain. 2013;29(7):621-2.

[14] Lefaucheur JP. Use of repetitive transcranial magnetic stimulation in pain relief. Exper. Rev. Neurother. 2008; 8(5): 799-808.

[15] Lefaucheur JP., Drouot X., Ménard-Lefaucheur I., Keravel Y., Nguyen JP. Motor cortex rTMS in chronic neuropathic pain: pain relief is associated with thermal sensory perception improvement. J. Neurol. Neurosurg. Psychiatry 2008; 79(9): 1044-9.

[16] Lefaucheur JP. The use of repetitive transcranial magnetic stimulation (rTMS) in chronic neuropathic pain. Neurophysiol. Clin. 2006; 36(3): 117-24.

[17] Leung WW., Jones AY., Ng SS., Wong CY., Lee JF. Acupuncture transcutaneous electrical nerve stimulation reduces discomfort associated with barostat-induced rectal distension: a randomized-controlled study. World J Gastroenterol. 2013; 21;19(3): 381-8.

[18] Liebano RE., Vance CG., Rakel BA., Lee JE., Cooper NA., Marchand S., Walsh DM., Sluka KA.Transcutaneous electrical nerve stimulation and conditioned pain modulation influence the perception of pain in humans. Eur J Pain 2013; 6. S. 1532.

[19] Loh J., Gulati A. The Use of Transcutaneous Electrical Nerve Stimulation (TENS) in a Major Cancer Center for the Treatment of Severe Cancer-Related Pain and Associated Disability. Pain Med. 2013; 25.

[20] Magis D., Schoenen J. Advances and challenges in neurostimulation for headaches. Lancet Neurol 2012,11:708–19

[21] Martelletti P., Jensen RH., Antal A., Arcioni R., Brighina F., de Tommaso M., Franzini A., Fontaine D., Heiland M., Jürgens TP., Leone M., Magis D., Paemeleire K., Palmisani S., Paulus W., May A. Neuromodulation of chronic headaches: position statement from the European Headache Federation. The Journal of Headache and Pain 2013, 14:86

[22] Masopust V., Nežádal T. Occipital stimulation –first experiencies (In Czech), Bolest 2012, Suppl. 1,15: 17.

[23] Masopust V., Beneš V., Netuka D., Pollin B., Rokyta R., Stejskal V. The motor cortex stimulation in the treatment of chronic thalamic pain (in Czech). Bolest 2001; 4(2): 91-4.

[24] McNearney TA., Sallam HS., Hunnicutt SE., Doshi D., Chen JD.. Prolonged treatment with transcutaneous electrical nerve stimulation (TENS) modulates neuro-gastric motility and plasma levels of vasoactive intestinal peptide (VIP), motilin and interleukin-6 (IL-6) in systemic sclerosis. Clin Exp Rheumatol. 2013; 7.

[25] Medeiros LF., de Souza IC., Vidor LP., de Souza A., Deitos A., Volz MS., Fregni F., Caumo W., Torres IL. Neurobiological effects of transcranial direct current stimulation: a review. Front Psychiatry. 2012;3:110.Moreno-Duarte I., Morse L., Alam M., Bikson M., Zafonte R., Fregni F. Targeted therapies using electrical and magnetic neural stimulation for the treatment of chronic pain in spinal cord injury. J. Neuroimage.2013; 30. S1053.

[26] Nnoaham KE., Kumbang J. Transcutaneous electrical nerve stimulation (TENS) for chronic pain. Cochrane Database Syst Rev. 2008, 16(3)

[27] O'Connell NE., Cossar J., Marston L., Wand BM., Bunce D., De Souza LH., Maskill DW., Sharp A., Moseley GL. Transcranial direct current stimulation of the motor cortex in the treatment of chronic nonspecific low back pain: a randomized, double-blind exploratory study.Clin J Pain. 2013; 29(1):26-34.

[28] Rokyta R., Kršiak M., Kozák J. eds Pain – the monography of Algesiology, ISBN 978-80-87323-02-01 Tigis, Praha 2012, s.747.

[29] Rokyta R., Fricová J. Neurostimulation Methods in the Treatment of Chronic Pain.Physiol. Res. 2012, 61 (Suppl. 2); 23- 31.

[30] Rokyta R. The pathophysiology of acupuncture (in Czech) Acupunctura Bohemo Slovaca, 2010, 2-3; 16-22.

[31] Rokyta R. The new approaches in the treatment of chronic pain. Joint Conference of the Czech and Slovak Neuroscience Societies, Prague, 2009, 27.

[32] Stein C., Eibel B., Sbruzzi G., Lago PD., Plentz RD. Electrical stimulation and electromagnetic field use in patients with diabetic neuropathy: systematic review and meta-analysis. Rev Bras Fisioter. 2013; 17(2).

[33] Vance CG., Rakel BA., Blodgett NP., DeSantana JM., Amendola A., Zimmerman MB., Walsh DM., Sluka KA. Effects of transcutaneous electrical nerve stimulation on pain, pain sensitivity, and function in people with knee osteoarthritis: a randomized controlled trial. Phys Ther. 2012, 92(7):898-910

[34] Villamar MF., Wivatvongvana P., Patumanond J., Bikson M., Truong DQ., Datta A., Fregni F. Focal modulation of the primary motor cortex in fibromyalgia using 4×1-ring high-definition transcranial direct current stimulation (HD-tDCS): immediate and delayed analgesic effects of cathodal and anodal stimulation. J Pain.2013; 14(4): 371-83.

[35] Zhang X., Cao B., Yan N., Liu J., Wang J., Tung VO., Li Y. Vagus nerve stimulation modulates visceral pain-related affective memory. Behav Brain Res. 2013, 1;236(1): 8-15.

[36] ZIEMANN U: TMS induced plasticity in human cortex. Rev Neurosci.2004 15 : 253-66,

[37] Zimmer A., Greul F., Meißner W. Pain management in urology. Urologe A. 2013; 52(4):585-95.

Chapter 6

Intramuscular Stimulation (IMS)

Sang-Chul Lee and Young-Jae Kim

Additional information is available at the end of the chapter

http://dx.doi.org/10.5772/58565

1. Introduction

Chronic pain is common with relatively high incidence and low recovery rates [1]. Chronic pain can cause disability, mild to severe suffering and a serious problem to the health of the public. Chronic pain is localized to the musculoskeletal system in the majority of patients [2]. The most reported forms of chronic musculoskeletal pain are frequently back pain. However non-specific spinal disorders are not possible to identify a pathomorphological source of the problem despite a thorough diagnostic work-up such as simple radiography, computed tomography, magnetic resonance imaging, ultrasound, electromyography and nerve conduction test [1]. There are many potential causatives and aggravating factors associated with non-specific spinal disorders. Though laboratory and radiologic tests provide a myriad of information including the musculoskeletal and nerve system and give important clues for the diagnosis, structural abnormalities and clinical symptoms do not match commonly in clinical practice [3]. Unfortunately some patients do not improve despite administering conservative treatment and then the various interventional therapies, including medical treatment and/or surgery, and they find themselves in search of a more effective pain relief.

Deep dry needling is one of the alternative treatment modalities for these patients who do not respond to drug therapy and clinical intervention [4]. Previous clinical study demonstrated that dry needling into the trigger points (MTrPs) of myofascial pain syndrome is as effective as the injection of local anesthetics in inactivating them [5]. Especially, there appears to be growing interest in the intramuscular stimulation (IMS) for myofascial pain of radiculopathic origin developed by the Canadian physician Dr. Chan Gunn [6]. According to Gunn's approach, dry needling should be performed not only in muscle at the site of pain but also in the paraspinal muscles of the same spinal segment that innervates the painful muscles as causes and treatment targets of chronic pain. IMS is the technique for

INTECH
open science | open minds

© 2015 The Author(s). Licensee InTech. This chapter is distributed under the terms of the Creative Commons Attribution License (http://creativecommons.org/licenses/by/3.0), which permits unrestricted use, distribution, and reproduction in any medium, provided the original work is properly cited.

needle insertion and mechanical stimulation into trigger points or motor units of muscle belong to both anterior and posterior primary rami of spinal nerve root which require treatment.

In this chapter, we introduce IMS as an alternative and effective method for the management of chronic pain.

2. Basic background for IMS

Dry needling methods have empirically been developed to treat musculoskeletal disorders. In 1942, Dr. Janet Travell and colleagues firstly published the method by intramuscular infiltration with procaine hydrochloride [7]. The wider use of dry needling started after Lewit's publication [5], where it was emphasized that the needling effect was distinct from that of the injected substance and the effect of injections was primarily caused by the mechanical stimulation of myofascial trigger points (MTrPs) with the needle. In addition, in numerous randomized clinical trials [8-9], no difference was found between injections of different substances and dry needling in the treatment of MTrPs.

Several models of dry needling have developed during the last 3 decades. The radiculopathy model is based on empirical observations by Dr. Gunn[10], named IMS to distinguish this approach from other methods of dry needling. IMS technique is based on the premise that myofascial pain syndrome is always the result of peripheral neuropathy or radiculopathy, defined as a condition that causes disordered function in the peripheral nerve [6].

3. Radiculopathic model of IMS

In the radiculopathy model, based on Cannon and Rosenblueth's Law of Denervation Supersensitivity [11], denervated tissues develop supersensitivity. When a portion from a chain of nerve units is irritated, the receptor sensitivities to chemical stimuli in that point and the zones below it (muscles, skin, blood vessels, ligaments and tenoperiostea) become abnormally increased and these effects are maximized at the directly damaged sites [10]. The most common sites of supersensitivity are skeletal muscles. Indeed supersensitivity leads to muscle shortening when a nerve unit is injured, and by which myofascial pain syndrome is induced [10]. In the musculature, shortened muscles can physically cause a large variety of pain syndromes by its relentless pull on various structures [12] [Fig. 1] [Table 1]. Muscular evidence of radiculopathy is almost found in the distribution of both dorsal and ventral rami of affected segmental nerves. Shortening of the paraspinal muscles (particularly the multifidi muscles) innervated by dorsal ramus of affected segmental nerves leads to disk compression and narrowing of the intervertebral foramina, or direct pressure on the nerve root, which subsequently results in peripheral neuropathy and the development of supersensitive nociceptors and pain [Fig. 2].

http://dx.doi.org/10.5772/58565

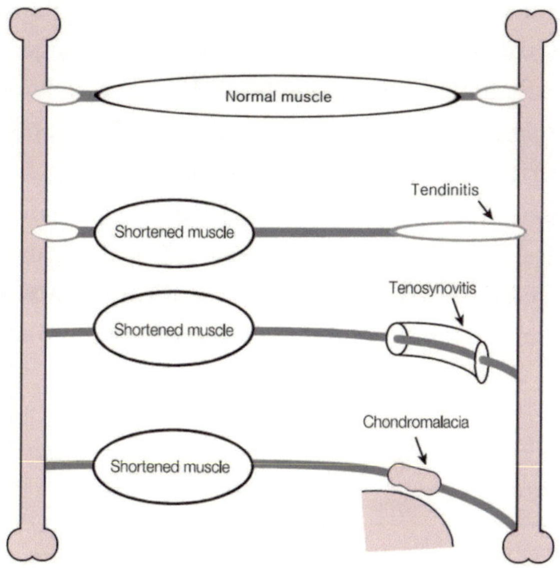

Figure 1. The shortened muscles cause the tendinitis, tenosynovitis and chondromalacia by increased traction at mechanically overloading the tendons and joints.

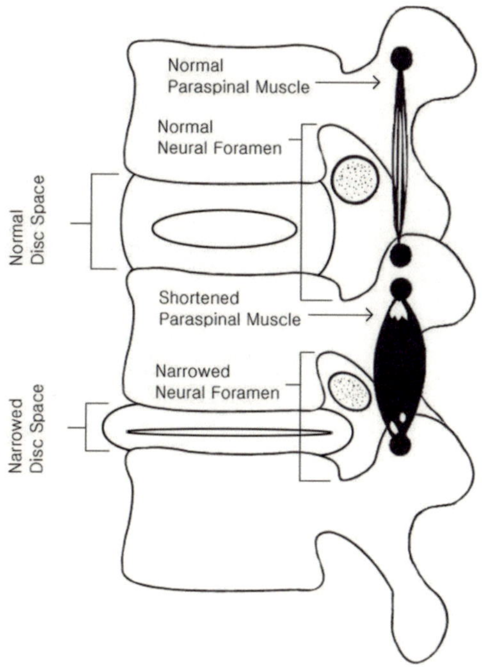

Figure 2. The shortened paraspinal muscles compress upon the nerve root by narrowed disc space and neural foramen.

Radiculoapthy can be often accompanied by partial denervation. Chronic attrition from the spondylosis is the most common among the causes of nerve damage, such as trauma, metabolic, degenerative, toxic, and other conditions [13]. The spondylosis has the structural disintegration and morphologic alterations that occur in the intervertebral disc, with pathoanatomical changes in surrounding structures. The spinal nerve root, because of its vulnerable position, is notably prone to injury from pressure, stretch, angulation, and friction due to pathoanatomical changes in spondylosis. Other causes of radiculopathy, such as arachnoiditis, neuroma, and intraspinal tumors are much less common. The spondylosis increases with age, and causes repeated major and minor injuries to a segment nerve leading to unresolved clinical residuals which may, or may not, produce pain [14].

Syndrome	Shortened muscle
Achilles tendonitis	Gastrocnemii, soleus
Bicipital tendonitis	Biceps brachii
Bursitis, pre-patellar	Quadriceps femoris
Capsulitis, frozen shoulder	All muscles acting on the shoulder
Carpal tunnel syndrome	pronator teres, the sublimis bridge, Trophedema in the forearm and carpal tunnel
Cervical fibrositis	Cervical paraspinal muscles
Chondromalacia patellae	Quadriceps femoris
De Quervain's tenosynovitis	Abductor pollicis longus, extensor pollicis brevis
Facet syndrome	Muscles acting across the facet joint
Fibromyalgia	Multisegmental (diffuse myofascial pain syndrome).
Hallux valgus	Extensor hallucis longus and brevis
Headaches- frontal	Upper trapezius, semispinalis capitis, occipitofrontalis
Headaches-temporal	Temporalis, trapezius
Headaches-vertex	Splenius capitis & cervicis, upper trapezius, semispinalis capitis, occipitofrontalis
Headaches-occipital	Sub-occipital muscles
Infrapatellar tendonitis	Quadriceps femoris
Intervertebral disc	Muscles acting across the disc space
Juvenile kyphosis and scoliosis	Unbalanced paraspinal scoliosis muscles (e.g., iliocostalis thoracis and lumborum)
Low back sprain	Paraspinal muscles
Plantar fascitis	Flexor digitorum brevis, lumbricals
Piriformis syndrome	Piriformis muscle
Rotator cuff syndrome	Supra-and infraspinati, teres minor, subscapularis
'Shin splints'	Tibialis anterior
Temporomandibular joint	Masseter, temporalis, pterygoids
Tennis elbow	Brachioradialis, carpi ulnaris, extensor carpi radialis brevis and longus, ext. digitorum, anconeus, triceps.
Torticollis (acute)	Splenius capitis & cervicis.

Table 1. Common myofascial pain syndromes caused by the shortened muscle syndrome

http://dx.doi.org/10.5772/58565

In addition, radiculopathy itself contributes to degenerative conditions. Neuropathy degrades the quality of collagen [15]. The amount of collagen in soft and skeletal tissues is also reduced. Because collagen lends strength to ligament, tendon, cartilage, and bone, neuropathy can expedite degeneration in weight-bearing and activity-stressed parts of the body which include the spine and joints.

Clinical features of radiculopathy differ from those of denervation such as loss of sensation and reflexes. The effects of radiculopathy vary according to the type of sensory, motor, autonomic, or mixed dysfunction and distribution of the nerve fibers involved.

4. Clinical features of radiculopathy

In radiculopathy, symptoms and signs are generally present in the territories of both posterior and anterior primary divisions of the affected nerve root. Clinical features of radiculopathy are projected to dermatomal, myotomal, and sclerotomal target structures supplied by the affected neural structure. The clinical characteristics can give rise to sensory, motor, autonomic, or mixed dysfunction.

Muscle shortening has painful spots on compression that are associated with hypersensitive palpable nodules in the taut band of skeletal muscle. The spots can cause tenderness, characteristic referred pain, motor dysfunction and autonomic phenomena. These can be tender, especially over motor points. Tender points can be found throughout the myotome and especially in paraspinal muscles.

Autonomic vasoconstriction of affected parts is colder in a noticeable manner. Increased permeability in blood vessels can lead to the trophedema that is edema in local subcutaneous tissue. The trophedema especially shows a characteristic feature like orange-peel skin over affected regions by rolling or squeezing an area of skin and subcutaneous tissue. The skin is tight and wrinkles absent. The consistency of subcutaneous tissue is firmer. The trophedema is not pitting to digital pressure, but to a blunt instrument pressure with the end of a matchstick. Excessive sweating as sudomotor activity may follow painful movements. The pilomotor reflex is often hyperactive and visible as goose-bumps in affected dermatomes.

The tendinous attachments to bone are thickened due to shortening muscle, which causes enthesopathy at the tenoperiosteal insertion.

5. Diagnosis for radiculopathy

The physical examination should always be preceded by a clinical history. It is important to inspect for any postural asymmetries, assess the range of motion for limitation, and examine the soft tissues for clinical features of radiculopathy. The spinal examination should be performed scrupulously according to segmental examination to elicit the signs that correspond to the affected spinal segments. The spinal segmental examination includes assessment for facet joint tenderness, tenderness to posteroanterior pressure on the spinous process, transverse pressure against the spinous process, and pressure against the interspinous ligamentum. This examination can identify the responsible spinal segments.

Because segmental radiculopathy primarily causes the significant changes in muscle, the examination of the segmental nerve supply to muscles is the clue to diagnosis. The changes in muscles are the most consistent increased muscle tone, tenderness over motor points and palpable taut bands, and result in restricting a range of joint motion. During examination according to the distribution of both dorsal and ventral rami of affected segmental nerves, each muscle must be palpated. Moreover, because many paraspinal muscles are compound and extend throughout most of the length of the vertebral column, the entire spine must be examined even when symptoms are localized to one region. The contracture caused by shortened muscles due to radiculopathy is invisible to X-rays, CT scans or MRI.

Laboratory and radiologic findings are generally not helpful for diagnosis of radiculopathy. Thermography reveals decreased skin temperature in affected dermatomes due to autonomic dysfunction. Other diagnostic observation is to find goose-bumps and orange-peel skin by rolling or squeezing an affected area. And the tenoperiosteal tenderness is present only when periosteal insertion is affected and is often painful to palpation only without giving the patient any pain spontaneously.

6. Technique for IMS

IMS is a system of dry needling that is based on a radiculopathy model for chronic pain. The key to IMS treatment is the release of muscle shortening. The fundamental Needling points for effective treatment are always situated to muscular motor points or musculotendinous junctions. These points generally coincide with palpable taut bands that are tender to digital pressure and are generally referred to as MTrPs. The muscles with tender points are generally shortened from contracture. Needling points generally belong to the same segmental level as presenting symptoms and signs. Tender points are distributed in a segmental or myotomal fashion, in muscles of both anterior and posterior primary rami which is indicative of radiculopathy. Practitioners purposely seek out tender and tight muscle bands in affected segments for needling.

The needles inserted in the plungers are made of a fine, flexible, solid and stainless steel like acupuncture needle [Fig 3, 4]. Its lengths are 4, 6, and 8 cm (diameter: 0.25, 0.3 and 0.4 mm respectively). The absolute size of needle is dependent on the muscle and the depth of the motor point being treated. IMS needles are longer, finer, and whippier than hypodermic needles and are particularly suited for deep muscle exploration. The plunger is sterilized by autoclaving.

When the needling point is identified, standard precautionary techniques for asepsis are followed (hands scrubbed, no gloves, and skin cleansed with alcohol). The thumb and index

http://dx.doi.org/10.5772/58565

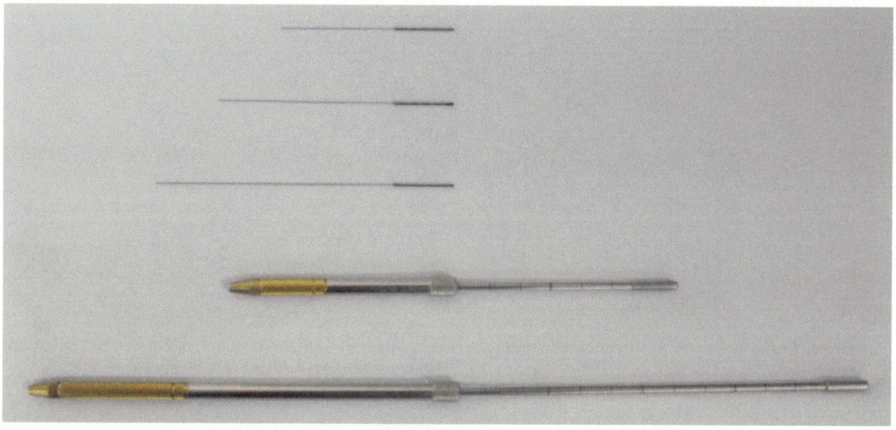

Figure 3. Types of needles and plungers according to the length of needles.

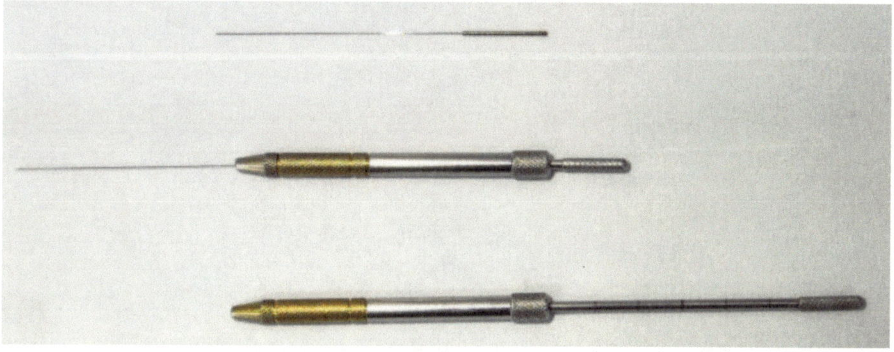

Figure 4. The needle is inserted in the plunger.

finger of the physician's nondominant hand holding plunger remain unmoved to guide the needle [Fig. 5]. The direction of needle insertions using plunger is perpendicular to the skin with the objective of penetrating the motor units. When the index finger of the physician's dominant hand on the non-needle end of plunger pushes the needle, it quickly penetrates the skin to 2 ~ 3 mm depth [Fig. 5 A]. And then IMS needle is followed several times by pecking and twirling movements [Fig. 5 B]. Therefore IMS allows stimulation of deeper motor units by using a manual plunger for inserting, pecking and twirling of the needle.

The fine, flexible needle transmits feed-back information on the nature and consistency of the tissues that it is penetrating. When the needle penetrates normal muscle, it meets with little hindrance. When it penetrates a contracted muscle, there is firm resistance, and the needle is grasped by the muscle. When an attempt is made to withdraw the needle, the grasp resists withdrawal. Leaving the grasped needle in situ for 5 to 20 minutes can lead to the release of a persistent contracture.

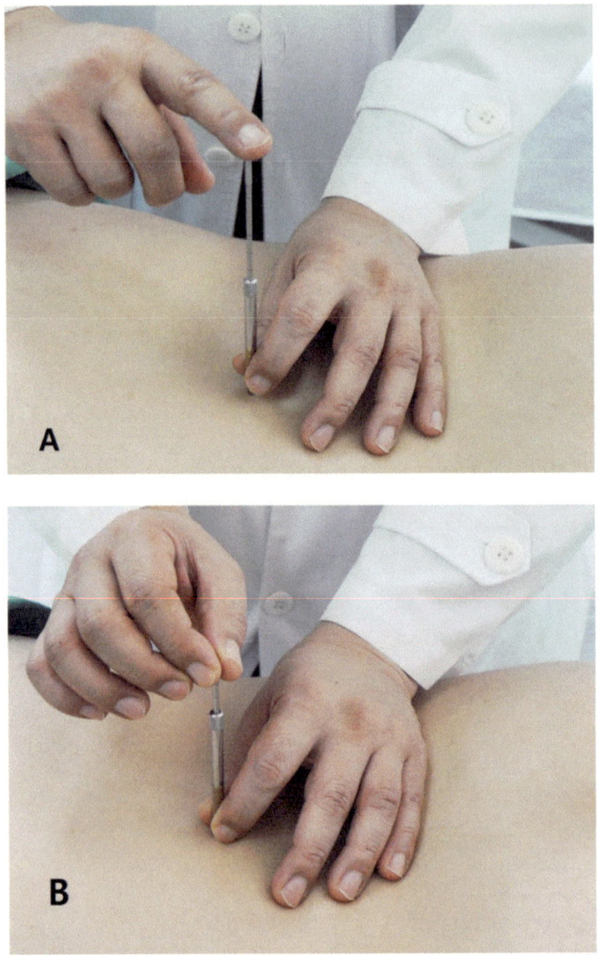

Figure 5. The technique of intramuscular stimulation. (A) Needle penetrates the skin. (B) Needle is pecked & rotated.

Following needling, muscle contracture, vasoconstriction and tenderness can disappear within seconds or minutes. Other signs, like trophedema may diminish more gradually, sometimes even taking days to disappear, but ultimately, all signs vanish following successful treatment.

7. The effect of IMS

There is limited evidence supporting that IMS has an overall treatment effect when compared with standardised care. The result of the meta-analysis searching all studies regardless of the language to include all the available clinical evidence on IMS included 5 randomized controlled trials (RCT) [16, 17]. The represented conditions had MPS of upper and lower half body, MPS of the upper trapezius muscle, chronic shoulder pain, tension-type headaches and chronic lower back pain. However, the large scale, good quality placebo controlled researches in IMS are needed for RCTs because of the limited sample size and poor quality of these studies.

Release of these muscles by stimulation of motor units with dry needling is usually necessary to restore joint range and relieve pain [10].Dry needling can cause a decrease in spontaneous electrical amplitude and subsequent relaxation via either a direct local electrical stimulus or via a reflex mechanism [18]. As the needle is introduced into muscle tissue, it can cause a shortened muscle to visibly fasciculate and subsequently relax [10]. In addition as the muscle is injured by the needle then a "current of injury" follows, this current of injury was first described in 1797 by Galvani. Injury potentials of several microamperes are generated and can persist and provide stimulation for days until the miniature wounds heal. It was demonstrated that denervation supersensitivity in animal muscle may be reduced or abolished by electrical stimulation [19].

In addition, twirling the needle causes muscle fibers cling to the needle to wind around its shaft. The rotation of a needle grasped by muscle shortening can produce intense stimulation. Unlike traction or manipulation, this stimulation is very precise and intense because the needle is precisely placed in a taut muscle band. Rotational motion is converted to linear motion which shortens the muscle fibers locally. This shortening of muscle fibers by twirling the needle activates muscle spindles and Golgi Tendon Organs and may cause subsequent muscle relaxation via local spinal reflexes. Therefore the needle rotation may induce neuroplastic changes as the pulling of collagen fibers and the transduction of the mechanical signal into fibroblasts can lead to a wide variety of cellular and extracellular events, including mechanoreceptor and nociceptor activation and eventually to neuropeptide liberation [20].

Needling also induces a sympatholytic effect that spreads throughout the body segment, releasing vasoconstriction. Pain in muscles, tendons and joints caused by excessive muscle tension is eased when the shortened muscles are relaxed. Subjective improvement can objectively be confirmed the increase in the motion of range, reduction of joint effusion and any decrease in muscle tenderness within minutes.

Dry needling delivers to the injured area the platelet-derived growth factor (PDGF) which induces deoxyribonucleic acid (DNA) synthesis and stimulates collagen formation [21].

One intervention of dry needle stimulation to a single MTrP evokes short term segmental antinociceptive effects [22]. MTrP stimulation by dry needling may evoke antinociceptive effects by modulating segmental mechanisms.

8. Adverse effect of IMS

No serious adverse effects were reported and the frequency of minor adverse effects occurred [23, 24, 25]. Several adverse effects associated specifically with dry needling include soreness after needling, local hemorrhages at the needling site and syncopal responses, and rarely reported a pneumothorax. Post-needling soreness is the most common due to local hemorrhages at the needling site and can be prevented by sufficient compression after treatment [26].

In addition, the thinner pointed-tipped IMS needles used for inserting trigger points can induce less tissue injuries than the thick and hollow needles with a beveled and cutting edge.

9. Difference between IMS and Acupuncture

IMS differs from chinese traditional acupuncture using superficial dry needling [table 2]. Unlike chinese traditional acupuncture, IMS requires a medical examination searching for early signs of radiculopathy, the knowledge of anatomy and a medical diagnosis, and uses neuroanatomical points that are found in a segmental pattern, instead of using traditional acupuncture points that is non-scientific meridians.

	Intramuscular stimulation	**Acupuncture**
Theory	Western medicine's understanding of the neurophysiology of pain and a greater knowledge of anatomy, muscle balancing and biomechanics	An ancient Chinese philosophy into non-scientific meridians
Diagnosis	Medical examination, and laboratory and X-ray test	Inspection and pulse diagnosis
needle placement	Into deep muscles	Into the superficial or subcutaneous tissues
Needling techniques	Pecking and twirling movements with plunger	Straight insertion
Treatment site	Motor points of the shortened muscle, and its corresponding spinal segment	pre-mapped out points in the body and meridians
Effect of treatment	Subjective and objective effects are usually experienced right after the treatment	Any effects are not experienced.

Table 2. The difference between IMS and Acupuncture

10. Conclusion of IMS

Many patients suffering from chronic pain have associated musculoskeletal pain which is not readily detectable with laboratory and radiologic tests. This pain may be due to both peripheral and central sensitization mechanisms. A radiculopathy model is offered to explain these syndromes. This model enables many apparently dissimilar musculoskeletal pain syndromes to be grouped under one etiologic classification such as radiculopathy. IMS is an alternative system of dry needling for treatment of chronic pain based on neurophysiologic concepts.

http://dx.doi.org/10.5772/58565

Author details

Sang-Chul Lee[1] and Young-Jae Kim[2]

1 Department of Anesthesiology and Pain Medicine, Seoul National University, Seoul, South Korea

2 Department of Anesthesiology and Pain Medicine, Busan Paik Hospital, College of Medicine, Inje University, Busan, South Korea

References

[1] Balagué F, Mannion AF, Pellisé F, Cedraschi C. Non-specific low back pain. Lancet 2012; 379: 482-91.

[2] Manchikanti L, Boswell MV, Singh V, Derby R, Fellows B, Falco FJ, et al. Comprehensive review of neurophysiologic basis and diagnostic interventions in managing chronic spinal pain. Pain Physician. 2009 ;12: E71-120.

[3] Elliott AM, Smith BH, Hannaford PC, Smith WC, Chambers WA. The course of chronic pain in the community: results of a 4-year follow-up study. Pain. 2002;99:299-307.

[4] Gunn CC. Dry needling of muscle motor points for chronic low back pain. Spine 1980; 5: 279-91.

[5] Lewit K. The needle effect in the relief of myofascial pain. Pain 1979;6:83-90.

[6] Gunn CC. Radiculopathic pain: diagnosis and treatment of segmental irritation or sensitization. J Musculoskelet Pain 1997;5:119-34.

[7] Travell J, Rinzler S, Herman M. Pain and disability of the shoulder and arm: treatment by intramuscular infiltration with procaine hydrochloride. JAMA 1942;120:417–22.

[8] Hong CZ. Lidocaine injection versus dry needling to myofascial trigger point. The importance of the local twitch response. Am J Phys Med Rehabil 1994;73:256–63.

[9] Cummings TM, White AR. Needling therapies in the management of myofascial trigger point pain: a systematic review. Arch Phys Med Rehabil 2001;82:986–92.

[10] Gunn CC. The Gunn approach to the treatment of chronic pain. 2nd Ed. New York: Churchill Livingstone; 1996:1–19

[11] Cannon WB, Rosenblueth A. The supersensitivity of denervated structure, a law of denervation. New York, MacMillan. 1949, pp 136-71

[12] Gunn CC: The mechanical manifestations of neuropathic pain. Annals of Sports Medicine 1990;5:138-141.

[13] Gunn CC. Prespondylosis and some pain syndrome following denervation supersensitivity. Spine 1978; 5: 185-92.

[14] Sola, AE: Treatment of myofasical pain syndromes. Advances in Pain Research and Therapy. Edited by C Benedetti, CR Chapman, and G Morrica. Raven Press, New York, 1984, Vol. 7, pp. 467-85.

[15] Klein L, Dawson MH, Heiple KG: Turnover of collagen in the adult rat after denervation. J Bone Jt Surgery ;59A:l065-7.

[16] Lim SM, Seo KH, Cho B, Ahn K, Park YH. A systematic review of the effectiveness and safety of intramuscular stimulation therapy. J Korean Med Assoc 2011;54:1070–80.

[17] Couto C, de Souza IC, Torres IL, Fregni F, Caumo W. Paraspinal stimulation combined with trigger point needling and needle rotation for the treatment of myofascial pain: a randomized sham-controlled clinical trial. Clin J Pain 2014;30:214–23.

[18] Chen J T, Chung K C, Hou C R, Kuan C R, Chen C R, Hong C Z. Inhibitory effect of dry needling on spontaneous electrical activity recorded from myofascial trigger points of rabbit skeletal muscle. Am J Phys Med Rehabil 2001;80:729-35.

[19] Lomo T, Massoulie J, Vigny M: Stimulation of denervated rat soleus muscle with fast and slow activity patterns induces different expression of acetylcholinesterase molecular forms. J Neurosci 1985;5:1180-7.

[20] Audette JF, Wang F, Smith H. Bilateral activation of motor unit potentials with unilateral needle stimulation of active myofascial trigger points. Am J Phys Med Rehabil 2004;83:368–74.

[21] Ross R, Vogel A. The platelet-derived growth factor. Cell 1978;4.203-10.

[22] Srbely JZ, Dickey JP, Lee D, Lowerison M. Dry needle stimulation of myofascial trigger points evokes segmental anti-nociceptive effects. J Rehabil Med 2010;42:463-8.

[23] Ga H, Choi JH, Park CH, Yoon HJ. Dry needling of trigger points with and without paraspinal needling in myofascial pain syndromes in elderly patients. J Altern Complement Med 2007;13:617–24.

[24] Huguenin L, Brukner PD, McCrory P, Smith P, Wajswelner H, Bennell K. Effect of dry needling of gluteal muscles on straight leg raise: a randomised, placebo controlled, double blind trial. Br J Sports Med 2005;39:84 –90.

[25] Simons DG, Travell JG, Simons LS. Travell & Simons' Myofascial Pain and Dysfunction: The Trigger Point Manual, vol 1: Upper Half of Body, 2nd ed., Baltimore: Williams & Wilkins, 1999:5.

http://dx.doi.org/10.5772/58565

[26] Kalichman L, Vulfsons S. Dry needling in the management of musculoskeletal pain J Am Board Fam Med 2010;23:640-6.

Chapter 7

Post Dural Puncture Headache – We Can Prevent It

Fuzhou Wang

Additional information is available at the end of the chapter

http://dx.doi.org/10.5772/57408

1. Introduction

Although modern anesthesiology has made great progress in the last decades, neuraxial anesthesia (NA) is still the keynote of regional blockade [1]. NA is popular for its effectiveness in producing anesthesia for providing excellent intraoperative neuromuscular paralysis and in generating analgesia for relieving postoperative pain if continuously infused [2, 3]. As the NA techniques are used popularly in clinic, post dural puncture headache (PDPH), a common iatrogenic complication resulted from post-spinal taps or accidental dural puncture (ADP) subsequent to epidural block, is frequently reported [4] and becomes a challenge to health caregivers [5]. Although the incidence of PDPH in research volunteers is ~6% [6], in patients for whom the NA is for clinical purposes the prevalence of PDPH ranges from 10% to over 80% in different aged patients underwent either epidural or spinal or combined block [7].

Investigations on the risk factors of PDPH revealed that female, age, perpendicular bevel orientation [8], previous history of PDPH [9], repeated dural puncture [10], needle gauge and design [11], and pregnancy [12] are factors substantially related with the occurrence of PDPH. The leakage of cerebrospinal fluid (CSF) was considered as the major cause of PDPH [13], whereas its real etiology is unknown. These procedure- and nonprocedure-related factors in combination determine the patterns of development of PDPH. Several procedures and methods were identified effective in treating and reducing the incidence of PDPH based on the knowledge of procedure-related factors, but whether could we prevent this morbid prior to its occurrence?

Techniques developed based on how to reduce CSF leakage are classified into either preventive or therapeutic ones. Although the results from the differently designed studies were inconsistent [4], one consensus on this topic reached is that we can prevent, at least in part, PDPH with currently available methods. Small size pencil point spinal needle [14, 15], parallel bevel orientation [8], liquid use for the loss of resistance (LOR) in epidural puncture [16], and

INTECH
open science | open minds

© 2015 The Author(s). Licensee InTech. This chapter is distributed under the terms of the Creative Commons Attribution License (http://creativecommons.org/licenses/by/3.0), which permits unrestricted use, distribution, and reproduction in any medium, provided the original work is properly cited.

prophylactic epidural blood patch [17, 18] are preventive considerations in reducing PDPH. Therapeutically, intrathecal saline injection [19, 20], repeatable epidural blood patch [21], and compensatory intrathecal catheterization for drug or fluid administration [22] are means treating the on-going PDPH. Although the effectiveness of these methods is changing in different population at different ages under different clinical procedures, they are still promising for our patients.

Beside abovementioned procedure-related techniques, emerging pharmacological data support the use of analgesics. The most recent systematic review and meta-analysis [23] revealed that morphine, cosyntropin, and aminophylline are effective for reducing the incidence of PDPH with any severity, but dexamethasone on the contrary increases the risk of PDPH. For fentanyl, caffeine, and indomethacin, no conclusive evidence reached in the effectiveness and safety for preventing and treating PDPH due to the design quality and low power of the available studies. In consideration of the contribution of high body mass index (BMI) [24] and non-smoking [25] to PDPH, we thus cannot only attribute PDPH to CSF leakage. Caregivers need take careful consideration of the methods listed in this chapter to prevent and improve the clinical outcomes of this iatrogenic morbid because of its multifactorial originality.

2. History and epidemiology

First epidural blockade was reported by an American physician Dr. James Leonard Corning in 1885 [26]. The actual history of spinal anesthesia can be traced back to 1888 by German physician Dr. Heinrich Irenaeus Quincke and 1889 by Britain physician Dr. Walter Essex Wynter aspirated CSF from patients with meningitis for lowering intracranial pressure [27-29]. In 1898, Dr. Karl August Bier from Germany performed first elective spinal anesthesia for surgery [30, 31]; at the same time, Dr. Bier and his assistant they themselves experienced spinal anesthesia, and reported plus another four patients (6/9) with PDPH symptoms [32]. Since that time, analgesics, hydration, and bed rest became the basic constitutes in treating PDPH [33]; however there were still some 40% cases showed no response to these therapeutics. From the early 1970s, anesthesiologists began to use epidural blood patch (EBP) to treat severe PDPH. Until 1990, EBP was first recommended by official guideline [34].

Over the past one century, the incidence of PDPH was sharply decreased from ~70% to ~1% [35], whereas the recently reported occurrence of PDPH is still seeing a big difference in various clinical settings from different regions when diverse techniques were used in patients with different ages. A Nordic survey found the incidence of ADP in Obstetric setting is 1% [36], and 73% of the ADP patients developed PDPH [37]. The incidence of PDPH in Obstetric in Middle East is 2-4.6% [14, 38], 22.7% in Western Africa [39], 16.9% in Southeast Asia [40], 16.6% in North Europe [41], and 6% in North America [42, 43]. In non-Obstetric patients, about 18% patients developed PDPH after spinal anesthesia [44], however a lower incidence (4%) was then reported in the next year by the same group [45]. In the earlier time, another group from Denmark reported the occurrence of PDPH was 7.3% in patients underwent different types of surgeries below the diaphragm after spinal anesthesia [46]. In orthopedic patients, about 1.6% experienced PDPH after continuous spinal anesthesia (CSA) or combined spinal epidural anesthesia (CSE) in South America [47]. In patients who underwent placement of an intrathecal drug delivery system (IDDS), 23% developed PDPH [48]. About 11-30.9% children with malignant disease attended for diagnostic or therapeutic lumbar puncture experienced PDPH [49, 50].

3. Risk factors

Clinical and epidemiological studies support a connection between PDPH and certain demographic factors. For adult, the frequency of PDPH was less in older age patients (51-75 years) than younger age comparisons (30-50 years) [51]. Children younger than 13 years rarely get PDPH [49, 52], but that does occur with increasing frequency in adolescents and are similar to those seen in adults [53]. To child younger than 13 years and adult older than 50 years, they have less PDPH incidence than their peers that largely may be related to the reduced CSF pressure [54, 55]. While there are some inconsistencies upon gender as an independent risk factor for the development of PDPH, a recent meta-analysis confirmed the declaration that the odds of developing a PDPH were significantly lower for male than nonpregnant female subjects with an odds ratio (OR), 0.55 and 95% confidence interval (95% CI), 0.44-0.67 [56]. Lower weight is found to be strongly associated with the higher incidence of PDPH [24] and cumulating evidence showed an inverse relationship between BMI and PDPH [57, 58] suggesting that heavier patients in general have higher intra-abdominal pressure, which in turn raises intra-epidural pressure and prevents cerebrospinal fluid from leaking when ADP occurs. New survey revealed that taller height, reduced pre-procedure intravenous hydration and lower systolic blood pressure (SBP) are novel risk factors that contribute to the pathogenesis of PDPH [59]. Although the incidence of PDPH from different countries, an indicator of racial difference, seems to be different [14, 38-43], the race itself looks unlike an independent risk factor for the PDPH that was observed in the same study [60]. Interesting findings showed that smokers had a considerably reduced rate of PDPH in comparison with non-smokers suggesting an inhibitory effect of tobacco smoking on PDPH that may be associated with the stimulation role of nicotine in dopamine neurotransmission [25].

In a more recent study, severe headache after lumbar puncture and sitting position were confirmed as predicting factors of the occurrence of PDPH, and in further sitting sampling position, history of depression, multiple effort of lumbar puncture, and high perceived stress during the procedure were found to be significantly associated with a longer duration of PDPH [61]. In the same study, migraineurs showed no change at the risk of developing PDPH compared to the non-headache subjects, and epidural puncture does not trigger migraine attacks [61]. However, there was report showing that patients had a history of chronic or recurrent headache has more chance in nearly 60% to develop PDPH than those without such a history [62]. For the multiple effort of lumbar puncture that indicates the inexperience in such clinical procedures increases the possibility of PDPH [6], but in contrast, other studies found no different between experienced and inexperienced practitioners, nor does between multiple and single dural puncture [63].

Although the leakage of CSF is regarded as the major cause of PDPH, the volume of CSF removed and its role in causing PDPH is unclear. Davignon and Dennehy reported that removal of 15-20 ml of CSF reliably caused headaches [64], but Kuntz *et al.* did not find such a causal relationship [65]. So it is hard to draw a conclusion from the available data that volume change in CSF causes PDPH. In clinical practice, the volume usually removed during diagnostic lumbar punctures or spinal anesthesia is less than 5ml that means it is not likely to be a significant factor for the PDPH. However, we cannot exclude the possibility that chronic leakage of CSF over more than 15 ml after ADP or spinal anesthesia is causative for the PDPH (see detailed pathophysiology of CSF leakage below).

Prophylactic treatment with 8 mg of dexamethasone not only increases the severity and incidence of PDPH, but is also ineffective in decreasing the prevalence of intra-operative nausea and vomiting during cesarean section indicating that dexamethasone treatment is a significant risk factor for the development of PDPH [66]. Nonetheless, hydrocortisone *i.v.* (100 mg in 2 ml 8 hourly for 48 h) was found effective in reducing PDPH following spinal anesthesia [67] suggesting that glucocorticoid with different potency and half life of action may possess different function in PDPH prevention and therapy.

Pregnancy is considered as a particular factor that relates to PDPH due to the young age, female, sometimes sitting position, pregnancy-associated depression and anxiety, and the special popularity of regional anesthesia in this population [68-70], but a meta-analysis showed that pregnancy itself does not increase the risk of PDPH [71]. For some cases of PDPH, we cannot exclude some other co-founding factors including fatigue, sleep deprivation, and night work that lead to higher incidence of ADP in clinical personnel when performing epidural analgesia. Table 1 summarizes the risk factors of PDPH.

Convincing risk factors
Young age
Female
Lower BMI
Taller height
Reduced pre-procedure intravenous hydration
Lower SBP
Non-smoking
Sitting position
History of depression
History of chronic or recurrent headache
High stress during the procedure

Multiple lumbar puncture
Dexamethasone therapy
Non-convincing risk factors
Experience level of personnel
Volume of CSF removed
Pregnancy itself
Fatigue, sleep deprivation, or night work
BMI: body mass index; SBP: systolic blood pressure; CSF: cerebrospinal fluid

Table 1. Risk factors of PDPH.

4. Anatomy of meninges

There three membranes, known as that cover the spinal cord lying within the vertebral canal. The outermost layer is the dura mater, a non-adherent, dense, and tough fibrous sheath closely applied to the inner layer of bone surrounding the spinal canal. Between the dura and the walls of the spinal canal is a potential imaginary space, the epidural space or cavum epidurale, which normally occupied by a small amount of by loose areolar tissue, fat, and the anterior and posterior plexuses of the vertebral veins. Dura mater is attached above to the margin of the foramen magnum, to the axis, and to the third cervical vertebra, and below to the level of the second sacral vertebra. In normal, a potential space known as the subdural space exists between dura mater and arachnoid mater, a thin and delicate membrane lies closely beneath the dura mater. Beneath the arachnoid mater is the pia mater that intimately applied to the spinal cord. Both the arachnoid and pia mater are continuous with the arachnoid and pia surrounding the brain. There is a space between the arachnoid mater and pia mater: the subarachnoid space, which normally is filled with CSF.

The conventional conception for the structure of spinal dura mater is that it is of elastic and collagen fibers running in the longitudinal direction. Based on this, clinical studies found the PDPH incidence is less in patients who underwent spinal anesthesia during which the dura mater was cut with a perpendicular orientation to the direction of the spinal dura fibers than those with parallel bevel orientation [8, 72]. But a more extensive electron microscopic study challenged this traditional conception of the of the anatomy of the spinal dura mater, they found that the dura mater is consisted of collages fibers that are arranged in several layers parallel to the surface, and each layer does not arranged in any specific orientation [73]. Moreover, the thickness of the posterior dura mater demonstrates big difference within and between individuals suggesting that perforation at thicker dura is less likely to result in CSF leakage than the thin dura because the thicker the dura mater, the easier the retraction after perforation, and this inter- or intra-individual variation in dural mater thickness may be an unpredictable variable affecting the management of dural puncture [74, 75].

5. Physiology of CSF

CSF secretion in adults varies between 400 to 600 ml per day, i.e. 0.28-0.42 ml/min, and about 60%-75% of CSF is produced by the choroid plexuses of the lateral ventricles and the *tela choroidea* of the third and fourth ventricles. The total volume of CSF in the adult is ~150 ml, of which 125ml distributes in cranial and spinal subarachnoid spaces and 25 ml in the ventricles. Therefore, CSF is renewed four to five times every 24 hours in young adults. CSF circulation is a dynamic phenomenon that pulses in response to the systolic pulse wave in choroidal arteries. Ageing-related cerebral atrophy and reduction in CSF turnover enlarge the CSF compartment markedly, and aging-associated slowing down of the CSF renewal all may explain the reason why aged population had a lower incidence of PDPH [51].

CSF pressure, one part of the intracranial pressure, is the result of a dynamic equilibrium between CSF secretion, absorption and resistance to flow. Physiological values of CSF pressure vary according to individuals and study methods between 13 and 20 cmH_2O in adults and 4 and 6 cmH_2O in infants [76]. In the lumbar region in the supine position, CSF pressure ranges between 5 and 15 cmH_2O, and this pressure can increase to over 40 cmH_2O when on the vertical position [77]. In the prone position, CSF pressure changes from 8 to 21 cmH_2O, but in lateral decubitus position it reduces to 7-17 cmH_2O [78]. Besides, the normal range for lumbar CSF pressure in children is 10 to 28 cmH_2O when measured in a flexed lateral decubitus position [79]. CSF pressure is determined by parenchymal and venous pressures. Increased SBP exerts negative feedback on choroidal secretion by decreasing the pressure gradient across the blood-CSF barrier and by reducing cerebral perfusion pressure.

6. Pathophysiology of CSF leakage and pathological mechanisms

CSF leak is defined as the escape of CSF from any tear or hole in the meninges. The direct consequence of CSF leak is the drop of CSF volume and then the pressure. It is not that clear for the causal relation between CSF leak and PDPH pathogenesis, however the explanatory theory on the role of CSF leak in PDPH onset is still widely accepted. Leakage of the CSF is the most common cause of spontaneous intracranial hypotension [77]. Theoretically, lumbar puncture-induced CSF leak is consisted of two phases: acute and chronic phases. The acute phase is largely resulted from the abrupt outflow of CSF from the broken within minutes to several hours, during which the CSF pressure dives down to a lower level (~3-4 cmH_2O) that eventually leads to shifts of intracranial contents and gravitational traction on pain sensitive structures, which worsens when the patient is upright and is relieved on lying down [80]. The chronic phase refers to a stage of which started from the formation of the new CSF pressure balance (several hours to one day after dural puncture) to the complete resolution from the puncture (1-6 weeks). This phasic alteration in CSF leakage can explain, at least in part, why the onset of PDPH in some patients occur 1 to 7 days after ADP, but some appeared 12 days post puncture [81]. In addition, the loss of CSF may activate adenosine receptors that subsequently dilate intracranial arteries and veins and then clinical manifestations of PDPH [82]. Based on the findings that pregnancy and the immediate postpartum period are associated with the lowest CSF density [83] and the particular high incidence of PDPH in Obstetric setting [68-70], the CSF density change during the chronic leakage of CSF was also considered as a potential reason of the PDPH.

For some patients they showed "crushing" postural headache without abnormal diagnostic lumbar puncture and computed tomography (CT) angiogram suggesting that the conventional understanding on the pathogenesis of PDPH based on the over-rigorous pooled analyses needs to be reconsidered [80]. In fact, the occurrence of PDPH has its own pathological bases. For the cranial innervations, studies showed that the dura mater is heavily innervated and most likely cause intense pain [84], and abnormal distention of intracranial nerve and extracerebral blood vessels all can consequently activate the trigeminal nervous system that were thought to be the origins of headache [85]. Functional immunohistochemistry found that neuropeptides and nitric oxide synthase (NOS) are expressed in the nerve fibers of the supratentorial dura mater and the structural alterations of nitroxidergic axons innervating blood vessels of the dura mater support the idea that nitric oxide (NO) is involved in the induction of headache [86]. Therefore further studies are needed on the relationship among dura mater innervations, expression of neuropeptides and NOS, and PDPH.

Artemin, a member of the glial cell line-derived neurotrophic factor family, is a vasculature-derived growth factor shown to regulate migration of sympathetic neuroblasts and targeting of sympathetic innervation [87]. Recent evidence supports the role of artemin in cold pain [88] and inflammatory pain [89]. Moreover, the expression of artemin was detected in the smooth muscle of dural vasculature, and its receptor GFRα3 was found present in nerve fibers that closely associated with tyrosine hydroxylase (TH) or calcitonin gene-related peptide (CGRP) [90] suggesting that artemin is involved in dural afferent activity through modulating both primary afferent and sympathetic systems. In further, catecholaminergic nerve fibers innervate human cranial dura mater in density, and these nerve fibers are more abundant in the perivascular dural zone than in the intervascular zone at the basal region [91]. In collection, given TH functions as the precursor of catecholamine (norepinephrine and epinephrine) [92], a potential interaction exists among artemin, sympathetic regulation, and catecholaminergic transmission in nerves located in cranial dura mater, and this interaction may underlie the occurrence of PDPH.

Dural innervations are of importance as, like its cranial counterpart, the spinal dura mater and its nerve root sleeves may be a source of primary pain. Different types of nervous branches are given off to the spinal dura mater within the vertebral canal. The nerves in the spinal dura mater have already been described as nociceptive sensory fibers [93-96], and they also belong to sympathetic vasomotor [97, 98]. We hereby proposed that a tonic inhibition of the spinal and cranial dural nerves exists under normal CSF pressure, but this inhibition would be reduced or reversely activated by chronic leakage of CSF after lumbar puncture. However, such reduction in tonic inhibition or/and reverse activation of the dural nerves does not determine the occurrence of PDPH, which depends on the alteration extent of the tone that can evoke nociceptive activation, i.e. it should at least reach the activation threshold. Based on this hypothesis, it can partially explain why not all patients after ADP will develop PDPH [37]. Figure 1 depicts the potential pathological mechanisms of PDPH.

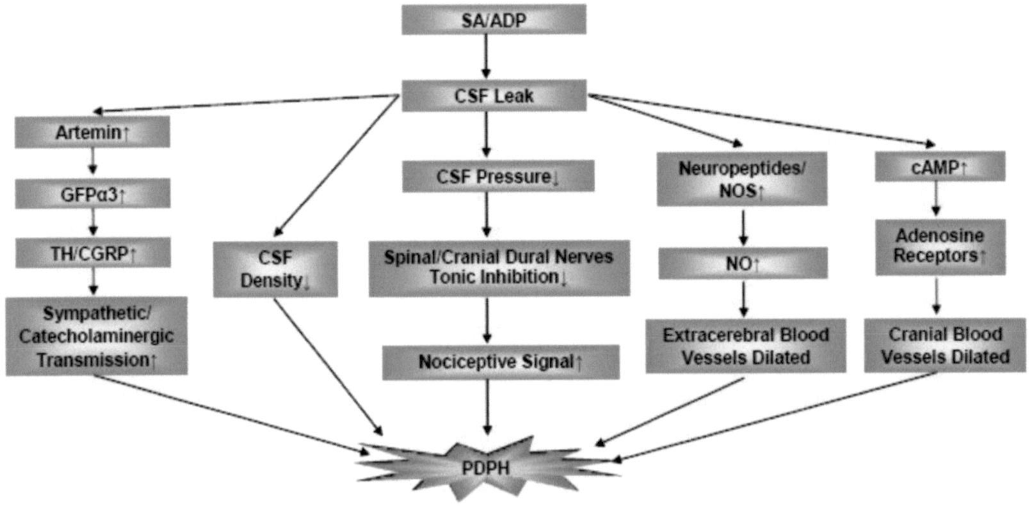

SA: spinal anesthesia; ADP: accidental dural puncture; CSF: cerebrospinal fluid; GFPα3: glial-cell-line-derived neurotrophic factor family receptor alpha-3; TH: tyrosine hydroxylase; CGRP: calcitonin gene related peptide; NOS: nitric oxide synthase; NO: nitric oxide; cAMP: cyclic adenosine monophosphate; PDPH: post-dural puncture headache.

Figure 1. Pathological mechanisms of the pathogenesis of PDPH.

7. Needle gauge and tip configuration

A huge body of evidence and systematic review support the view that the diameters of the needles that pierce the spinal dura mater and the tip design, cutting-edge or pencil-point, are two key facets that determine the eventual incidence of PDPH [99]. Of the same type needles, 29G (19%) compared with 25G Quincke needle (17%) led to no reduction of PDPH [44]. Similarly, both 25G and 26G Quincke needle had same incidence of PDPH (8-9%), but in comparison, 24G Sprotte non-cutting tip needle results in a significantly lower incidence (1.5%) [100]. Patients receiving spinal anesthesia with a 27G Quincke needle suffered significantly more frequently from PDPH (6.6%) than the 27G pencil-point needle controls (1.7%) [45]. In Obstetric women, 25G Quincke, 27G Quincke and 27G Whitacre spinal needles produce 8.3%, 3.8% and 2.0% of PDPH, respectively [14], and 10% in the 25G Quincke and none in the 24G Gertie Marx spinal needle [101]. For the non-Obstetric patients, the incidences of PDPH for 27G Quincke and 27G Whitacre spinal needles were 2.7% and 0.37%, respectively [102].

However, in 33% patients reported PDPH, no statistically significant differences were found between Spinocan 22G sharp bevel needles or Whitacre 22G pencil point needle [103]. For 26G Eldor spinal needles, it was found to be better (0%) than 25G Quincke spinal needle (8.3%) for Cesarean sections to decrease the incidence of PDPH [104]. In pediatric patients, 5% in the 26G Atraucan and 4% in the 27G Whitacre spinal needle developed PDPH after spinal anesthesia for subumbilical surgery [105], and pencil point needle causes less PDPH compared to cutting point needle: 0.4% versus 4.5%, respectively [15]. Vallejo and colleagues compared the incidence of PDPH in five spinal needles and found that the PDPH were 5%, 8.7%, 4%, 2.8%, and 3.1% for 26G Atraucan, 25G Quincke, 24G Gertie Marx, 24G Sprotte, and 25G Whitacre needles, respectively in Obstetric patients [106]. Table 2 summarizes the incidence of PDPH after different spinal needles.

Needle	Incidence of PDPH	Tip Configuration	Showcase
Atraucan	5% (26G)	Combination Quincke-pencil point bevel	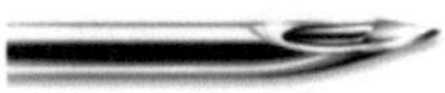
Eldor	0% (26G)	Double hole pencil point	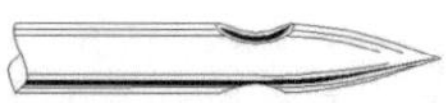
Gertie Marx	0%-4% (24G)	Single port pencil point	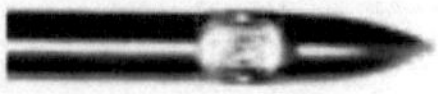
Quincke	2.7%-19% (29G-25G)	Cutting edge	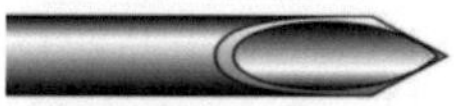
Spinocan	39% (22G)	Cutting edge	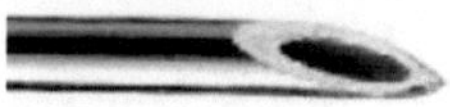
Sprotte	1.5%-2.8% (24G)	Single port pencil point	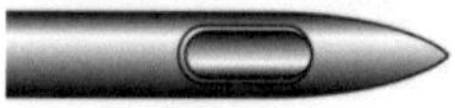
Whitacre	0.37%-39% (22G-27G)	Single port pencil point	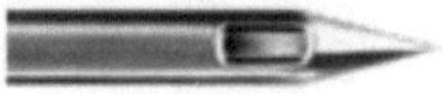

Table 2. Incidence of PDPH after different spinal needles.

8. Therapeutic strategy

The occurrence of PDPH resulted from ADP or spinal anesthesia is completely unavoidable, although we can reduce its incidence via various preventive means. Therefore, health care-givers need familiar with all potential therapeutic strategies, and treat them following different treatment protocols that are divided into four steps: conservative treatment (1st step), aggressive medical treatment (2nd step), conventional invasive management (3rd step), and aggressive invasive management (4th step) [4]. Table 3 summarizes the 4-step therapeutic maneuvers for PDPH.

8.1. First step: Conservative treatment

Initially, conservative methods are recommended for the treatment of PDPH largely because of its self-limiting property. The use of abdominal binder for PDPH patients is mainly based on its pressure transmission from the increased pressure of abdominal cavity to CSF pressure [106]. Although no powerful evidence supports this hypothesis, and the CSF pressure can change along with the intra-abdominal pressure [107], it is uncertain the consequently increased CSF pressure at early period of lumbar puncture would push more CSF exit from the broken. Conventionally, it has been suggested that PDPH would be less common if patients routinely have a period of bed rest after dural puncture because about 1-70% patients after the puncture experienced postural headache. In addition, giving supplementary fluids additional to the normal dietary intake can restore the loss of CSF. Although the degree of CSF leak does not correlate with the severity of the symptoms in a PDPH [40], it is assumed that improvements in the ratio of CSF production to CSF leak will improve the clinical picture. Dehydration can result in a decrease in CSF production [108]. However, if a patient is appropriately hydrated, and the rate of CSF production is normal, there is no evidence that overhydration will increase the rate of CSF production any further. For both bed rest and hydration, the most recent systematic review did not find convincing evidence supporting the routine bed rest after dural puncture is beneficial for the prevention of PDPH onset, and also it is still unclear whether vigorous intravenous fluid supplementation has any prophylactic or therapeutic benefit in alleviating PDPH [109].

Due to the ethical consideration, pre-operative communication will let the patients know that PDPH is a common iatrogenic complication, and the subsequent problems include the inability to perform daily activities, an extended length of stay (LOS) at hospital, and a higher visiting rate to the emergency room after discharge. All these will raise patients' anxiety to their possibly miserable experiences after regional anesthesia, and the psychological stress will be exacerbated if PDPH eventually occurred. Therefore, psychological support will help PDPH patients more precisely understand: 1) PDPH is a self-terminating process; 2) many medical procedures can alleviate and treat PDPH; 3) active cooperation with clinicians will promote resolution; 4) keep normal diet; and 5) think solutions with faith but not with fear. So try to comfort or reassure PDPH patients psychologically will enhance their confidence to the treatments, and improve the outcomes [110].

Symptomatic analgesia was also used as the conservative management of PDPH. Oral acetaminophen (1000 mg) along with fluid administration was suggested [4, 111], whereas the actual effect is unknown. Prophylactic administration of acetaminophen (500 mg)-caffeine combination did not prevent PDPH [112]. Non-steroidal anti-inflammatory drugs (NSAIDs), the most popular over-the-counter drugs for analgesia also can be used for PDPH treatment [32]. Antiemetics combined with other analgesics were suggested for headache or migraine, but whether such medication performs effective function in PDPH is not elucidated. Dexamethasone, a traditional anti-inflammatory glucocorticoid, is found possessing antiemetic effect for postoperative patients [113], and also was used in migraine treatment [114], but for PDPH no convincing evidence was found [23]. Erol reported that gabapentin, a gamma-aminobutryic acid (GABA) analog, significantly reduced pain, nausea and vomiting compared to ergotamine/caffeine combinations in patients with PDPH [115] suggesting that gabapentin exerts function in PDPH patients through both analgesic and antiemetic effect.

8.2. Second step: Aggressive medical treatment

Aggressive medical treatments that include subarachnoid catheter left *in situ*, occipital nerve block, intravenous methylxanthines, and symptomatic therapies are recommended once the conservative management was not that effective in treating PDPH. Leaving a subarachnoid catheter *in situ* after spinal anesthesia or ADP has at least three benefits: 1) mechanical blockade of the CSF leak: intrathecal (*i.t.*) catheter left *in situ* for 24 h closes the hole in the arachnoid dura preventing the leakage of CSF; 2) indirect inflammation: catheter-evoked inflammatory responses helping closing the broken; 3) therapeutic administration: convenient drug or fluid infusion or injection through the emplaced catheter for postoperative analgesia or artificial CSF supplementation. This is particularly effective in reducing the incidence of PDPH (~14%) after ADP with large gauge epidural needles than those without catheter placement (70-85%) [22]. Of this technique, Kuczkowski and Benumof composed a 5-step protocol for PDPH prevention and treatment following ADP [22], and their subsequent investigation on it proved more effective than ever in conquering the incidence of PDPH to 6.6% [116]. Similarly, subsequent catheter placement into the epidural space after ADP in cesarean delivery and leaving the catheter for postoperative analgesia for 36-72 h reduced the incidence of PDPH significantly (7.1% compared to 58% in non-catheterized patients) [117]. However, attention needs to be paid on this procedure due to the potential risk of catheter-associated infection [118] and cauda equina syndrome [119, 120]. In addition, placement of the catheter needs informed consent and should be reconsidered for it causes discomfort especially when prolonged retention is intended [32].

Since the first case has been reported on the successful treatment of PDPH with occipital nerve block (ONB) [121], several other PDPH patients from different institutes were presented after treatment with ONB [122, 123]. The sensory fibers of the greater occipital nerve (GON) originate from the C2 and C3 segments of the spinal cord, and its cutaneous sensory distribution extends over the posterior part of the head, spreading anteriorly to the vertex towards the area supplied by the ophthalmic division of the trigeminal nerve [124]. The lesser occipital nerve (LON) arises from the lateral branch of the ventral ramus of the second cervical nerve. Near the cranium it perforates the deep fascia, and is continued upward along the side of the head behind the auricula, supplying the skin and communicating with the GON [125]. In migraine patients, a unilateral greater ONB can initiate an inhibitory process that shuts down several symptom generators which alleviates allodynia first then headache [126]). Moreover, physical compression of LON causes migraine [127]. In PDPH patients, nerve stimulator-guided bilateral blockade of the GON and LON were found effective in controlling PDPH symptoms [128].

Methylxanthines, a group of derivatives of xanthine, act on adenosine receptors nonselectively as antagonists that in turn lead to vasoconstriction, which exactly negate the compensatory cerebral vasodilation that occurs in response to loss of CSF volume, a theoretical cause that has been implicated in the pathogenesis of PDPH [82]. In addition, methylxanthines can activate sodium-potassium pumps [129] that are involved in the regulation of CSF production [130], which may finally lead to headache relief. There are three major methylxanthines include aminophylline, caffeine, and theophylline that are widely used in patients who suffered PDPH. In a randomized trial, 1 mg/kg aminophylline *i.v.* given immediately after umbilical cord clamping significantly reduced the incidence of PDPH from 23.3% (no aminophylline injection) to 5% in Cesarean patients underwent spinal anesthesia, and the severe headache after 48 hours was also markedly lower (3%) than the control (11%) [131]. Although caffeine was considered as a potential drug in relieving PDPH, but currently available evidence does not endorse its therapeutic value for PDPH because no valid pharmacological rationale for this drug exists, which majorly due to the clinical trials are few in number, small in sample size, weak or flawed in methodology, and non-effectiveness, contradictory, and even confliction in results [132]. Furthermore, prophylactic oral multidose caffeine-paracetamol also cannot prevent PDPH [112] suggesting that the use of caffeine in PDPH treatment needs to be evaluated carefully and herein I do not recommend it. However, oral theophylline was found effective in treating PDPH painful symptom [133], and studies compared the analgesic efficacy of theophylline infused *i.v.* to placebo found the therapy significantly decreased the painfulness of PDPH and it was suggested as an easy, rapid, minimally invasive, an effective treatment for PDPH [134]. If methylxanthines are ready to use in managing PDPH, the side effects for these types of drugs should be bear in mind like the central nervous system (CNS) stimulation, seizures, gastric irritation, and cardiac dysrhythmia when patients had psychiatric history, gastroenterological and cardiovascular problems [135, 136].

Beside abovementioned analgesics in the conservative treatment, more potent pharmacological analgesics are recommended in this aggressive medical treatment phase. Cosyntropin, an adrenocorticotropic hormone (ACTH) analog with less antigenic than the naturally occurring hormone, was used successfully to treat PDPH. Cosyntropin functions through: 1) stimulating the adrenal cortex to secrete glucocorticoids, mineralocorticoids, and androgens; 2) activating adenyl cyclase, which increases intracellular cAMP that can promote CSF production; and 3) increasing β-endorphins in the CNS which subsequently leads to an increase in the pain threshold. The doses of cosyntropin changed from 0.25 mg to 1.0 mg *i.v.* or intramuscularly (*i.m.*), and the headache was controlled by 80%-100%, and incidence of PDPH and the need of EBP were reduced, and the time from ADP to occurrence of PDPH was prolonged [137-141]. The side effects of ACTH administration include infection, mood elevation, and intracranial hemorrhage [142].

Although epinephrine was initially regarded as a vasoconstrictor in neuraxial analgesia, its analgesic effect in the spinal cord is rarely investigated in human being. Accumulating data support the analgesic role of spinal noradrenergic transmission in various pain conditions [143]. Controversial results were reported for the possible effect of epinephrine added into local anesthetics and opioids on the incidence of PDPH. Using continuous intrathecal patient-controlled analgesia (PCA) consisting fentanyl, bupivacaine and epinephrine completely prevented the occurrence of PDPH in Cesarean patients after ADP [144], but other studies did not find correlation between occurrence of PDPH and type of local anesthetics or additives including epinephrine and opioids [145]. Opioids are still the mainstay of pain management, and intrethecal morphine was also found to be effective in controlling PDPH [23]. While dexamethasone was found no beneficial to PDPH patients, and even is a risk factor for the development of PDPH [66], hydrocortisone *i.v.* (100 mg in 2 ml 8 hourly for 48 h) on the contrary was found effective in reducing PDPH following spinal anesthesia [67].

Gabapentin and pregabalin are two GABA analogs that have been reported to be useful in the management of epilepsy and neuropathic pain. For PDPH patients, increasing number of cases were reported after successful treatment with gabapentin or pregabalin [146-150]. Sumatriptan, a serotonin type 1-D receptor agonist, was reported effective in the treatment of PDPH, with complete resolution of symptoms [151], but Connelly *et al.* did not find significant relief in headache [152]. Methergine is used widely in the management of refractory headache and migraine [153, 154], and also it was found to be an effective drug in alleviate PDPH [155], although the actual efficacy of its single use in this context is not sure [156]. The antidepressant mirtazapine has a net positive effect on noradrenergic neurotransmission, and was reported effective in relieving PDPH [157]. In sum, although these satellite cases treated with above-mentioned medications showed effective in managing PDPH, their clinical application needs to be evaluated substantially before prescribed for PDPH.

8.3. Third step: Conventional invasive management

When medical therapies in the step 2 fail for relief of PDPH and when the symptoms of PDPH is debilitating or severe, management should move on to procedural invasive therapies. The most widely used conventional invasive procedure is blood patch, and some alternative materials like hydroxyethyl starch and saline will be discussed if EBP is contraindicated. EBP is a treatment of choice for PDPH with high success rate and low incidence of complications [158].

8.3.1. Theoretical basis of EBP

As early 1960s, Gormley found that the incidence of PDPH in patients with "bloody taps" were comparably lower than those with only saline taps [159], and then the thought of EBP began to develop. Until 1970, the use of EBP became popular, and in 1990, first official guideline recommended EBP for PDPH treatment [34]. Theoretically, EBP is assumed to work by increasing CSF pressure and stimulating fibrin and platelet formation, and secondly, the introduced blood into the epidural space will clot and exerts tamponade effect by occluding the perforation that subsequently will prevent further leakage of CSF.

8.3.2. EBP technique

EBP has the same technique as the epidural anesthesia. Modern epidural kits are disposable and are sterilized package that includes all equipments and drugs without preservative. The epidural needle (usually Tuohy needle) is typically 16-18G, 8cm long with surface markings at 1cm intervals, and has a blunt bevel with a 15-30 degree curve at the tip (the Huber tip). Wings attached at the junction of the needle shaft with the hub, which allow better control of the needle as it is advanced. In general, a traditional glass syringe with an easily slide plunger is used to identify the epidural space. The newer commercially available disposable epidural packs contain a plastic syringe with a plunger that has very low resistance. For EBP, there is no need to use epidural catheter for continuous medication.

To identify the epidural space, several methods can be used like loss of resistance (LOR) and hanging drop technique. Of the hanging drop technique, it has been abandoned by modern anesthesia. Given the reports on the better anesthesia quality and the possible complications of large amounts of air injected into the epidural space and surrounding structures [160], therefore the LOR to saline is preferred in EBP. Even though the EBP technique can be performed with the patient either in the sitting or lateral decubitus position, the latter is the preference due to the sitting position causes more incidence of PDPH [78]. On this position, the patient should be encouraged to adopt a curled up position, as this tends to open the spaces between the spinous processes and facilitates the identification of the intervertebral spaces. After the back has been prepared with sterile solution and draped in sterile fashion, the desired level is selected.

There are two approaches for the epidural needle insertion: midline or paramedian approach. The midline approach needs insert the epidural needle through the supraspinous ligament, and then advance the needle into the interspinous ligament, until distinct sensation of increased resistance is felt as the needle passes into the ligamentum flavum. For the paramedian approach, the inserting point of the epidural needle is 1-2 cm lateral to the spinous processes, and then insert and advance the needle perpendicularly to the skin until the lamina or pedicle is encountered, and then redirect it approximately 30° cephalad and 15° medially in an attempt to "walk the needle" off the lamina, at which point the needle should be in close proximity to the ligamentum flavum. After felt the resistance from the ligamentum flavum, the needle is then advanced further using LOR to saline.

8.3.3. Contraindications of EBP

Although the performance of EBP has the same contraindications that normally apply to epidural anesthesia, it also has some particular concerns. General absolute contraindications include: 1) patient refusal; 2) coagulopathy; 3) therapeutic anticoagulation; 4) skin infection at injection site; 5) localized sepsis in lumbar area; 6) raised intracranial pressure; 7) hypovolemia; 8) unexplained neurological symptoms; 9) active neurological disease; and 10) generalized sepsis. General relative contraindications include: 1) uncooperation; 2) pre-existing neurological disorders; 3) fixed cardiac output states; 4) anatomical abnormalities of vertebral column; and 5) prophylactic low dose heparin. Particular contraindications of EBP: 1) raised white cell count and pyrexia; 2) human immunodeficiency virus (HIV)-positive patients with other active bacterial or viral illnesses; 3) oncology (EBP in these patients may raises the potential for seeding the neuraxis with neoplastic cells).

Special attention should be paid when anticoagulants are used: 1) full anticoagulation with warfarin or standard heparin is absolute contraindication to EBP; 2) partial anticoagulation with low molecular weight heparin (LMWH) or low dose warfarin (International Normalized Ratio, INR < 1.5) is relative contraindication; 3) for low dose standard heparin (Minihep), wait for 4 h after a dose before performing EBP, and it should not be given until 1 h following blood patch; 4) allow a 12 h interval between LMWH administration and EBP; 5) NSAIDs including aspirin do not increase the risk of epidural hematoma; 6) avoid EBP for 24 h when fibrinolytic and thrombolytic drugs are used, and check clotting prior to needle insertion; 7) EBP needs avoid when patients were diagnosed thrombocytopenia especially when the platelet count is less than 100 000/mm^3.

8.3.4. EBP procedures

Once the EBP was determined to be applied, following procedures should be scheduled.

1. Give a full explanation of the cause of the headache, the reasons for performing an EBP, the technique, potential hazards and anticipated success rate;
2. Obtain informed consent;
3. Move patient to fully equipped work area;
4. Undertake under the direct supervision of a consultant or senior physician in the operating room with an assistant;
5. Lie flat for an hour before the EBP procedure (that may improve its efficacy by reducing the volume of CSF in the extradural space);
6. Secure *i.v.* access for fluid titration;
7. Two operators are required, both scrubbed, gowned and masked;
8. Position patient in lateral position;
9. Operator 1: sterilize skin over back, drape and perform epidural puncture at the same level as previous puncture or one level below;
10. Operator 2: simultaneously sterilize skin over antecubital fossa, drape and perform venepuncture withdrawing 20 ml of blood;
11. Blood is handed to operator 1 who injects blood via epidural needle until either the patient complains of a tightness in the buttocks or lower back, or until 20 ml is injected;
12. If back or leg pain (due to arachnoid irritation) occurs, stop injecting and wait a few seconds. If pain persists, abandon procedure. If a catheter has been used, remove it immediately after injection is complete;
13. Inject remaining blood into blood culture bottles for culture and sensitivity;
14. Nurse patient supine for 1-2 h, then mobilize cautiously;
15. Keep the patient under close review. If symptoms have not completely resolved, refer to consultant, and a repeat blood patch may be required;
16. Record procedures in medical book;
17. Refer the patient visit anesthetic clinic 2-4 weeks.

8.3.5. Distribution of the blood patch

No consensus reached as to the precise volume of blood required for EBP, but it is now recognized that the 2-3 ml of blood originally described by Gormley [159] is inadequate, and that 20-30 ml of blood is more likely to ensure success. However there was successful case treated with larger volumes of blood up to 60 ml in patients with spontaneous intracranial hypotension [161].

Several studies reported the distribution of the blood patch in the epidural space using radiolabelled red blood cells [162] or magnetic resonance imaging (MRI) scanning [163]. After injection, the blood spread caudally and cephalad regardless of the direction of the bevel of the needle, and also the blood can reach to the anterior epidural space circumferentially, and also can pass into the paravertebral space. When injecting 14 ml of blood, the highest level it can reach is six spinal segments, and caudally three segments. It is presumed that the compression of the thecal space that elevates the subarachnoid pressure for the first 3 h contributes to the rapid resolution of the headache. About 7-13 h after the EBP, there will be a thick layer of mature clot over the dorsal part of the thecal sac formed due to the procoagulant effect of CSF [164, 165].

8.3.6. PDPH outcomes of EBP

The reported success rate of the EBP technique is 70-98% if carried out more than 24 h after the dural puncture [36, 166]. Kokki et al. reported that EBP performed later than 48h following lumbar puncture or ADP is effective in parturients with postdural puncture symptoms [167]. If the first EBP failed to relieve the headache, repeated EBP can be used with the same success rate each. In a randomized controlled trial (RCT) in which a "sham" procedure was assigned as the comparison to the EBP, 11 out of 12 patients (92%) reported successful relief for the first EBP application, and the twelfth being relieved by a second procedure, whereas the sham-treated patients reported no benefit from the procedure (168). In another RCT, the respective successful rates of EBP and conservative treatments were 42% and 10% at day 1, and 84% and 14% at day 7 in PDPH patients. For those without recovery, the severity of headache was mild in all EDBP patients, but moderate or severe in conservatively treated patients (169). If the headache persists or debilitates after several attempts, other invasive maneuvers should be considered as appeared in the step 4.

8.3.7. Complications of EBP

While EBP is an effective treatment with a low complication rate, it is also an invasive method that can cause permanent neurological sequelae such as early and late back pain, radiculopathy, spinal-subdural hematoma, spinal-epiarachnoid hematoma, intrathecal hematoma, arachnoiditis, and infection. In consideration of headache as a common symptom of PDPH and cerebral venous thrombosis (CVT), therefore it is hard to distinguish them especially after EBP [170-175] suggesting that it should be carefully evaluated before EBP was planned in patients with altered coagulation state (see above *Contraindications of EBP*), and when possible treatments that would affect the coagulation were ready to be given. Besides, rare cases were reported that EBP may cause epidural scarring that eventually results in slow spread of epidural local anesthetics, unilateral block and low efficacy if later epidural block was performed [176].

8.3.8. Prophylactic EBP

There were studies suggesting the use of prophylactic EBP in preventing PDPH, but the data were conflicting. Reported cases including patients underwent post-myelogram [177], and spinal anesthesia and ADP with an epidural needle [178, 179], have confirmed the benefit of prophylactic patching. Nonetheless, other studies found prophylactic EBP cannot decrease the incidence of PDPH or reduce the need for criteria-directed therapeutic epidural patch for parturients after ADP, but it can shorten the duration of PDPH symptoms [18]. One possible explanation for the failure of EBP is that the pressure gradient between the thecal and epidural space may be high enough immediately after blood injection which leads to patch separation from the site of the perforation. Therefore a greater volume of blood may be needed to produce a successful patch [32].

8.3.9. EBP for Jehovah's Witness

Due to Biblical interpretation principles, Jehovah's Witness patients do not authorize even autologous transfusions because blood removed from the body lost the continuity [180]. In the early time, alternative methods like epidural saline or Dextron were suggested [181]. Until 2003, Silva Lde *et al.* reported a closed system, through which two Jehovah's Witness patients with PDPH were treated successfully with autologous EBP [182]. Since then several cases were reported treated with the closed system successfully [183-185]. For this system, in brief, it includes two serum catheters cut in 60 cm segments, one two-way connection, one three-way tap and one 20 ml syringe. The system was assembled to allow one connection to venepuncture needle (20G), one connection to the three-way tap, and the remaining two ways were connected to a 20 ml syringe and to the other serum catheter segment, which would be connected to the epidural needle. After approval by the ethical committee, and informed consent by the patient, the system was filled with saline (6 ml). After epidural puncture and intravenous puncture, the already described system was connected to the epidural needle. Occluding the epidural needle way by moving three-way tap, 20 ml venous blood was aspirated to the syringe and venous catheter way was occluded. Then, epidural needle way was opened and syringe's content was injected in the epidural space. After removal of the epidural needle and system, venous access was maintained for fluid infusion. Patient remained at rest for 2 h and discharged with the recommendation to visit the clinic in case of recurrence.

8.3.10. Alternative maneuvers to EBP

For PDPH patients with absolute contraindications, alternative methods are suggested. In theory, epidural injection of other materials like saline or hydroxyethyl starch (HES) would produce the same mass effect, and restore normal CSF dynamics. Advocates of the epidural saline patch [32] include: 1) a single 30 ml bolus of epidural saline after development of headache; 2) 10-120 ml of saline injected as a bolus via the caudal epidural space; 3) 1.0-1.5 l of epidural Hartmann's solution over 24 h, starting on the first day after dural puncture; 4) 35 ml/h of epidural saline or Hartmann's solution for 24-48 h. However, large volume of saline should be avoided in case intraocular hemorrhages through a precipitous rise in intracranial pressure [186]. Kara et al. reported a successful pediatric case with PDPH treated with epidural saline patch [187]. Epidural HES patch was also found effective in treating PDPH when patients contraindicated to EBP like bacteremia and leukemia [188, 189]. Although there were successful cases managed with other epidural materials, it is still not conclusive for their clinical use due to the lack of high quality evidence.

8.4. Forth step: Aggressive and invasive management

When epidural patch with blood, saline or HES failed to resolve the headache, the diagnosis needs to be reevaluated and more aggressive methods can be considered. These invasive managements only apply to those with persistent, severe and debilitating headache after treatment using above means in the step 3.

Fibrin glue, also known as fibrin sealant, is a biological adhesive made up of fibrinogen and thrombin that are applied to the tissue sites to glue them together or block bleed by creating a fibrin clot [190]. Fibrin glue is used frequently in repairing cranial dural perforations to block CSF leak after intradural procedures [191]. There are successful PDPH cases treated with epidural fibrin glue injected through percutaneous CT guidance or blindly in patients [192, 193] and animal models [194]. Moreover, the effectiveness of fibrin glue in sealing the hole and stopping the leakage of CSF has been studies using *in vitro* model of postdural puncture leakage and got supportive results for its application under this condition [195]. However, conflicting cases reported that such artificial formulation had a risk of the development of aseptic meningitis [196], and in further it has been warned against the application of fibrin glue when they were used in CNS because fibrin glue contains tranexamic acid (t-AMCA) which may cause severe nervous complications [197].

Surgery was considered as the last option for the treatment of PDPH if all abovementioned methods failed to resolve it. Neurosurgical procedure can be performed to identify and suture the hole in dura mater under the operating microscope. In one refractory PDPH patient in whom the headache lasted over two year, surgical repair successfully resolved the headache immediately, and the patient was rapidly mobilized from bed without orders for bed rest or any further precautions [198]. Before performing surgeries, the exact location of the CSF leak should be identified. Several medical diagnostic techniques are currently available to help detect the CSF leakage: dynamic CT myelography for fast-flow CSF leak, delayed CT myelography or magnetic resonance myelography for slow-flow leak.

9. Preventive strategy

Although the effectiveness of the prophylactic EBP is controversial [18, 176, 177], there are studies found advocating role for other strategies in reducing the incidence of PDPH. Deliberate intrathecal saline injection (5 ml) before spinal administration of hyperbaric bupivacaine as a preventive approach is an effective and simple way to minimize PDPH in patients undergoing cesarean section (the incidence is 2% versus 16% without prophylactic saline) [20]. Subsequent spinal catheterization with epidural catheter following ADP can be used to prevent extra leakage of CSF, and then prevents PDPH [22, 116, 199]. Preventive epidural morphine 3mg given after the end of anesthesia and another 3 mg given on the following day reduced the incidence of PDPH from 48% to 12% [200]. Preventive administration of cosyntropin after ADP in parturients was associated with significant reduction in the incidence of PDPH and need for EBP and significant prolongation of the time from ADP to occurrence of PDPH [141]. Orally used prophylactic frovatriptan 2.5 mg/diet for 5 days markedly decreased the occurrence of PDPH [201]. Other methods like prophylactic administration of caffeine, magnesium, aminophylline, dexamethasone, or intravenous fluid infusion all cannot reduce the incidence of PDPH [202, 203].

10. Recommendations for clinicians

The occurrence of PDPH is determined by multiple factors including patient's demographic variables, caregiver's aspects, procedure-related factors, and post-accidental strategies. It is unclear which of them weighs over the others and what the accurate weight for each factor is in contributing to the onset of the headache. An arbitrary predictive curve of the incidence of PDPH to its risk factors herein is modeled and depicted in Figure 2 to show the association between the headache and different risk factors, and also give a potential prediction of the PDPH occurrence. In this model, each risk factor is scored "1", and all currently identified risk factors are summed up and in total get a scoring "10". Of the PDPH incidence changes from "0" to "100". For example, a 24-year non-smoking full-term pregnant woman with depression history was assigned to spinal anesthesia for Cesarean section by a third-year resident under the supervision by his consultant, so this woman had a risk scoring of "6", and the probability for the PDPH occurrence is ~32%.

Risk factor	Scoring
Young age	1
Female	1
Lower BMI	1
Taller height	1
Non-smoking	1
History of depression	1
History of chronic or recurrent headache	1
Experience level of personnel	1
Pregnancy itself	1
Fatigue, sleep deprivation, or night work	1
Total	**10**

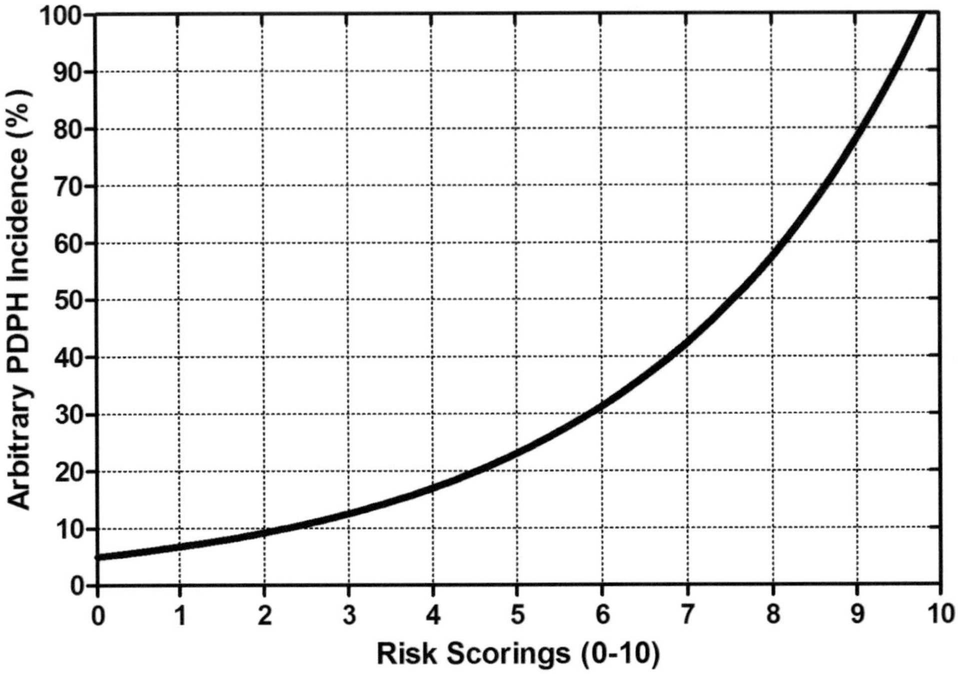

Figure 2. PDPH risk predictive curve.

Beside the risk predictive model, we need bear in mind following recommendations before and during performing spinal anesthesia.

1. Soothe patients psychologically to release stress;
2. Advance corresponding knowledge of the health care personnel;
3. Be energetic and active when performing procedures;
4. Hydrate patients prior procedures at least 500 ml;
5. Stabilize blood pressure at individual's physiological level;
6. Use lateral decubitus position for procedures;
7. Avoid repeat attempts of lumbar puncture;
8. No dexamethasone any time;
9. Reduce the volume of CSF withdrawn.

For the strategies after spinal anesthesia or ADP, refer to Table 3 for the therapeutic means and section 9 for the preventive maneuvers.

Conservative treatment (1st step)
Abdominal binder
Bed rest
Intravenous hydration
Psychological support
Symptomatic analgesia
Acetaminophen
Antiemetics
Dexamethasone
Gabapentin
Non-steroidal anti-inflammatory drugs (NSAIDs)
Aggressive medical treatment (2nd step)
Intravenous methylxanthines
Aminophylline
Caffeine
Theophylline
Occipital nerve block
Symptomatic therapies
Adrenocorticotropic hormone (ACTH) *i.v.*, *i.m.*
Epinephrine *i.t.*
Hydrocortisone *i.v.*
Methergine *i.v.*
Mirtazapine *o.l.*
Opioids *i.t.*
Pregabalin/Gabapentin *i.v.*, *o.l.*
Sumatriptan *s.c.*
Subarachnoid catheter left *in situ*
Conventional invasive management (3rd step)
Epidural blood patch (EBP)
Epidural saline patch
Epidural hydroxyethyl starch patch
Aggressive and invasive management (4th step)
Epidural fibrin glue
Invasive surgery

i.m.: intramascular; i.t.: intrathecal; i.v.: intravenous; o.l.: oral; s.c.: subcutaneous

Table 3. Therapeutic strategies for PDPH.

11. Concluding remarks

As a well known iatrogenic complication, PDPH has its special morbidity that affects patient's daily life, even though it carries self-terminating characteristic. Based on its particular risk factors and special pathophysiological concerns, many preventive and therapeutic methods are developed, although they need to be verified by further quality studies. While we cannot find a once-for-all method for the perplexing headache, we can individually assess the patient and predict the risk of PDPH using the arbitrary predictive model in combination with the prior-procedure preventive strategies. The key to avoid such an annoying morbid is to bear all associated concerns in mind and keep alert when facing a patient ready to spinal anesthesia or epidural puncture, and actively seek and carry out effective remediation once PDPH occurred. Yes, PDPH, we can prevent it only if we paid our attention carefully on this issue.

Acknowledgements

This work is supported by the National Natural Scientific Foundation of China (NSFC, 30901397 and 81371248), Nanjing Municipal Outstanding Young Scientist in Medical Science Development (JQX12009), and Nanjing Municipal Grant for Medical Science Development (ZKX10018).

Author details

Fuzhou Wang[1,2]

1 Department of Anesthesiology and Critical Care Medicine, The Affiliated Nanjing Maternity and Child Health Care Hospital, Nanjing Medical University, Nanjing, China

2 Division of Neuroscience, The Bonoi Academy of Science and Education, Winston-Salem, NC, USA

References

[1] Barbosa FT, Castro AA, de Miranda CT. Neuraxial anesthesia compared to general anesthesia for procedures on the lower half of the body: systematic review of systematic reviews. Revista Brasileira de Anestesiologia 2012;62(2) 235-243.

[2] Cwik J. Postoperative considerations of neuraxial anesthesia. Anesthesiology Clinics 2012;30(3) 433-443.

[3] Walker SM, Yaksh TL. Neuraxial analgesia in neonates and infants: a review of clinical and preclinical strategies for the development of safety and efficacy data. Anesthesia & Analgesia 2012;115(3) 638-662.

[4] Bezov D, Ashina S, Lipton R. Post-dural puncture headache: Part II--prevention, management, and prognosis. Headache 2010;50(9) 1482-1498.

[5] Gaiser RR. Postdural puncture headache: a headache for the patient and a headache for the anesthesiologist. Current Opinion in Anaesthesiology 2013;26(3) 296-303.

[6] de Almeida SM, Shumaker SD, LeBlanc SK, Delaney P, Marquie-Beck J, Ueland S, Alexander T, Ellis RJ. Incidence of post-dural puncture headache in research volunteers. Headache 2011;51(10) 1503-1510.

[7] Bezov D, Lipton RB, Ashina S. Post-dural puncture headache: part I diagnosis, epidemiology, etiology, and pathophysiology. Headache 2010;50(7) 1144-1152.

[8] Amorim JA, Gomes de Barros MV, Valença MM. Post-dural (post-lumbar) puncture headache: risk factors and clinical features. Cephalalgia 2012;32(12) 916-923.

[9] Amorim JA, Valença MM. Postdural puncture headache is a risk factor for new postdural puncture headache. Cephalalgia 2008;28(1) 5-8.

[10] Seeberger MD, Kaufmann M, Staender S, Schneider M, Scheidegger D. Repeated dural punctures increase the incidence of postdural puncture headache. Anesthesia & Analgesia 1996;82(2) 302-305.

[11] O'Connor G, Gingrich R, Moffat M. The effect of spinal needle design, size, and penetration angle on dural puncture cerebral spinal fluid loss. American Association of Nurse Anesthetists Journal 2007;75(2) 111-116.

[12] Kuczkowski KM. Post-dural puncture headache in the obstetric patient: an old problem. New solutions. Minerva Anestesiologica 2004;70(12) 823-830.

[13] Westbrook JL, Uncles DR, Sitzman BT, Carrie LE. Comparison of the force required for dural puncture with different spinal needles and subsequent leakage of cerebrospinal fluid. Anesthesia & Analgesia 1994;79(4) 769-772.

[14] Shaikh JM, Memon A, Memon MA, Khan M. Post dural puncture headache after spinal anaesthesia for caesarean section: a comparison of 25 g Quincke, 27 g Quincke and 27 g Whitacre spinal needles. Journal of Ayub Medical College Abbottabad 2008;20(3) 10-13.

[15] Apiliogullari S, Duman A, Gok F, Akillioglu I. Spinal needle design and size affect the incidence of postdural puncture headache in children. Paediatric Anaesthesia 2010;20(2) 177-182.

[16] Heesen M, Klöhr S, Rossaint R, van de Velde M, Straube S. Can the incidence of accidental dural puncture in laboring women be reduced? A systematic review and meta-analysis. Minerva Anestesiologica 2013; 79(10) 1187-1197.

[17] Duffy PJ, Crosby ET. The epidural blood patch. Resolving the controversies. Canadian Journal of Anaesthesia 1999;46(9) 878-886.

[18] Scavone BM, Wong CA, Sullivan JT, Yaghmour E, Sherwani SS, McCarthy RJ. Efficacy of a prophylactic epidural blood patch in preventing post dural puncture headache in parturients after inadvertent dural puncture. Anesthesiology 2004;101(6) 1422-1427.

[19] Charsley MM, Abram SE. The injection of intrathecal normal saline reduces the severity of postdural puncture headache. Regional Anesthesia and Pain Medicine 2001;26(4) 301-305.

[20] Faridi Tazeh-Kand N, Eslami B, Ghorbany Marzony S, Abolhassani R, Mohammadian K. Injection of intrathecal normal saline in decreasing postdural puncture headache. Journal of Anesthesia 2013; Doi: 10.1007/s00540-013-1683-8

[21] Boonmak P, Boonmak S. Epidural blood patching for preventing and treating postdural puncture headache. The Cochrane Database of Systematic Reviews 2010;(1) CD001791.

[22] Kuczkowski KM, Benumof JL. Decrease in the incidence of post-dural puncture headache: maintaining CSF volume. Acta anaesthesiologica Scandinavica 2003;47(1) 98-100.

[23] Basurto Ona X, Uriona Tuma SM, Martínez García L, Solà I, Bonfill Cosp X. Drug therapy for preventing post-dural puncture headache. The Cochrane Database of Systematic Reviews 2013;(2) CD001792.

[24] Singh S, Chaudry SY, Phelps AL, Vallejo MC. A 5-year audit of accidental dural punctures, postdural puncture headaches, and failed regional anesthetics at a tertiary-care medical center. ScientificWorldJournal 2009;9 715-722.

[25] Dodge HS, Ekhator NN, Jefferson-Wilson L, Fischer M, Jansen I, Horn PS, Hurford WE, Geracioti TD. Cigarette smokers have reduced risk for post-dural puncture headache. Pain Physician 2013;16(1) E25-E30.

[26] Corning JL. Spinal anaesthesia and local medication of the cord. New York Medical Journal 1885; 42 483-485.

[27] Wynter WE. Four cases of tubercular meningitis in which paracentesis was performed for the relief of fluid pressure. The Lancet 1891; 1 981-982.

[28] Quincke HI. Ueber hydrocephalus. Verhandlung des Congress Innere Medizin (X) 1891; 321-339.

[29] Quincke HI. Die lumbalpunction des Hydrocephalus. Berlin Klinik Wochenschrift 1891; 28 929-233.

[30] Bier A. Versuche über Cocainisirung des Rückenmarkes (Deutsch). Deutsch Zeitschrift für Chirurgie 1899; 51 361.

[31] Marx GF. The first spinal anesthesia. Who deserves the laurels? Regional Anesthesia 1994;19(6) 429-430.

[32] Turnbull DK, Shepherd DB. Post-dural puncture headache: pathogenesis, prevention and treatment. British Journal of Anaesthesia 2003;91(5) 718-729.

[33] Mosavy SH, Shafei M. Prevention of headache consequent upon dural puncture in obstetric patient. Anaesthesia 1975;30(6) 807-809.

[34] Guidelines for the practice of obstetric anaesthesia in Nottingham. Queen's Medical Centre Nottingham, NHS Trust. June 1990. 1st Version.

[35] Waise S, Gannon D. Reducing the incidence of post-dural puncture headache. Clinical Medicine 2013;13(1) 32-34.

[36] Darvish B, Gupta A, Alahuhta S, Dahl V, Helbo-Hansen S, Thorsteinsson A, Irestedt L, Dahlgren G. Management of accidental dural puncture and post-dural puncture headache after labour: a Nordic survey. Acta anaesthesiologica Scandinavica 2011;55(1) 46-53.

[37] Van de Velde M, Schepers R, Berends N, Vandermeersch E, De Buck F. Ten years of experience with accidental dural puncture and post-dural puncture headache in a tertiary obstetric anaesthesia department. International Journal of Obstetric Anesthesia 2008;17(4) 329-335.

[38] Srivastava V, Jindal P, Sharma JP. Study of post dural puncture headache with 27G Quincke & Whitacre needles in obstetrics/non obstetrics patients. Middle East Journal of Anesthesiology 2010;20(5) 709-717.

[39] Imarengiaye C, Ekwere I. Postdural puncture headache: a cross-sectional study of incidence and severity in a new obstetric anaesthesia unit. African Journal of Medicine and Medical Science 2006;35(1) 47-51.

[40] Tejavanija S, Sithinamsuwan P, Sithinamsuwan N, Nidhinandana S, Suwantamee J. Comparison of prevalence of post-dural puncture headache between six hour- supine recumbence and early ambulation after lumbar puncture in thai patients: A randomized controlled study. Journal of the Medical Association of Thailand 2006;89(6) 814-820.

[41] L'ubuský M, Berta E, Procházka M, Marek O, Kudela M. Development of incidence of post-dural puncture headache in patients undergoing caesarean section in spinal anaesthesia at the Department of Obstetrics and Gynecology in Olomouc during 2003-2004. Casopis Lékaru Ceských 2006;145(3) 204-208.

[42] Baysinger CL, Pope JE, Lockhart EM, Mercaldo ND. The management of accidental dural puncture and postdural puncture headache: a North American survey. Journal of Clinical Anesthesia 2011;23(5) 349-360.

[43] Berger CW, Crosby ET, Grodecki W. North American survey of the management of dural puncture occurring during labour epidural analgesia. Canadian Journal of Anaesthesia 1998;45(2) 110-114.

[44] Schmittner MD, Terboven T, Dluzak M, Janke A, Limmer ME, Weiss C, Bussen DG, Burmeister MA, Beck GC. High incidence of post-dural puncture headache in patients with spinal saddle block induced with Quincke needles for anorectal surgery: a randomised clinical trial. The International Journal of Colorectal Disease 2010;25(6) 775-781.

[45] Schmittner MD, Urban N, Janke A, Weiss C, Bussen DG, Burmeister MA, Beck GC. Influence of the pre-operative time in upright sitting position and the needle type on the incidence of post-dural puncture headache (PDPH) in patients receiving a spinal saddle block for anorectal surgery. The International Journal of Colorectal Disease 2011;26(1) 97-102.

[46] Lybecker H, Møller JT, May O, Nielsen HK. Incidence and prediction of postdural puncture headache. A prospective study of 1021 spinal anesthesias. Anesthesia & Analgesia 1990;70(4) 389-394.

[47] Imbelloni LE, Gouveia MA, Cordeiro JA. Continuous spinal anesthesia versus combined spinal epidural block for major orthopedic surgery: prospective randomized study. Sao Paulo Medical Journal 2009;127(1) 7-11.

[48] Neuman SA, Eldrige JS, Qu W, Freeman ED, Hoelzer BC. Post dural puncture headache following intrathecal drug delivery system placement. Pain Physician 2013;16(2) 101-107.

[49] Wee LH, Lam F, Cranston AJ. The incidence of post dural puncture headache in children. Anaesthesia 1996;51(12) 1164-1166.

[50] Lowery S, Oliver A. Incidence of postdural puncture headache and backache following diagnostic/therapeutic lumbar puncture using a 22G cutting spinal needle, and after introduction of a 25G pencil point spinal needle. Paediatric Anaesthesia 2008;18(3) 230-234.

[51] Wadud R, Laiq N, Qureshi FA, Jan AS. The frequency of postdural puncture headache in different age groups. Journal of the College of Physicians and Surgeons-Pakistan 2006;16(6) 389-392.

[52] Bolder PM. Postlumbar puncture headache in pediatric oncology patients. Anesthesiology 1986;65(6) 696-698.

[53] Ylonen P, Kokki H. Epidural blood patch for management of postdural puncture headache in adolescents. Acta anaesthesiologica Scandinavica 2002;46(7) 794-798.

[54] Tobias JD. Postdural puncture headache in children - etiology and treatment. Clinical Pediatrics 1990;33(2) 110 -113.

[55] Tourtellotte WW, Henderson WG, Tucker RP, Gilland O, Walker JE, Kokman E. A randomized, double-blind clinical trial comparing the 22 versus 26 gauge needle in production of the post-lumbar puncture syndrome in normal individuals. Headache 1972;12(2) 73-78.

[56] Wu CL, Rowlingson AJ, Cohen SR, Michaels RK, Courpas GE, Joe EM, Liu SS. Gender and post-dural puncture headache. Anesthesiology 2006;105(3) 613-618.

[57] Peralta FM, Chalifoux LA, Stevens CD, Higgins N. Obese parturients and the incidence of postdural puncture headache after unintentional dural puncture. Anesthesiology 2011; A341.

[58] Faure E, Moreno R, Thisted R. Incidence of postdural puncture headache in morbidly obese parturients. Regional Anesthesia 1994;19(5) 361-363.

[59] Chong YFV, Tan K. A survey of lumbar puncture complications and their risk factors: the influence of height, intravenous hydration and systolic blood pressure on post-dural puncture headache. Neurology 2012; 78 (Meeting Abstracts 1) P04.250.

[60] Leibold RA, Yealy DM, Coppola M, Cantees KK. Post-dural-puncture headache: characteristics, management and prevention. Annals of Emergency Medicine 1993;22(12) 1863-1870.

[61] van Oosterhout WP, van der Plas AA, van Zwet EW, Zielman R, Ferrari MD, Terwindt GM. Postdural puncture headache in migraineurs and nonheadache subjects: a prospective study. Neurology 2013;80(10) 941-948.

[62] Clark JW. Substance P concentration and history of headache in relation to postlumbar puncture headache: towards prevention. Journal of Neurology, Neurosurgery & Psychiatry 1996;60 (6) 681-683.

[63] Flaatten H, Krakenes J, Vedeler C. Post-dural puncture related complications after diagnostic lumbar puncture, myelography and spinal anesthesia. Acta Neurologica Scandinavica 1998;98(6) 445-451.

[64] Davignon KR, Dennehy KC. Update on postdural puncture headache. International Anesthesiology Clinics 2002;40(4) 89-102.

[65] Kuntz KM, Kokmen E, Stevens JC, Miller P, Offord KP, Ho MM. Post-lumbar puncture headaches: experience in 501 consecutive procedures. Neurology 1992;42(10) 1884-1887.

[66] Yousefshahi F, Dahmardeh AR, Khajavi M, Najafi A, Khashayar P, Barkhordari K. Effect of dexamethasone on the frequency of postdural puncture headache after spinal anesthesia for cesarean section: a double-blind randomized clinical trial. Acta Neurologica Belgica 2012;112(4) 345-350.

[67] Alam MR, Rahman MA, Ershad R. Role of very short-term intravenous hydrocortisone in reducing postdural puncture headache. Journal of Anaesthesiology Clinical Pharmacology 2012;28(2) 190-193.

[68] Choi PT, Galinski SE, Lucas S, Takeuchi L, Jadad AR. Examining the evidence in anesthesia literature: a survey and evaluation of obstetrical postdural puncture headache reports. Canadian Journal of Anaesthesia 2002; 49(1) 49-56.

[69] Kuczkowski KM. Post dural puncture headache, intracranial air and obstetric anesthesia. Anaesthesist 2003; 52(9) 798-800.

[70] Choi PT, Galinski SE, Takeuchi L, Lucas S, Tamayo C, Jadad AR. PDPH is a common complication of neuraxial blockade in parturients: a meta-analysis of obstetrical studies. Canadian Journal of Anaesthesia 2003;50(5) 460-469.

[71] Morewood GH. A rational approach to the cause, prevention and treatment of postdural puncture headache. Canadian Medical Association Journal 1993;149(8) 1087-1093.

[72] Runza M, Pietrabissa R, Mantero S, Albani A, Quaglini V, Contro R. Lumbar dura mater biomechanics: experimental characterization and scanning electron microscopy observations. Anesthesia & Analgesia 1999;88(6) 1317-1321.

[73] Reina MA, de Leon-Casasola OA, Lopez A, De Andres J, Martin S, Mora M. An in vitro study of dural lesions produced by 25-gauge Quincke and Whitacre needles evaluated by scanning electron microscopy. Regional Anesthesia and Pain Medicine 2000;25(4) 393-402.

[74] Reina MA, López-García A, Dittmann M, de Andrés JA. Structural analysis of the thickness of human dura mater with scanning electron microscopy. Revista Española de Anestesiología y Reanimación 1996;43(4) 135-137.

[75] Reina MA, López García A, de Andrés JA, Sellers F, Arrizabalaga M, Mora MJ. Thickness variation of the dural sac. Revista Española de Anestesiología y Reanimación 1999;46(8) 344-349.

[76] Sakka L, Coll G, Chazal J. Anatomy and physiology of cerebrospinal fluid. European Annals of Otorhinolaryngology, Head and Neck Diseases 2011;128(6) 309-316.

[77] Kuczkowski KM. Post-dural puncture headache in pregnant women: What have we learned? Revista Colombiana de Anestesiología 2006; 34 267-272.

[78] Schwartz KM, Luetmer PH, Hunt CH, Kotsenas AL, Diehn FE, Eckel LJ, Black DF, Lehman VT, Lindell EP. Position-related variability of CSF opening pressure measurements. AJNR American Journal of Neuroradiology 2013;34(4) 904-907.

[79] Ellis R III. Lumbar cerebrospinal fluid opening pressure measured in a flexed lateral decubitus position in children. Pediatrics 1994;93(4) 622-623.

[80] Hatfalvi BI. Postulated mechanisms for postdural puncture headache and review of laboratory models. Clinical experience. Regional Anesthesia 1995;20(4) 329-336.

[81] Reamy BV. Post-epidural headache: how late can it occur? The Journal of the American Board of Family Medicine 2009;22(2) 202-205.

[82] Fearon W. Post-lumbar puncture headache. P&S Medical Review1993.

[83] Richardson MG, Wissler RN. Density of lumbar cerebrospinal fluid in pregnant and nonpregnant humans. Anesthesiology 1996;85(2) 326-330.

[84] Kemp WJ III, Tubbs RS, Cohen-Gadol AA. The innervation of the cranial dura mater: neurosurgical case correlates and a review of the literature. World Neurosurgery 2012;78(5) 505-510.

[85] Cumberbatch MJ, Williamson DJ, Mason GS, Hill RG, Hargreaves RJ. Dural vasodilation causes a sensitization of rat caudal trigeminal neurones in vivo that is blocked by a 5-HT1B/1D agonist. British Journal of Pharmacology 1999;126(6) 1478-1486.

[86] Knyihár-Csillik E, Tajti J, Chadaide Z, Csillik B, Vécsei L. Functional immunohistochemistry of neuropeptides and nitric oxide synthase in the nerve fibers of the supratentorial dura mater in an experimental migraine model. Microscopy Research and Technique 2001;53(3) 193-211.

[87] Damon DH, Teriele JA, Marko SB. Vascular-derived artemin: a determinant of vascular sympathetic innervation? American journal of physiology-Heart and Circulatory Physiology 2007;293(1) H266-H273.

[88] Lippoldt EK, Elmes RR, McCoy DD, Knowlton WM, McKemy DD. Artemin, a glial cell line-derived neurotrophic factor family member, induces TRPM8-dependent cold pain. The Journal of Neuroscience 2013;33(30) 12543-12552.

[89] Thornton P, Hatcher JP, Robinson I, Sargent B, Franzén B, Martino G, Kitching L, Glover CP, Anderson D, Forsmo-Bruce H, Low CP, Cusdin F, Dosanjh B, Williams W, Steffen AC, Thompson S, Eklund M, Lloyd C, Chessell I, Hughes J. Artemin-GFRα3 interactions partially contribute to acute inflammatory hypersensitivity. Neuroscience Letters 2013;545 23-28.

[90] McIlvried LA, Albers K, Gold MS. Distribution of artemin and GFRalpha3 labeled nerve fibers in the dura mater of rat: artemin and GFRalpha3 in the dura. Headache 2010;50(3) 442-450.

[91] Cavallotti D, Artico M, De Santis S, Iannetti G, Cavallotti C. Catecholaminergic innervation of the human dura mater involved in headache. Headache 1998;38(5) 352-355.

[92] Fernstrom JD, Fernstrom MH. Tyrosine, phenylalanine, and catecholamine synthesis and function in the brain. Journal of Nutrition 2007;137(6 Suppl 1) 1539S-1548S.

[93] Edgar MA, Nundy S. Innervation ofthe spinal dura mater. Journal of Neurology, Neurosurgery & Psychiatry 1966; 29 530-534.

[94] Edgar MA, Ghadially JA. Innervation of the lumbar spine. Clinical Orthopaedics and Related Research 1976; 115 35-41.

[95] Cyriax J. Dural pain. The Lancet 1978; 1 919-921.

[96] Sekiguchi Y, Konnai Y, Kikuchi S, Sugiura Y. An anatomic study of neuropeptide immunoreactivities in the lumbar dura mater after lumbar sympathectomy. Spine (Phila Pa 1976). 1996;21(8) 925-930.

[97] Bridge CJ. Innervation of spinal meninges and epidural structures. The Anatomical Record 1959; 133 553-561.

[98] Konnai Y, Honda T, Sekiguchi Y, Kikuchi S, Sugiura Y. Sensory innervation of the lumbar dura mater passing through the sympathetic trunk in rats. Spine (Phila Pa 1976) 2000;25(7) 776-782.

[99] Halpern S, Preston R. Postdural puncture headache and spinal needle design. Metaanalyses. Anesthesiology 1994;81(6) 1376-1383.

[100] Ross BK, Chadwick HS, Mancuso JJ, Benedetti C. Sprotte needle for obstetric anesthesia: decreased incidence of post dural puncture headache. Regional Anesthesia 1992;17(1) 29-33.

[101] Imarengiaye CO, Edomwonyi NP. Evaluation of 25-gauge Quincke and 24-gauge Gertie Marx needles for spinal anaesthesia for caesarean section. East African Medical Journal 2002;79(7) 379-381.

[102] Santanen U, Rautoma P, Luurila H, Erkola O, Pere P. Comparison of 27-gauge (0.41-mm) Whitacre and Quincke spinal needles with respect to post-dural puncture headache and non-dural puncture headache. Acta Anaesthesiologica Scandinavica 2004;48(4) 474-479.

[103] Luostarinen L, Heinonen T, Luostarinen M, Salmivaara A. Diagnostic lumbar puncture. Comparative study between 22-gauge pencil point and sharp bevel needle. The Journal of Headache and Pain 2005;6(5) 400-404.

[104] Tabedar S, Maharjan SK, Shrestha BR, Shrestha BM. A comparison of 25 gauge Quincke spinal needle with 26 gauge Eldor spinal needle for the elective Caesarian sections: insertion characteristics and complications. Kathmandu University Medical Journal 2003;1(4) 263-266.

[105] Kokki H, Turunen M, Heikkinen M, Reinikainen M, Laisalmi M. High success rate and low incidence of headache and neurological symptoms with two spinal needle designs in children. Acta Anaesthesiologica Scandinavica 2005;49(9) 1367-1372.

[106] Kuczkowski KM. The management of accidental dural puncture in pregnant women: what does an obstetrician need to know? Archives of gynecology and obstetrics 2007;275(2) 125-131.

[107] Bloomfield GL, Ridings PC, Blocher CR, Marmarou A, Sugerman HJ. Effects of increased intra-abdominal pressure upon intracranial and cerebral perfusion pressure before and after volume expansion. Journal of Trauma 1996;40(6) 936-943.

[108] Laterra J, Keep R, Betz LA, Goldstein GW. Blood-brain-cerebrospinal fluid barriers (Chapter 36). Basic Neurochemistry: Molecular, Cellular and Medical Aspects. 6th edition. Eds. Siegel GJ, Agranoff BW, Albers RW, Fisher SK, Uhler MD. Philadelphia: Lippincott-Raven; 1999.

[109] Arevalo-Rodriguez I, Ciapponi A, Munoz L, Roqué I Figuls M, Bonfill Cosp X. Posture and fluids for preventing post-dural puncture headache. The Cochrane Database of Systematic Reviews 2013;(7) CD009199.

[110] Mehta S, Rajaram S, Goel N. Postdural puncture headache. Advances in obstetrics and gynecology (Vol. 3). Jaypee Brothers Medical Publisher, 2011; p143-p146.

[111] Caple C. Lumbar puncture: complications and after-care. Evidence-Based Care Sheet. Cinahl Information Systems. 2012; p1-p2.

[112] Esmaoglu A, Akpinar H, Uğur F. Oral multidose caffeine-paracetamol combination is not effective for the prophylaxis of postdural puncture headache. Journal of Clinical Anesthesia 2005;17(1) 58-61.

[113] Allen TK, Jones CA, Habib AS. Dexamethasone for the prophylaxis of postoperative nausea and vomiting associated with neuraxial morphine administration: a systematic review and meta-analysis. Anesthesia & Analgesia 2012;114(4) 813-822.

[114] Soleimanpour H, Ghafouri RR, Taheraghdam A, Aghamohammadi D, Negargar S, Golzari SE, Abbasnezhad M. Effectiveness of intravenous dexamethasone versus propofol for pain relief in the migraine headache: a prospective double blind randomized clinical trial. BMC Neurology 2012;12 114.

[115] Erol DD. The analgesic and antiemetic efficacy of gabapentin or ergotamine/caffeine for the treatment of postdural puncture headache. Advances in Medical Sciences 2011;56(1) 25-29.

[116] Kuczkowski KM. Once a post-dural puncture headache patient--always post-dural puncture headache patient: an update. Acta Anaesthesiologica Belgica 2005;56(1) 23.

[117] Cesur M, Alici HA, Erdem AF, Silbir F, Celik M. Decreased incidence of headache after unintentional dural puncture in patients with cesarean delivery administered with postoperative epidural analgesia. Journal of Anesthesai 2009;23(1) 31-35.

[118] Bevacqua BK, Slucky AV, Cleary WF. Is postoperative intrathecal catheter use associated with central nervous system infection? Anesthesiology 1994;80(6) 1234-1240.

[119] Rigler ML, Drasner K, Krejcie TC, Yelich SJ, Scholnick FT, DeFontes J, Bohner D. Cauda equina syndrome after continuous spinal anesthesia. Anesthesia & Analgesia 1991;72(3) 275-281.

[120] Moore JM. Continuous spinal anesthesia. American Journal of Therapeutics 2009;16(4) 289-294.

[121] Matute E, Bonilla S, Gironés A, Planas A. Bilateral greater occipital nerve block for post-dural puncture headache. Anaesthesia 2008;63(5) 557-558.

[122] Akin Takmaz S, Unal Kantekin C, Kaymak C, Başar H. Treatment of post-dural puncture headache with bilateral greater occipital nerve block. Headache 2010;50(5) 869-872.

[123] Hamzehzadeh S, Eng C, Tran T. Occipital nerve blockade successfully treats patient with suspected post-dural puncture headache (PDPH). Regional Anesthesia and Pain Medicine Spring 2011. http://www.asra.com/display_spring_2011.php?id=137.

[124] Mueller O, Hagel V, Wrede K, Schlamann M, Hohn HP, Sure U, Gaul C. Stimulation of the greater occipital nerve: anatomical considerations and clinical implications. Pain Physician 2013;16(3) E181-E189.

[125] Madhavi C, Holla SJ. Triplication of the lesser occipital nerve. Clinical Anatomy 2004;17(8) 667-671.

[126] Young W, Cook B, Malik S, Shaw J, Oshinsky M. The first 5 minutes after greater occipital nerve block. Headache 2008;48(7) 1126-1128.

[127] Seo BF, Jung SN, Sohn WI, Kwon H. Lymph node compression of the lesser occipital nerve: a cause of migraine. Journal of Plastic, Reconstructive & Aesthetic Surgery 2011;64(12) 1657-1660.

[128] Naja Z, Al-Tannir M, El-Rajab M, Ziade F, Baraka A. Nerve stimulator-guided occipital nerve blockade for postdural puncture headache. Pain Practice 2009;9(1) 51-58.

[129] Lindinger MI, Willmets RG, Hawke TJ. Stimulation of Na+, K(+)-pump activity in skeletal muscle by methylxanthines: evidence and proposed mechanisms. Acta Physiologica Scandinavica 1996;156(3) 347-353.

[130] Speake T, Whitwell C, Kajita H, Majid A, Brown PD. Mechanisms of CSF secretion by the choroid plexus. Microscopy Research and Technique 2001;52(1) 49-59.

[131] Sadeghi SE, Abdollahifard G, Nasabi NA, Mehrabi M, Safarpour AR. Effectiveness of single dose intravenous aminophylline administration on prevention of post dural puncture headache in patients who received spinal anesthesia for elective cesarean section. World Journal of Medical Sciences 2012;7(1) 13-16.

[132] Halker RB, Demaerschalk BM, Wellik KE, Wingerchuk DM, Rubin DI, Crum BA, Dodick DW. Caffeine for the prevention and treatment of postdural puncture headache: debunking the myth. Neurologist 2007;13(5) 323-327.

[133] Schwalbe SS, Schifmiller MW, Marx GF. Theophylline for PDPH. Anesthesiology 1991; 75 A1082.

[134] Ergün U, Say B, Ozer G, Tunc T, Sen M, Tüfekcioglu S, Akin U, Ilhan MN, Inan L. Intravenous theophylline decreases post-dural puncture headaches. Journal of Clinical Neuroscience 2008;15(10) 1102-1104.

[135] Boison D. Methylxanthines, seizures, and excitotoxicity. Handbook of Experimental Pharmacology 2011;(200) 251-266.

[136] Riksen NP, Smits P, Rongen GA. The cardiovascular effects of methylxanthines. Handbook of Experimental Pharmacology 2011;(200) 413-437.

[137] Kshatri AM, Foster PA. Adrenocorticotropic hormone infusion as a novel treatment for postdural puncture headache. Regional Anesthesia 1997; 22(5) 432-434.

[138] Carter BL, Pasupuleti R. Use of intravenous cosyntropin in the treatment of postdural puncture headache. Anesthesiology 2000;92(1) 272-274.

[139] Cánovas L, Barros C, Gómez A, Castro M, Castro A. Use of intravenous tetracosactin in the treatment of postdural puncture headache: our experience in forty cases. Anesthesia & Analgesia 2002;94(5) 1369.

[140] Ghai A, Wadhera R. Adrenocorticotrophic hormone-is a single dose sufficient for post-dural puncture headache? Acta Anaesthesiologica Scandinavica 2007; 51 266.

[141] Hakim SM. Cosyntropin for prophylaxis against postdural puncture headache after accidental dural puncture. Anesthesiology 2010;113(2) 413-420.

[142] Ambrogio AG, Pecori Giraldi F, Cavagnini F. Drugs and HPA axis. Pituitary 2008;11(2) 219-229.

[143] Pertovaara A. Noradrenergic pain modulation. Progress in Neurobiology 2006;80(2) 53-83.

[144] Cohen S, Amar D, Pantuck EJ, Singer N, Divon M. Decreased incidence of headache after accidental dural puncture in caesarean delivery patients receiving continuous postoperative intrathecal analgesia. Acta Anaesthesiologica Scandinavica 1994;38(7) 716-718.

[145] Etezadi F, Yousefshahi F, Khajavi M, Tanha FD, Dahmarde AR, Najafi A. Post dural puncture headache after cesarean section, a teaching hospital experience. Journal of Family and Reproductive Health 2012; 6(1) 17-21.

[146] Torres D. Gabapentin and PDPH. Acute Pain 2007; 9(2) 93.

[147] Lin YT, Sheen MJ, Huang ST, Horng HC, Cherng CH, Wong CS, Hot ST. Gabapentin relieves post-dural puncture headache--a report of two cases. Acta Anaesthesiologica Taiwanica 2007;45(1) 47-51.

[148] Wagner Y, Storr F, Cope S. Gabapentin in the treatment of post-dural puncture headache: a case series. Anaesthesia and Intensive Care 2012 Jul;40(4) 714-718.

[149] Zencirci B. Postdural puncture headache and pregabalin. Journal of Pain Research 2010;3 11-14.

[150] Huseyinoglu U, Huseyinoglu N, Hamurtekin E, Aygun H, Sulu B. Effect of pregabalin on post-dural-puncture headache following spinal anesthesia and lumbar puncture. Journal of Clinical Neuroscience 2011;18(10) 1365-1368.

[151] Carp H, Singh PJ, Vadhera R, Jayaram A. Effects of the serotonin-receptor agonist sumatriptan on post-dural puncture headache: report of six cases. Anesthesia & Analgesia 1994;79(1) 180-182.

[152] Connelly NR, Parker RK, Rahimi A, Gibson CS. Sumatriptan in patients with post-dural puncture headache. Headache 2000;40(4) 316-319.

[153] Graff-Radford SB, Bittar GT. The use of methylergonovine (Methergine) in the initial control of drug induced refractory headache. Headache 1993;33(7) 390-393.

[154] Saper JR, Evans RW. Oral methylergonovine maleate for refractory migraine and cluster headache prevention. Headache 2013;53(2) 378-381.

[155] Hakim S, Khan RM, Maroof M, Usmani H, Huda W, Jafri F. Methylergonovine maleate (methergine) relieves postdural puncture headache in obstetric patients. Acta Obstetricia et Gynecologica Scandinavica 2005;84(1) 100.

[156] Alici HA, Cesur M, Erdem AF, Ingec M, Bebek Z. Is methergine alone sufficient in relieving postdural puncture headache? Acta Obstetricia et Gynecologica Scandinavica 2006;85(5) 632-633.

[157] Sheen MJ, Ho ST. Mirtazapine relieves postdural puncture headache. Anesthesia & Analgesia 2008;107(1) 346.

[158] Sandesc D, Lupei MI, Sirbu C, Plavat C, Bedreag O, Vernic C. Conventional treatment or epidural blood patch for the treatment of different etiologies of post dural puncture headache. Acta Anaesthesiologica Belgica 2006;57 55-56.

[159] Gormley JB. Treatment of post-spinal headache. Anesthesiology 1960; 21 565-566.

[160] Sanford CL 2nd, Rodriguez RE, Schmidt J, Austin PN. Evidence for using air or fluid when identifying the epidural space. American Association of Nurse Anesthetists Journal. 2013;81(1) 23-28.

[161] Pleasure SJ, Abosch A, Friedman J, Ko NU, Barbaro N, Dillon W, Fishman RA, Poncelet AN. Spontaneous intracranial hypotension resulting in stupor caused by diencephalic compression. Neurology 1998;50(6) 1854-1857.

[162] Szeinfeld M, Ihmeidan IH, Moser MM, Machado R, Klose KJ, Serafini AN. Epidural blood patch: evaluation of the volume and spread of blood injected into the epidural space. Anesthesiology 1986; 64(6) 820-822.

[163] Beards SC, Jackson A, Griffiths AG, Horsman EL. Magnetic resonance imaging of extradural blood patches: appearances from 30 min to 18 h. British Journal of Anaesthesia 1993; 71(2) 182-8.

[164] DiGiovanni AJ, Galbert MW, Wahle WM. Epidural injection of autologous blood for ostlumbar-puncture headache. II. Additional clinical experiences and laboratory investigation. Anesthesia & Analgesia 1972; 51(2) 226-232.

[165] Cook MA, Watkins-Pitchford JM. Epidural blood patch: a rapid coagulation response. Anesthesia & Analgesia 1990; 70(5) 567-568.

[166] Abouleish E, Vega S, Blendinger I, Tio TO. Long-term follow-up of epidural blood patch. Anesthesia & Analgesia 1975; 54(4) 459-463.

[167] Seebacher J, Ribeiro V, LeGuillou JL, Lacomblez L, Henry M, Thorman F, Youl B, Bensimon G, Darbois Y, Bousser MG. Epidural blood patch in the treatment of post dural puncture headache: a double blind study. Headache 1989; 29(10) 630-632.

[168] van Kooten F, Oedit R, Bakker SL, Dippel DW. Epidural blood patch in post dural puncture headache: a randomised, observer-blind, controlled clinical trial. Journal of Neurology, Neurosurgery and Psychiatry 2008; 79(5) 553-558.

[169] Kokki M, Sjövall S, Keinänen M, Kokki H. The influence of timing on the effectiveness of epidural blood patches in parturients. International Journal of Obstetric Anesthesia 2013;22(4) 303-309.

[170] Kueper M, Goericke SL, Kastrup O. Cerebral venous thrombosis after epidural blood patch: coincidence or causal relation? A case report and review of the literature. Cephalalgia 2008;28(7) 769-773.

[171] Ghatge S, Uppugonduri S, Kamarzaman Z. Cerebral venous sinus thrombosis following accidental dural puncture and epidural blood patch. International Journal of Obstetric Anesthesia 2008;17(3) 267-270.

[172] Borum SE, Naul LG, McLeskey CH. Postpartum dural venous sinus thrombosis after postdural puncture headache and epidural blood patch. Anesthesiology 1997;86(2) 487-490.

[173] Barrett J, Alves E. Postpartum cerebral venous sinus thrombosis after dural puncture and epidural blood patch. The Journal of Emergency Medicine 2005;28(3) 341-342.

[174] Jungmann V, Werner R, Bergmann J, Daum J, Wöhrle JC, Dünnebacke J, Silomon M. Postpartum cerebral venous sinus thrombosis after epidural anaesthesia. Anaesthesist 2009;58(3) 268-272.

[175] Collier CB. Blood patches may cause scarring in the epidural space: two case reports. International Journal of Obstetric Anesthesia 2011;20(4) 347-351.

[176] Gutterman P, Bezier HS. Prophylaxis of postmyelogram headaches. Journal of Neurosurgery 1978; 49 869-871.

[177] Colonna-Romano P, Shapiro BE. Unintentional dural puncture and prophylactic epidural blood patch in obstetrics. Anesthesia & Analgesia 1989; 69(4) 522-523.

[178] Agerson AN, Scavone BM. Prophylactic epidural blood patch after unintentional dural puncture for the prevention of postdural puncture headache in parturients. Anesthesia & Analgesia 2012;115(1) 133-136.

[179] Benson KT. The Jehova's Witness patient: considerations for the anesthesiologist. Anesthesia & Analgesia 1989; 69(5) 647-656.

[180] Bearb ME, Pennant JH. Epidural blood patch in a Jehovah's Witness. Anesthesia & Analgesia 1987;66(10) 1052.

[181] Silva Lde A, de Carli D, Cangiani LM, Gonçalves Filho JB, da Silva IF. Epidural blood patch in Jehovah's Witness: two cases report. Revista Brasileira de Anestesiologia 2003;53(5) 633-639.

[182] Jagannathan N, Tetzlaff JE. Epidural blood patch in a Jehovah's Witness patient with post-dural puncture cephalgia. Canadian Journal of Anaesthesia 2005;52(1) 113.

[183] Pérez Ferrer A, Martínez B, Gredilla E, de Vicente J. Epidural blood patch in a Jehovah's witness. Revista Española de Anestesiología y Reanimación 2005;52(6) 374-375.

[184] Tanaka T, Muratani T, Kusaka Y, Minami T. Epidural blood patch for intracranial hypotension with closed system in a Jehovah's Witness. Masui 2007;56(8) 953-955.

[185] Clark CJ, Whitwell J. Intraocular haemorrahge after epidural injection. BMJ 1961; I 1612-1613.

[186] Kara I, Ciftci I, Apiliogullari S, Arun O, Duman A, Celik JB. Management of postdural puncture headache with epidural saline patch in a 10-year-old child after inguinal hernia repair: a case report. Journal of Pediatric Surgery 2012;47(10) e55-e57.

[187] Vassal O, Baud MC, Bolandard F, Bonnin M, Vielle E, Bazin JE, Chassard D. Epidural injection of hydroxyethyl starch in the management of postdural puncture headache. International Journal of Obstetric Anesthesia 2013;22(2) 153-155.

[188] Chassard D, Vassal O. Epidural injection of hydroxyethyl starch in the management of postdural puncture headache. International Journal of Obstetric Anesthesia 2013; 22(4) 353-354.

[189] Dhillon S. Fibrin sealant (evicel® [quixil®/crosseal™]): a review of its use as supportive treatment for haemostasis in surgery. Drugs 2011;71(14) 1893-1915.

[190] Chauvet D, Tran V, Mutlu G, George B, Allain JM. Study of dural suture watertightness: an in vitro comparison of different sealants. Acta Neurochirurgica (Wien) 2011;153(12) 2465-2472.

[191] Gentili ME. Epidural fibrin glue injection stops postdural puncture headache in patient with long-term intrathecal catheterization. Regional Anesthesia and Pain Medicine 2003;28(1) 70.

[192] Crul BJ, Gerritse BM, van Dongen RT, Schoonderwaldt HC. Epidural fibrin glue injection stops persistent postdural puncture headache. Anesthesiology 1999;91(2) 576-577.

[193] García-Aguado R, Gil F, Barcia JA, Aznar J, Hostalet F, Barberá J, Grau F. Prophylactic percutaneous sealing of lumbar postdural puncture hole with fibrin glue to prevent cerebrospinal fluid leakage in swine. Anesthesia & Analgesia 2000;90(4) 894-898.

[194] Gil F, García-Aguado R, Barcia JA, Guijarro E, Hostalet F, Tommasi-Rosso M, Grau F. The effect of fibrin glue patch in an in vitro model of postdural puncture leakage. Anesthesia & Analgesia 1998;87(5) 1125-1158.

[195] Schlenker M, Ringelstein EB. Epidural fibrin clot for the prevention of post-lumbar puncture headache: a new method with risks. Journal of Neurology, Neurosurgery & Psychiatry 1987;50(12) 1715.

[196] Schlag MG, Hopf R, Redl H. Convulsive seizures following subdural application of fibrin sealant containing tranexamic acid in a rat model. Neurosurgery 2000;47(6) 1463-1467.

[197] Pouskoulas CD, Taub E, Ruppen W. Successful treatment of post-dural-puncture headache with surgical dura repair two years after spinal anesthesia. Cephalalgia 2013; 33(15) 1269-1271.

[198] Jadon A, Chakraborty S, Sinha N, Agrawal R. Intrathecal catheterization by epidural catheter: management of accidental dural puncture and prophylaxis of PDPH. Indian Journal of Anaesthesia 2009;53(1) 30-34.

[199] Al-Metwalli RR. Epidural morphine injections for prevention of post dural puncture headache. Anaesthesia 2008; 63(8) 847-850.

[200] Bussone G, Tullo V, d'Onofrio F, Petretta V, Curone M, Frediani F, Tonini C, Omboni S. Frovatriptan for the prevention of postdural puncture headache. Cephalalgia 2007;27(7) 809-813.

[201] Zajac K, Zajac M, Hładki W, Jach R. Is there any point in pharmacological prophylaxis of PDPH (post-dural puncture headache) after spinal anaesthesia for Caesaren section? Przeglad lekarski 2012;69(1) 19-24.

[202] Doroudian MR, Norouzi M, Esmailie M, Tanhaeivash R. Dexamethasone in preventing post-dural puncture headache: a randomized, double-blind, placebo-controlled trial. Acta Anaesthesiologica Belgica 2011;62(3) 143-146.

Chapter 8

Analgesia for the Trunk: A Comparison of Epidural, Thoracic Paravertebral and Transversus Abdominis Plane Blocks

Linda Le-Wendling, Julia DeLoach,
Allison Haller and Barys Ihnatsenka

Additional information is available at the end of the chapter

http://dx.doi.org/10.5772/57403

1. Introduction

Major open upper and lower abdominal surgery, such as pancreaticoduodenectomy, abdominal aortic surgery, bowel resection, gastric bypass, gynecologic surgery and liver resection results in major morbidity for patients, including moderate to severe pain in the acute postoperative period.

Data on postoperative pain after surgery consistently shows moderate-to-severe pain in the first 24 hours after surgery with traditional systemic analgesic techniques, such as intravenous or intramuscular opioids, patient-controlled opioid analgesia, and multimodal analgesia with opioids combined with acetaminophen, NSAIDs, neuropathic agents, and ketamine [1, 2, 3]. In fact, moderate-to-severe pain can persist for 3 days after surgery [4]. In addition, specific multimodal analgesic techniques may be contraindicated depending on patient history, such as the use of NSAIDs in patients with renal dysfunction.

Pain following open abdominal surgery comprises both incisional pain and visceral pain. Interestingly, incisional pain may be reduced with the use of local anesthetics deposited around the incision site, and the use of wound catheters have been noted to reduce opioid consumption by about 30% [5]. However, the use of wound catheters does not allow for analgesia of the abdominal muscles beneath the incision nor the pain emanating from the viscera, which still results in substantial amounts of opioid consumption. Approximately 25-150 mg intravenous morphine equivalents are required to provide adequate analgesia in the first 24 to 48 hours after surgery [6, 7]. Even the use of systemic local anesthetics, such as

INTECH
open science | open minds

© 2015 The Author(s). Licensee InTech. This chapter is distributed under the terms of the Creative Commons Attribution License (http://creativecommons.org/licenses/by/3.0), which permits unrestricted use, distribution, and reproduction in any medium, provided the original work is properly cited.

intraoperative lidocaine infusions, has only been documented to improve pain scores by small increments in open abdominal surgery (4-10mm NRS) [8].

Despite opioid use, moderate-to-severe pain with coughing and mobilization continues to remain high in the first 72 hours after surgery, though with significant improvement after 24 hours. In addition, use of opioids may result in significant side effects such as hypoventilation, sedation, gastric dysmotility, and nausea and vomiting, which can worsen patient recovery [9, 10].

Regional anesthesia and analgesia can be used to significantly reduce postoperative pain scores and spare the use of systemic opioids. Regional anesthesia can be performed at the neuraxis (epidural), the nerve root (paravertebral), and the peripheral nerve (transversus abdominis plane) level. Local anesthetic deposition at these sites will selectively block nerve conduction and result in different analgesic and side effect profiles. This chapter will examine the role of each of these regional anesthetic techniques for postoperative analgesia, explain the procedure and offer pearls to improve the success of analgesia, discuss the benefits and potential complications of the use of each of these modalities, as well as review the literature and current evidence for their use in the postoperative period.

2. Thoracic Epidural Analgesia (TEA)

TEA is demonstrated to be a superior analgesic modality for major abdominal surgery. Unfortunately, it is not without risk of complications and side effects. More importantly, successful implementation of TEA requires additional technical skills and resources (equipment), appropriate education and training of physicians and support staff, as well as a well-defined framework for management (standing orders for infusion and management of side effects). Its role in postoperative care may even be more important in light of the evidence showing that it not only improves patient satisfaction due to excellent pain control, but also may have many other positive effects on postoperative outcomes (see below).

When approaching a patient undergoing major abdominal surgery, the actual procedure itself is but a small part of the process. A thorough discussion of indications and contraindications and counseling of the patient on possible complications and side effects should be performed. Once the decision is made to proceed with thoracic epidural analgesia, there are multiple decisions to be made to optimize analgesia, such as optimal level of thoracic epidural placement, patient positioning, amount and type of sedation, testing of epidural catheter for intravascular and intrathecal location, optimal bolus regimen, and optimal maintenance regimen. In addition, assessment of efficacy of the block and troubleshooting inadequate epidural blockade is crucial for improved patient pain relief and satisfaction.

http://dx.doi.org/10.5772/57403

3. Dermatomes and innervation of the viscera

Pain associated with major abdominal surgery can be divided into somatic pain and visceral pain. Therefore, when performing epidural analgesia, both the abdominal wall innervation and the afferent visceral innervation, must be targeted to provide optimal analgesia.

The innervation of the abdominal wall has a segmental dermatomal distribution and is supplied by the anterior and lateral cutaneous branches of the ventral rami of the seventh to twelfth intercostal nerves (T7-12). To provide analgesia to the abdominal wall using the least amount of analgesics in the epidural space, the optimal location for epidural placement is a thoracic epidural placed at the level of the mid-thoracic spine (T7-9) for upper abdominal surgery and low thoracic spine (T10-12) for lower abdominal surgery.

Lumbar epidural placement for thoracic surgery, although possibly providing some analgesic benefit, will result in unnecessarily higher requirements for local anesthetic and opioid dosages in the epidural space with a resultant increase in the incidence of side effects such as lower extremity weakness (lower extremities receive their sensory and motor innervation from the lumbar and sacral roots), and urinary retention.

Visceral pain does contribute to a smaller, but still substantial, portion of postoperative surgical pain. It is usually short lived with the exception of pancreatic surgery and is much less intense then somatic pain. Unfortunately, innervation of the viscera is complex. Visceral afferent fibers travel alongside both sympathetic and parasympathetic efferent nerves of the autonomic nervous system. Therefore, epidural analgesia will unlikely completely cover all visceral afferent pain fibers for affected organs.

Visceral organ	Innervation
Stomach/pancreas	Celiac ganglia (T5-9)
Liver	Celiac ganglia (T5-9) Phrenic ganglia (C3-5) Vagus nerve (CN XI)
Small and large intestine	Celiac ganglia (T5-9) Superior mesenteric ganglia (T9-12) Inferior mesenteric ganglia (L1-2) Vagus nerve (CN XI)
Kidneys and ureters	Least and lesser thoracic nerves (T10-12) Vagus nerve (CN XI)
Pelvic viscera	T11-L4
Bladder	Pelvic splanchnic nerves (S2-4) Upper lumbar splanchnic nerves (L1-2)

Table 1. Visceral innervation

Because of the complicated innervation of the viscera and the relatively smaller number of afferent fibers as compared to cutaneous innervation, the decision on the optimal level to place the continuous epidural blockade is mainly determined by the location of the incision on the abdominal wall.

Failure to achieve optimal analgesia with an epidural technique may be caused by several reasons; one, incorrect determination of nerve root level that is responsible for the pain (an example being the placement of a lumbar epidural for surgery of the abdomen), and two, inability to place the catheter in the epidural space despite choosing the correct level of placement. The first reason is less crucial because epidural spread of injectate will allow some degree of forgiveness in placement of the epidural catheter a few levels from the desired level. Occasionally a predominantly unilateral epidural sensory distribution can occur due to anatomical issues (rare) or due to exit of the epidural catheter through the neuroforamina. Even despite optimal placement of the epidural catheter, analgesia could be suboptimal due to inappropriate dosing, pump failure or pharmacy delays. Because epidural dosing is somewhat empirical, frequent follow up is required for optimization, and top ups or patient-controlled epidural analgesia may be necessary to achieve improved pain control. Occasionally, epidural dosing is limited by the patient's inability to tolerate hypotension or other side effects. And finally, inadvertent dislodgment of catheter will result in failure of this analgesic modality.

4. Identifying the epidural space

Inability to identify the epidural space is a significant source of failure for TEA with major abdominal surgery. Compared to the lumbar epidural space, the thoracic epidural space, though more continuous, is variable in its width, roughly 7.5 mm in the upper thoracic region and 4.1 mm at T11-12 [11]. Approaches to placement of continuous TEA blocks consist of midline or paramedian approaches, both with drawbacks. The midline approach is performed with the needle entry point at the midline of the spinous processes, thus minimizing need for medial or lateral needle angulation. The paramedian approach is performed with a needle entry point lateral to midline and can be used to avoid bony contact with the spinous processes for ease of access to the epidural space.

The midline approach allows for minimal medial-to-lateral displacement of the needle. In young patients with minimal loss of disk height, and at the upper and lower thoracic region where the spinous processes are not as angulated, the midline approach is relatively simple to perform. Between T5 and T9, the spinous processes are more angulated, and midline approaches require greater cephalad angulation of the needle and greater needle depths to successfully identify the epidural space. If the needle entry point is not optimal, identification of the epidural space may be extremely difficult (Figure 1). In addition, the ligamentum flavum does not fuse midline in all patients, such that the feeling of resistance as the needle traverses this structure is not reliably noted, resulting in a more subtle change in resistance during the loss of resistance technique. Lirk and colleagues noted that the incidence of midline ligamentum flavum gaps is 2-5% at the level of T6 to T9, 17.9% at T9 to T10, and approximately 30% at T10 to T12 [12]. Successful midline approach depends on optimal patient position to "open up" the space between spinous processes, so it may be less suitable when positioning is limited (such as when TEA is performed postoperatively in a patient in severe pain). Also, steep needle angulations will require greater needle depths, even in less obese patients. Unlike the paramedian approach where depth is predictable once lamina is contacted, the midline approach requires experience to estimate the potential depth. Midline approaches in patients with rotation of the spine or a patient in a lateral decubitus position may be difficult for the novice as the needle trajectory may deviate away from the interspinous ligament, resulting in a false loss of resistance.

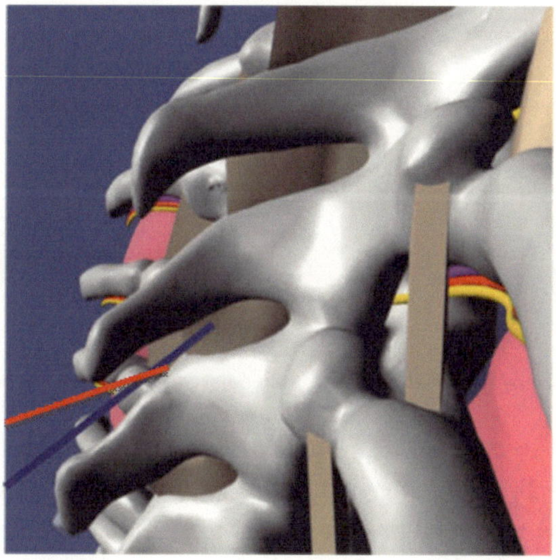

Figure 1. Two spinous processes with needle entry point at superior aspect (red line) and inferior aspect (blue line) of the space between spinous processes showing that the inferior aspect results in more successful placement midline

The paramedian approach allows for shallower needle depths, less cephalad needle angulation, and more consistency in the presence of the ligamentum flavum when compared to the midline approach. In addition, the lamina is utilized as a reliable deep marker for the identification of the epidural space. This approach is also less dependent on optimal patient positioning and is usually technically easier when done with the patient in the lateral decubitus position. However, determination of optimal medial angulation of the needle may be difficult and the thickness of ligamentum flavum decreases the further lateral the approach. Therefore, ideally, the needle tip should enter the epidural space as close to midline as possible. Traditionally, needle insertion occurs approximately 1 cm lateral to the spinous process, and how medial of an angle the needle is directed depends on the depth of the epidural space (Figure 2).

If medial angulation is too great, the needle may cross midline to the contralateral side, resulting in not only a false loss of resistance, but also complications such as pneumothorax. The extra manipulation along the transverse dimension adds a degree of difficulty to the

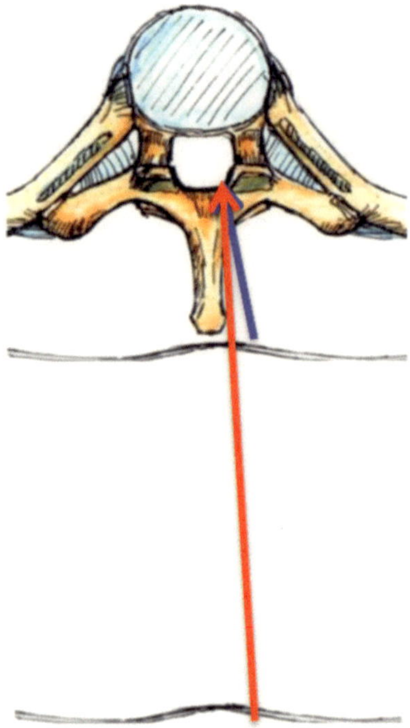

Figure 2. Obese patient and skinny patient and anticipated medial needle angulation

paramedian approach. An alternative approach to minimize the need for medial angulation is a paraspinous approach, where the needle entry point is only slightly lateral (~3mm) to the spinous process. In this technique, no or minimal medial angulation is required and the spinous process can be avoided along the needle trajectory (Figure 3).

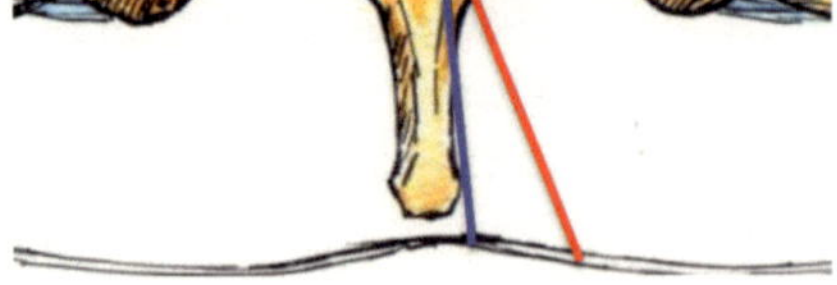

Figure 3. Paraspinous approach, blue line demonstrates the trajectory of the paraspinous process, red line demonstrates trajectory of a paramedian approach with more medial angulation of the needle

5. Using live fluoroscopy, existing CT scan imaging and ultrasound to guide needle depth and entry point

Live fluoroscopy can be helpful in patients with difficult spine anatomy, but is impractical due to availability of equipment and concerns about radiation exposure.

The use of existing CT scan imaging to determine the depth of the epidural space can give the proceduralist a more informed expectation of depth of needle insertion, leading to higher success rates (Figure 4). Indeed, estimates of needle depth are more accurate when using a paramedian approach with a needle trajectory where the needle requires minimal angulation. The optimal needle insertion point on the skin occurs when a needle that is perpendicularly oriented in the parasagittal plane to the skin is advanced, the tip lies on the superior surface of the lamina, such that only a slight cephalad angulation is required to access the interlaminar space.

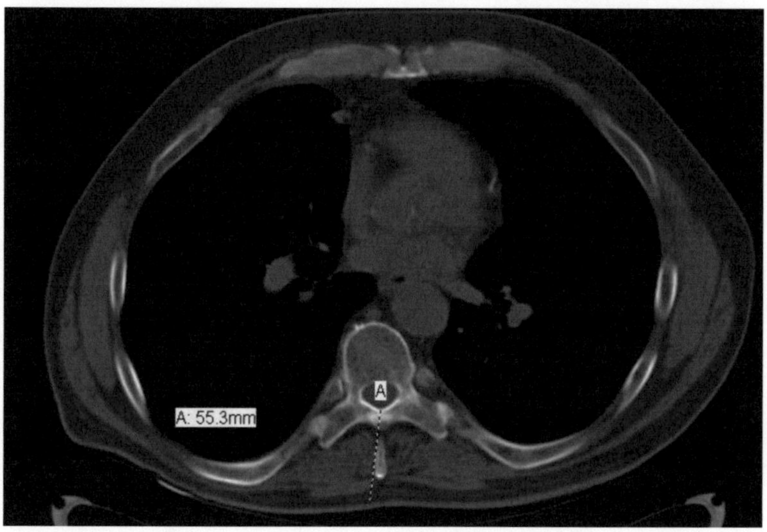

Figure 4. Measurement of depth of epidural space on CT scan

Another imaging modality that may assist with improved success of epidural space identification includes the use of ultrasound. When oriented in a transverse plane, the ultrasound may allow the proceduralist to determine midline accurately in patients whose landmarks are not palpable. The parasagittal view may be used to identify the correct level of insertion and the superior and inferior border of the lamina, to identify the optimal site of needle entry (Figure 5).

Alternatively the inferior border of the transverse process may be used as a second landmark to estimate a skin projection of the optimal spot on the lamina for initial needle placement for subsequent "walk off" into the epidural space. Ultrasound may also assist in determining the depth of the lamina and epidural space. However, care must be taken not to apply too much pressure to the ultrasound probe on the skin, leading to a falsely shallow estimated distance.

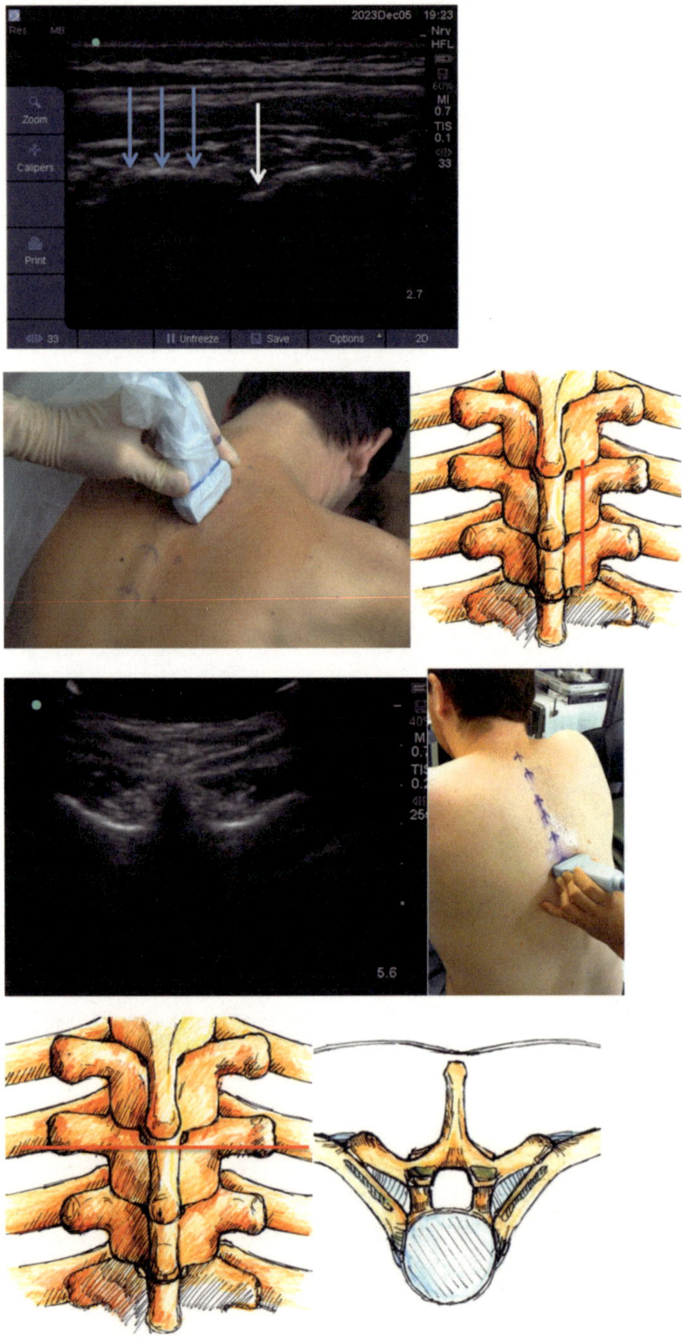

Figure 5. Ultrasound images of the spinous process, lamina and transverse processes; a. parasagittal view of the lamina, blue arrows indicate lamina, white arrow indicates interlaminar space, b. diagram showing the orientation of ultrasound probe for parasagittal view of the lamina line), c. transverse view of the spinous process, lamina, and transverse processes, d. diagram showing the orientation of the ultrasound probe for the transverse view of the spine (red line)

Ultrasound may also help to determine the largest interspace for ease of access. Although ultrasound imaging may assist with determining optimal location to proceed with epidural catheter placement, live ultrasound-guided needle placement is not widely used in clinical practice due to the need for an extra set of hands to stabilize the probe and concerns regarding the unknown effect of inadvertent transference of ultrasound gel into epidural space.

6. Indications and contraindications

Indications for use of TEA include major open abdominal surgery in which moderate-to-severe pain is expected to last more than 24 hours. This can include open procedures such as abdominal aortic aneurysm repair, Whipple procedures, bowel surgery, large ventral hernia repair, cholecystectomy, major gynecologic surgery, nephrectomy, and cystectomy. Surgeries such as pheochromocytoma resection, in which catecholamine surges may result in life-threatening blood pressure and heart rate swings may also benefit from the use of TEA to blunt the catecholamine release to surgical stimulation. Hepatectomy results in significant pain. However, the use of epidural anesthesia should be balanced against the need to reduce bleeding at the surgical site using measures such as volume restriction. Although most patients with hepatic surgery tend to be hypercoagulable postoperatively, large liver resections may result in a reduced ability to produce vitamin K dependent factors for coagulation and subsequent potential for excessive risk of catastrophic bleeding in the spinal canal with possible spinal cord compression.

There is a subset of patients that particularly benefit from the use of TEA. Patients with pulmonary comorbidities and patients with obstructive sleep apnea may benefit from the opioid sparing effects of TEA and the decreased risk of respiratory depression. In patients with chronic pain or who consume high dose opioids and are tolerant to opioids, TEA may allow for more effective analgesia.

Contraindications to TEA have been traditionally labeled as absolute and relative. Absolute contraindications to TEA include placement of neuraxial block at the peak effect of a potent anticoagulant or when the patient is at risk of bleeding due to other reasons such as profound thrombocytopenia or hemophilia, patient refusal, and localized infection along the trajectory of the needle. Frequently, the medical decision to perform a TEA is not as straightforward, and the risk-to-benefit ratio must be determined to provide the patient with a more thorough informed consent.

Relative contraindications to TEA include placing the epidural in patients who are febrile or immunosuppressed or in patients who have a true local anesthetic allergy, metastatic lesions to the spine, intracranial hypertension, planned postoperative anticoagulation, severe hypovolemia, aortic stenosis, neurologic disorders such as multiple sclerosis, or in patients at risk of masking unrelated complications (patients with multiple traumatic injuries who require frequent neurologic assessment of the lower extremity or patients at risk for anterior spinal cord syndrome after open thoracoabdominal aneurysm repair). With regards to the febrile patient, more concerning is whether elevated temperatures are a result of bacteremia and if traumatic needle placements may introduce pathogens directly into the subarachnoid space and place the patient at risk for meningitis. Observational studies of lumbar punctures in febrile patients have not demonstrated increased risk of meningitis, though expert opinion recommends caution with neuraxial procedures in patients with bacteremia.

Despite thorough preoperative planning and weighing of the benefits and risks of TEA, difficult scenarios may still arise. For example, an epidural that is placed preoperatively in a patient with no contraindication for neuraxial blockade who develops an intraoperative myocardial infarction and requires an anti-platelet agent or thrombin inhibitor after placement of a coronary stent presents a difficult situation in which clinical judgment as to the optimal postoperative management of the epidural catheter is tested.

7. Benefits and effectiveness

Thoracic epidural anesthesia and analgesia can result in significantly lower pain scores at rest and with movement during major open abdominal aortic surgery [13]. This degree of analgesia was found to last until postoperative day 3. The benefits of TEA extend beyond patient comfort and analgesia. The authors also noted a decreased incidence of myocardial infarction, acute respiratory failure and continued need for postoperative mechanical ventilation, gastrointestinal complications and renal complications.

Blockade of the cardiac sympathetic fibers arising from T1 to T5 has been demonstrated to reduce heart rate, mean arterial pressure and myocardial contractility. This reduction in cardiac work results in decreased myocardial oxygen consumption. Coronary insufficiency, demonstrated by electrocardiography, echocardiography, and angiography, is reduced by TEA [14].

Interestingly, although blockade of sympathetic fibers may result in predominant parasympathetic tone and lead to increased bronchomotor activity of the lungs, asthmatic episodes have decreased with use of TEA. This is speculated to be due to reduced afferent input. In addition, the use of epidural analgesia spares the amount of opioids required to achieve adequate analgesia, reducing opioid-related side effects, most notably sedation and respiratory depression.

The stress response to major surgical insult has been shown to be reduced by predominantly blocking the efferent and afferent pathways to the adrenal medulla. A thoracic epidural blockade of T6 to L1 results in a blunted catecholamine response and decreased cortisol levels [14].

Improved gut motility with the use of TEA has been documented to reduce postoperative ileus in bowel surgery by approximately 12 hours [15]. This improved gut motility may be attributed

http://dx.doi.org/10.5772/57403

to the reduced sympathetic tone and sparing of the parasympathetic tone (vagus nerve) in the gastrointestinal tract as well as reduction in postoperative opioids, which have been known to cause gastric dysmotility. In addition, blockade of the splanchnic nerves T6-L1 may reduce vascular resistance, allowing for pooling of blood in the gut [14]. If systemic blood pressures are maintained, this can result in improved perfusion of the bowel mucosa.

New exciting data about the possible reduction of cancer recurrence with intraoperative dosing and postoperative maintenance of thoracic epidural catheters after different types of oncologic surgery is appearing in the literature. However, at this time, most human data is retrospective in nature.

8. Side effects

The side effects of continuous epidural infusion are mostly specific to the medications used. Most commonly, local anesthetic and opioids are delivered through the epidural space, and their combined use allows for improved analgesia with less doses of each.

Local anesthetic in the epidural compartment results in a sympathectomy. Vasodilation, especially of the splanchnic circulation, results in a relative reduction in preload as the intravascular volume is redistributed, resulting in hypotension. This effect is especially noticeable in patients who undergo bowel preps in anticipation of surgery of the gastrointestinal tract, who are already intravascularly depleted prior to epidural placement. In addition, dense concentrations of local anesthetic will also result not only in blockade of pain but in sensory and motor changes. Although sensory changes may be even desired, motor changes may detrimentally affect the patient. Low thoracic epidurals have the ability to anesthetize the muscles of the lower extremity. Proximal motor function, such as hip flexion, can be affected if epidural spread reaches the upper lumbar roots. Midthoracic epidural catheter placements with low volume infusions of local anesthetic will mostly affect intercostal and abdominal muscles. The motor effects on these muscles have not appreciatively affected the patient's ability to cough.

Respiratory depression and sedation can also occur [16]. Two types of respiratory depression, early and late, each with a different mechanism have been described. The most feared complication is delayed respiratory depression that may occur 12-24 hours after epidural administration of hydrophilic opioids (morphine) due to rostral migration of the drug into the cerebral spinal fluid, which can be especially concerning if patient's ventilation status is not closely monitored. With use of more lipophilic opioids such as sufentanil in the epidural space, plasma concentrations may increase shortly after bolus administration of the drug and reach levels high enough to cause systemic effects with early respiratory depression [17, 18]. Overall, respiratory depression with use of opioid medications is higher with the intravenous as opposed to the epidural route of administration.

Urinary retention appears to be related more to local anesthetic and less to opioid use. Post-void residuals were noted to be more affected by epidural bupivacaine as opposed to epidural fentanyl, even at the thoracic epidural level [19]. Despite this effect, the absence of a bladder catheterization in a patient with an epidural infusion of low concentration local anesthetic and opioid has not resulted in an increased need for repeat catheterization of the bladder. In addition, the early removal of bladder catheters has resulted in a decreased incidence of urinary tract infections [20].

	Opioids	**Local Anesthetics**
Respiratory	Depression	Usually no depression
Cardiovascular	No reduction in Blood Pressure	Postural hypotension Reduced heart rate w/ high block
Sedation	Yes	Mild/absent
Nausea/Vomiting	Yes	Uncommon
Pruritus	Yes	No
Motor	No effect	Block
Sensation	No effect	Block
Urinary retention	Yes	Yes
GI	Decreased motility	Increased motility

Table 2. Comparison of side effects of epidural opioid and local anesthetics

9. Epidural management

To provide safe care to the patient that will undergo TEA, the procedure is preferably performed 30-60 minutes prior to surgery with the patient optimally positioned in the sitting position and ASA monitors attached in a dedicated block area. Supplemental oxygen is provided and judicious sedation is given to allow for patient feedback and block assessment immediately after the procedure. Aseptic technique using sterile gown, gloves and mask as well as chloraprep skin disinfecting and draping is preferable to reduce the risk of infection. The use of soft-tipped epidural catheters is preferable to reduce the potential perforation of epidural veins and resistance to advancement when a false loss of resistance occurs. There is unlikely a clinical difference in the use of single or multiple orifice catheters. Advancement of the catheter to approximately 5 cm past the needle tip will allow for adequate, but not excessive length of the catheter and avoid the potential for knotting. Meticulous attention to taping with use of adhesives such as mastizol is important to prevent premature dislodgement of the catheter. Special tapes are available that have reduced the incidence of catheter migration (Sorbaview, Centurion Medical Products, Michigan).

After confirming lack of intravascular and subarachnoid placement of the catheter, dosing of the catheter with local anesthetics such as ropivacaine 0.5 or 0.75% could be used in 3-5 ml increments to achieve a band of anesthesia in the area of surgery. Smaller boluses (3 mL) or shorter acting agents (lidocaine) can be used when the risk of immediate hypotension (frail patient after bowel preparation) or risk for significant intraoperative bleeding is high. (Usually, a 3-5 ml test dose of lidocaine is enough to confirm epidural position and may result in 3-8 dermatomal levels of spread. Occasionally, intravenous fluid boluses or use of ephedrine (including subcutaneous or intramuscular injection) may be needed to maintain stable hemodynamics. Before the time of induction in the operating room, injection of 100 micrograms of fentanyl into the epidural space will provide analgesia without further effects on hemodynamics. The onset of epidural fentanyl is 10 minutes, and despite the fact that fentanyl is lipophilic, a large dose results in significant CSF concentrations. Additionally, the use of vasoconstrictors in the epidural space increases the fraction of fentanyl in the neuraxial space and provides segmental analgesia for several hours. Determining the patient response to the initial test dose and boluses allows the clinician to better anticipate the effects and determine the optimal postoperative epidural prescription. At the author's institution, the standard infusion is ropivacaine 0.2% at a basal rate of 6 to 8 ml per hour with a PCEA bolus of 4 ml every 30 minutes. All patients have standing orders for intravenous opioids as rescue analgesics. Infusions are immediately initiated at induction with top ups of ropivacaine 0.5% 30 minutes prior to emergence from anesthesia. Dedicated members of an Acute Pain Service assess the patients immediately after surgery for presence or absence of epidural analgesia and the need for further dosing of the epidural catheter. These assessments are performed by physicians who also review the patient's volume status and the need for additional fluids or vasopressors.

For the same volume and dose of local anesthetic, the effect is greater with the use of TEA than with lumbar epidural and definitely more than with thoracic paravertebral analgesia. Even a 3 ml test dose of lidocaine 1.5% with epinephrine 1:200, 000 can result in a 3-4 dermatome effect, as demonstrated by loss of the patient's ability to detect cold. The volume of local anesthetic infusion depends on the extent of the surgery. Bolus dosing leads to greater spread of volume in the epidural space as compared with basal infusion. Manual bolus usually results in better spread than bolus dosing through the pump due to higher injection pressures.

The optimal drug regimen in the epidural space would provide optimal analgesia and minimize the risks associated with the medications used. Due to the reduced risk of cardiovascular toxicity with improved sensory-motor differentiation, ropivacaine 0.2-0.3% is the preferred local anesthetic at the author's institution. Use of shorter duration local anesthetics may allow for faster titration of epidural effect, but may result in tachyphylaxis and rapid offset when discontinued and requires close nurse monitoring to reduce gaps in analgesia during bag changes. Bupivacaine is a good alternative, but results in greater motor blockade and makes assessment of whether lower extremity weakness is due to excess local anesthetic or epidural hematoma more difficult. Bupivacaine is less costly and can be safer when used only for infusions at low concentrations to avoid potentially catastrophic local anesthetic systemic toxicity (LAST).

Opioids may be used to reduce the local anesthetic dose required to provide analgesia. Higher concentrations of opioids may result in noticeable sedation and respiratory depression in patients and should be used with caution in elderly patients and patients with obstructive sleep apnea or other pulmonary comorbidities. Morphine, hydromorphone, fentanyl and sufentanil are all reasonable alternatives for epidural analgesia. The addition of systemic opioids or other sedatives in addition to the use of neuraxial opioids has resulted in significant respiratory depression and sedation and is discouraged for opioid naïve patients.

Unfortunately, there is no data for the ideal prescription or medication combination. Different institutions use different local anesthetics and opioids in different combinations at different concentrations. In general, the total dose is more important than the concentration. (Tables 3, 4, 5) The addition of epinephrine (usual concentration 2 mcg/ml) in the infusion decreases systemic absorption of drugs delivered epidurally and increases the transfer of the drugs to the subarachnoid space with improved analgesia.

Opioid	Bolus Dose	Onset	Peak	Duration	Infusion Dose	Lipid Solubility
Morphine	1-6mg	20-30mins	30-60mins	10-24hrs	0.1-0.75mg/hr	1
Hydromorphone	1-2mg	10-20mins	20-30mins	5-15hrs	0.1-0.5mg/hr	1.5
Fentanyl	25-100mcg	5-10mins	10-20mins	1-5hrs	25-100mcg/hr	800
Sufentanil	10-50mcg	5-10mins	10-15mins	1-5hrs	10-50mcg/hr	1800

Table 3. Epidural Opioids

Morphine
PO – 30mg
IM – 10mg
Epidural – 2-3mg
Intrathecal – 0.2-0.3mg

Table 4. Equianalgesic dose of morphine based on route of administration

Drug	Bolus dose	Lockout interval (min)	Background infusion
Morphine	0.2 mg	10 min	+/- 0.4 mg/hr
Hydromorphone	0.15-0.3 mg	15-30 min	
Fentanyl	15-50 mcg	5-15 min	+/- 50-100 mcg/hr
Sufentanil	4 mcg	6 min	+/- 8 mcg/hr

Table 5. Opioid analgesic prescription for TEA

http://dx.doi.org/10.5772/57403

Unfortunately, with the increased productivity and time constraints of a busy hospital setting, it is not uncommon to use standard manufacturer-prepared bags with predetermined mixtures of local anesthetics and opioids to provide easy and uninterrupted flow of drugs for continuous epidural analgesia. The use of standardized prescriptions also helps to minimize drug errors.

In the author's institution, the preference is to have only local anesthetic in the epidural infusion as a standard infusion with the delivery of opioids intravenously as a rescue analgesic. This allows for the flexibility by all services to provide for parenteral opioids without cumulative opioid effects from the epidural, and allows for satisfactory alternative analgesia should the TEA not provide complete coverage. In addition, in the opioid naïve patient, should the patient develop intolerable side effects from opioids, the time to symptom resolution after discontinuation of intravenous opioids is much shorter than with neuraxial opioids. Not uncommonly, patients achieve excellent analgesia with local anesthetics as the sole epidural medication with the addition of non-opioid adjuncts such as acetaminophen or non-steroidal anti-inflammatory agents. Most benefits of TEA are usually from the use of epidural local anesthetics and not opioids. Occasionally, patients, such as those with chronic pain, will need both epidural and intravenous opioids for optimal analgesia.

10. Discontinuation and step down analgesia

The optimal duration of epidural analgesia should include the period of time that expected pain would be moderate to severe in intensity. The avoidance of intravenous opioids may allow for earlier return of bowel function and reduce their negative effects, such as sedation and respiratory depression. Therefore, use of epidural analgesia until at least the third postoperative day, or until return of bowel function, allows optimization of this analgesia modality. Weaning trials should be attempted prior to removal to avoid premature discontinuation of the epidural. The severity of postoperative pain has many variables such as extent of surgery and the patient's tolerance of pain.

Analgesic adjuncts such as acetaminophen, non-steroidal anti-inflammatory drugs, and systemic opioids may be considered in addition to epidural analgesia. These medications can and should be considered on an individual basis depending on patient comorbidities such as pulmonary or renal dysfunction.

Patients with chronic pain who are on pre-existent opioid therapy require continuation of systemic opioids. In addition, pain outside of the distribution of the epidural spread, such as headache and low back pain, will not be improved by thoracic epidural analgesia, and systemic analgesics would be needed for patient comfort. The use of NMDA antagonists such as ketamine, anti-spasmodic agents, and benzodiazepines can be considered for the patient, but their use may lead to further central effects and worsening sedation.

Epidural management should be tailored to the individual patient to provide effective analgesia. Routine and frequent follow-up and adjustments of medications, concentrations, and volumes improve satisfaction with analgesia and is key to providing effective analgesia. In addition, consistent follow-up allows for early detection and management of complications.

11. Complications

Complications of TEA include post-dural puncture headache (PDPH) with inadvertent dural puncture. The rate of dural puncture is operator dependent. The incidence of PDPH after an inadvertent dural puncture with a large bore epidural needle is nearly 70-80% with the incidence of chronic headaches 28% [21]. Regardless, patients demonstrating signs of PDPH will have difficulties with ambulation and rehabilitation.

Unrecognized intrathecal catheter placement may result in high spinals. Neurologic injury from thoracic epidural placement is predominantly attributed to neuraxial hematoma or infection (meningitis or epidural abscess) although spinal cord ischemia, direct needle trauma or chemical toxicity also occur [22].

Because the increase in incidence of neuraxial hematomas after the introduction of the low-molecular weight heparin enoxaparin in the United States in 1993, guidelines on the placement of neuraxial blocks in the anticoagulated patient were introduced and updated periodically. These guidelines are based on existing cases of neuraxial hematomas and aid the physicians in determining the optimal time from anticoagulant dose to epidural placement and removal. Patients with higher susceptibility to neuraxial hematoma includes the elderly female patient, possibly from the increased incidence of spinal stenosis and reduced tolerance to similar volumes of blood near the spinal column. However, the incidence of neuraxial hematoma in a patient without abnormal hemostasis is low [23].

Major surgery negatively impacts postoperative immune status. Therefore, infectious risks such as localized infection and epidural abscess from epidural catheterization occur. While epidemiologic studies are few, a study in Denmark estimated the incidence of epidural abscess to be 1:1930 epidural catheters [24]. Adherence to aseptic technique and routine assessment of catheter site is imperative to avoid this complication.

12. Thoracic paravertebral analgesia

12.1. Anatomy

The paravertebral space is a potential space that, when filled with fluid (e.g. local anesthetic), becomes wedge-shaped. It is bordered by: anteriorly, the parietal pleura; medially, the posterolateral vertebral body, the vertebral disc, and the vertebral foramen and spinal nerve; posteriorly, the superior costotransverse ligament (SCTL); laterally, the posterior intercostal membrane and the intercostal space; superiorly/inferiorly, the heads and necks of the ribs. The SCTL runs obliquely from the transverse process superiorly to the rib below inferiorly. It is slightly more superficial superiorly and is slightly denser laterally (Figure 6).

The paravertebral spaces of the cervical and thoracic regions communicate, but there is unpredictable spread of local anesthetic. Large-volume (15-20 ml) boluses of local anesthetics will usually spread 1 or 2 levels cephalad and caudad but may remain within the level injected [25]. MRI study of the paravertebral spread of 20 ml of 1% mepivacaine with contrast demonstrated fairly consistent spread of contrast dye 1 level cephalad and 3 levels caudad to the

http://dx.doi.org/10.5772/57403

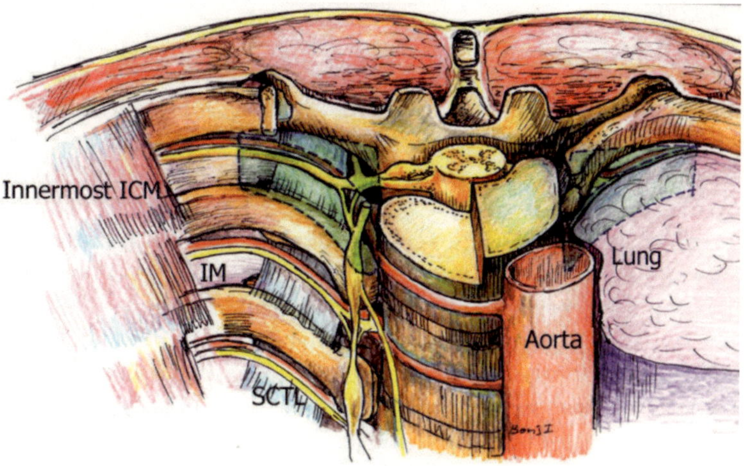

Figure 6. The median distance from skin to paravertebral space is 5.5 cm, with greater depth in the upper (T1-3) and lower (T9-12) thoracic regions (WR). Body habitus significantly influences the depth to this space, which can be measured using ultrasound.

level of injection. However, the number of sensory dermatomes affected by this block was highly variable [26]. If more than 4 levels of spread are desired, multiple injections should be performed to improve analgesic distribution of local anesthetic. For major abdominal surgery, bilateral paravertebral catheters should be used.

12.2. Technique

Multiple techniques may be used to identify the paravertebral space. Loss of resistance, nerve stimulation, and ultrasound may be used individually or in combination.

12.3. Identification of point of insertion

12.3.1. Palpation

The patient is ideally positioned seated with the neck and back flexed and the shoulders relaxed. Alternatively, the patient may be positioned lateral decubitus. The spinous processes of the thoracic vertebrae are level with the transverse process (TP) of the next lower vertebra. After palpation of the spinous process, the needle entry point should be made 2.5 cm lateral to the superior aspect of the spinous process. (As an example, a T7 paravertebral block is desired, then the needle entry point would be 2.5 cm lateral to the superior aspect of the T6 spinous process.) Landmark identification does not require any special equipment, however, there is considerable interpatient and intrapatient variability in the location of the TP relative to the spinous process. For example, the upper thoracic TPs are longer and have a more cephalad angulation. Needle insertion too medial can result in contact with the lamina, and too lateral insertion would put the needle in contact with the rib or pleura. Where TPs are angled more cephalad, standard landmark identification can result in needle placement between TPs, increasing the risk of pneumothorax.

12.3.2. Ultrasound (Figure 7)

Ultrasound can assist with accurate identification of the level to be blocked and assessment of depth from skin to the transverse process and to pleura. A linear, high-frequency probe can be used for thin patients and curvilinear, low frequency probes may be needed for larger patients. Once the level of entry is identified, the probe is placed in a transverse orientation such that the tip of the spinous process, lamina, transverse process and ribs are identified. The lateral aspect of the TP is centered on the screen and the skin is marked, representing the lateral entry point. Care should be taken not to tilt the probe excessively cephalad or caudad. The probe should be completely perpendicular to the skin with equal pressure on both ends of the probe. The probe is then placed in a parasaggital orientation approximately 5cm from midline and slid medially, looking for the transition from rib to TP, which should be where the lateral mark is made. The TP is more superficial than the rib and will be seen as a "step-up" on the screen. Ribs are also more rounded, and the TP have a square contour. The ultrasound is positioned such that the inferior aspect of the TP is centered. Again, the US probe must be perpendicular to the skin with equal pressure applied to both ends of the ultrasound probe. The skin is then marked where the center of the probe lies (at the inferior edge of the TP). This mark represents the vertical entry point for the needle. Release of excessive pressure from the probe allows for accurate determination of depth of TP and pleura from skin. Extension of the marks for lateral and vertical entry points should create an intersected point for optimal needle entry. The block may then proceed as described below using either loss of resistance or nerve stimulation as endpoints. Ultrasound can be especially useful in obese patients without palpable landmarks but image quality decreases with increasing depth to TPV space. Ultrasound used as a "rescue" technique can be limited if loss of resistance (LOR) to air is used from prior attempts due to image distortion from subcutaneous air.

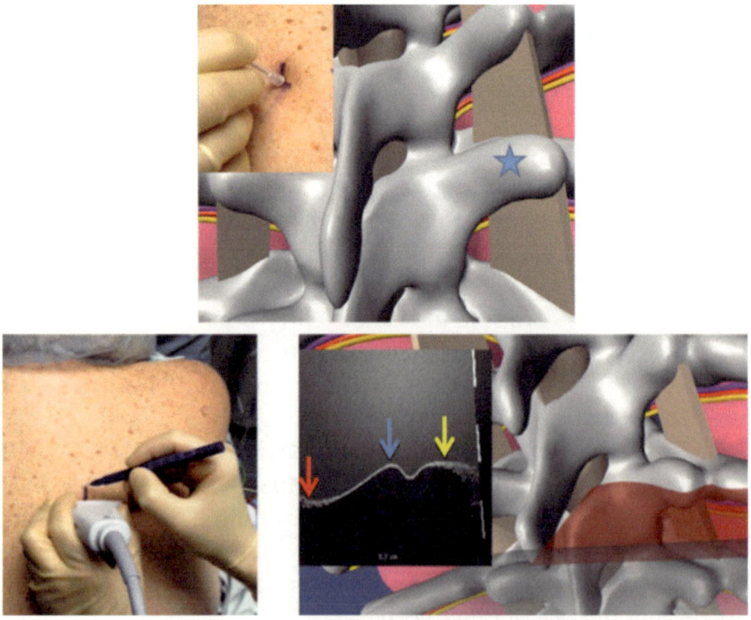

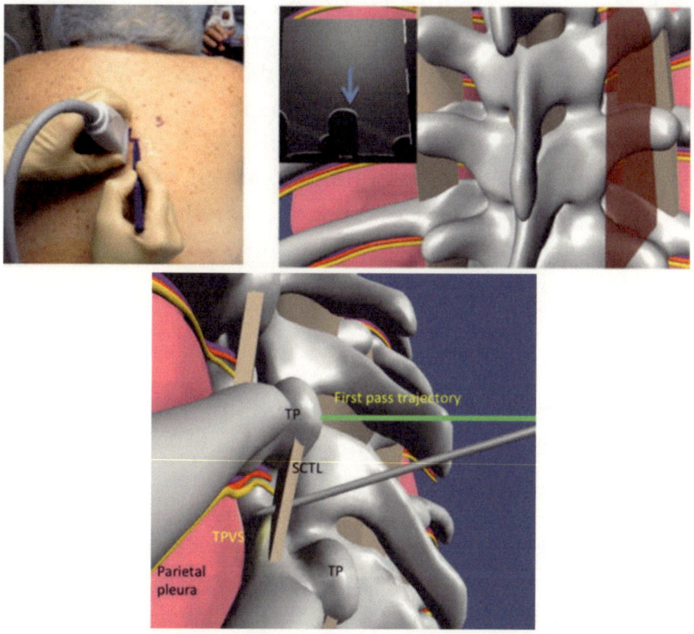

Figure 7. Ultrasound identification of transverse process: a. The star represents the desired entry point of the needle, which is directly over the transverse process, b. Initially, a transverse probe orientation allows the proceduralist to identify the most lateral aspect of the TP and where it contacts rib. Lamina (red arrow), lateral aspect of TP (blue arrow) and rib (yellow arrow) are shown. In the simulated image of the spine, the red shade represents the slice of tissue that is on the ultrasound image, c. Next, a parasaggital probe orientation allows visualization of the transverse processes. The inferior aspect of the TP is placed at the center of the length of the probe in anticipation of walking the needle caudad to the TP. Blue arrow designates desired point needle tip contact with bone. On ultrasound image, left is cephalad, right is caudad. In the simulated image of the spine, the red shade represents the slice of tissue that is seen on the ultrasound image. d. Placement of the initial needle tip on inferior aspect of the TP allows minimal needle angulation caudad to access TPV space.

13. Paravertebral space endpoints

13.1. Loss of resistance

The needle is advanced through the skin in the parasagittal plane until bone is contacted. Maintaining the needle in a strictly parasagittal direction decreases the risk of neuraxial complications, which are increased with medial angulation of the needle, and pneumothorax, which are more likely to occur with lateral needle angulation. With use of surface landmarks and palpation (instead of US) to identify surface landmarks, needle depth from skin to TP is not measured. This distance, however, may be anticipated, although estimates of needle depth may be less accurate if the proceduralist has had less experience. However, if bone (TP) is not contacted at an expected and appropriate depth, the needle is withdrawn and angled slightly cephalad, and if not, caudad, until contact with bone is made. In general, in the average 70kg patient, bone contact should occur at a depth of 2-4 cm. The authors, however, encourage the use of ultrasound to determine depth of TP and pleura to assist the proceduralist in more accurate estimations of TP, thoracic paravertebral space, and pleura to minimize both failures and excessively deep needle placements (pneumothorax). As the paravertebral space is approximately 1 cm deep to the TP, the needle is then grasped 1 cm from the skin, withdrawn to the subcutaneous tissue, and angled caudally. With a LOR syringe attached, the needle is advanced until LOR is attained, being careful not to advance beyond the depth marked by finger-grasp. Once the paravertebral space is entered and following negative aspiration of air, blood or cerebral spinal fluid, local anesthetic with epinephrine is injected and/or a catheter is threaded into the paravertebral space.

13.2. Nerve stimulator

Alternatively, nerve stimulation can be used as an endpoint. With a nerve stimulator set at 2 Hz frequency, 0.3 msec pulse duration and an amplitude of 3-5 mA, a stimulating needle is advanced as with the LOR technique. Paraspinal muscle contractions are frequently observed superficial to the TPV as the needle is advanced. These twitches are no longer observed once the needle advances through the superior costotransverse ligament into the paravertebral space. At this point intercostal muscle or abdominal muscle contractions can be observed, or palpated in the obese patient. In a fully awake or lightly sedated patient, a thumping sensation may be reported by the patient. The electrical current is then decreased to 0.8mA with small needle manipulations if necessary to retain desired muscle contraction. Local anesthetic is then injected or a catheter is inserted through the needle, but needle manipulation to maintain motor stimulation with a stimulating catheter is not necessary and may lead to increased risk of pleural puncture.

13.3. Ultrasound

For ultrasound assisted block placement, ultrasound may be used after LOR or nerve stimulation (NS) to confirm correct needle/catheter placement by observing anterior displacement of the parietal pleura as local anesthetic is injected. Ultrasound can also be used to confirm absence of pneumothorax after the procedure.

Ultrasound-guided placement, which means constant visualization of the needle during placement into the paravertebral space, requires greater skill and experience with ultrasound (Figure 8). There are two main orientations for holding the ultrasound probe, parasagittal and axial, as well as two approaches with the needle, in-plane and out-of-plane. The preferred technique at the authors' institution is a parasagittal probe orientation with the inferior and lateral aspect of the transverse process centered on the screen. Using an out-of-plane technique, the needle is advanced perpendicular to the skin about 2-3 mm from the probe with minimal medial angulation. Tissue deflection can be seen as the needle is advanced. The depth of the TP on the US screen is noted and the needle is advanced no further 5mm from the anticipated depth of TP, eliciting contact with bone. Then the US probe is placed down and the needle is walked off in a caudad direction as above. Alternatively, an oblique parasaggital view can be obtained (Figure 8) with the cephalad aspect of the probe just slightly medial and the caudad aspect of the probe slightly lateral. An in-plane approach can be utilized. However, needle visualization can be tricky, and this in-plane approach is recommended for more advanced proceduralists. In addition, the in-plane technique is more suitable for non-obese patients as image resolution at greater depths may be suboptimal.

14. Indications/Contraindications

Thoracic paravertebral analgesia may be used as an alternative to epidural analgesia for all surgery of the trunk. Unilateral thoracic paravertebral blocks may be performed for thoracotomy and breast surgery while bilateral thoracic paravertebral blocks can be performed for open abdominal surgery. Bilateral thoracic paravertebral blocks for hepatectomy allow for analgesia with a reduced incidence of sympathectomy. Bilateral thoracic paravertebral blocks can also be used as a backup plan for patients who are at a higher risk for epidural hematoma (anticoagulated patient) or for patients in which the epidural space cannot be identified. However, to achieve nearly the same analgesic distribution as epidural analgesia, a higher volume and more bolus dosing is usually required.

Contraindications to the use of thoracic paravertebral analgesia are similar to those of epidural analgesia, but with a lower (but not zero) risk of inadvertent dural puncture and epidural hematoma. Patient refusal and infection along the trajectory of the needle tract remain absolute contraindications.

Contraindication	Rationale
Severe coagulopathy	While the paravertebral space is distensible, it is not easily compressed if bleeding does occur
Systemic infection	Risk of introducing infection into the paravertebral space, especially when not or inadequately treated prior to anticipated TPV placement
Tumor along anticipated needle trajectory	Risk of tumor "seeding"
Previous ipsilateral thoracic surgery	Risk of altered tissue planes due to scarring, especially if use loss of resistance technique is planned

Table 6. Relative contraindications

15. Benefits/Efficacy

There is growing use of bilateral paravertebral nerve blocks as an alternative to neuraxial techniques for analgesia in patients in whom neuraxial catheters are contraindicated or difficult.

Due to the lower risk of hypotension compared to epidural from a decreased sympathectomy, continuous paravetebral blocks may be preferable when hemodynamic instability is antici-

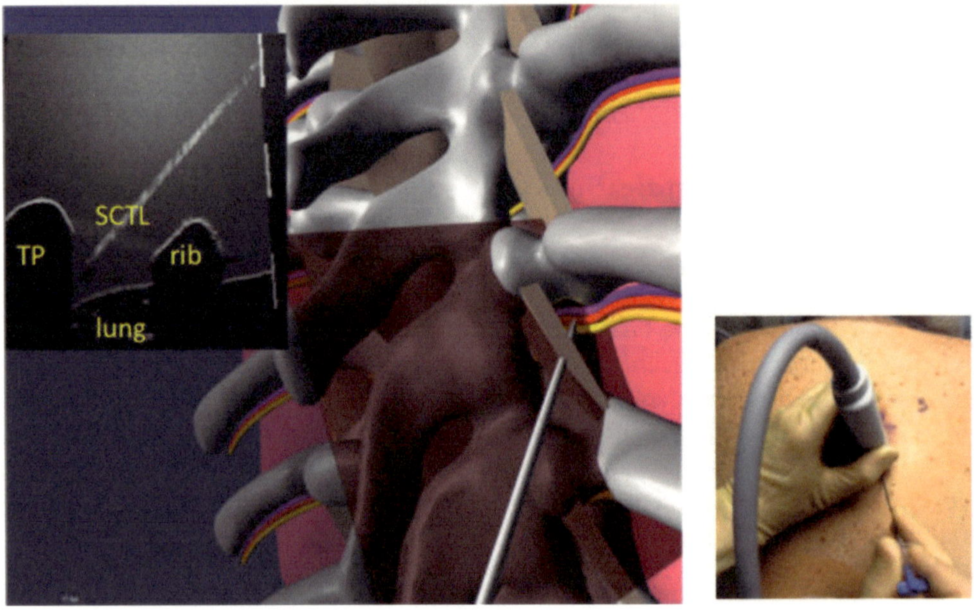

Figure 8. Live needle guidance for TPV block is an advanced technique and should be done only in individuals experienced in needle guidance under ultrasound. An oblique parasaggital view of the paravertebral space may improve visualization of the paravertebral space and pleura as well as an optimal needle trajectory.

pated (high surgical blood loss, hepatectomy). Bilateral thoracic paravertebral catheters can provide nearly similar pain control compared to thoracic epidural with decreased need for colloid infusion and vasoactive medications [27].

In patients undergoing total abdominal hysterectomy, both PVC and TAP catheters were found to be effective at reducing post-operative opioid requirements leading to reduction in opioid-induced side effects such as PONV, compared to control patients receiving opioids. Also, both patients with continuous TPV and TAP blocks had reduced pain scores and increased satisfaction compared to control patients [28].

In a meta-analysis of patients undergoing thoracotomy, PVC was found to significantly decrease pain scores and also to decrease pulmonary complications. The number-needed-to-treat to prevent one pulmonary complication was 4.2 ± 0.08. There was no benefit of epidural pain control versus systemic opioid analgesia with regards to pulmonary complications. Pain control with paravertebral catheters and epidural catheters was found to be comparable [29].

At the author's institution, although continuous bilateral TPV provides excellent analgesia in a subset of patients, higher volumes and bolus dosing of TPV catheters is required to achieve adequate spread of local anesthetic. Still, the analgesia does not appear as consistent as with TEA and the addition of subarachnoid morphine has been routinely used to improve analgesia. However, with high injection pressures from bolus dosing of TPV, epidural spread can be noted with TPV and improved analgesia is observed. Despite this fact, patients still appear to have higher requirements for systemic analgesics with bilateral continuous TPV as compared to TEA.

16. Side effects and complications

Side effects of thoracic paravertebral are less observed compared to TEA. A sympathectomy is not observed as frequently, although motor and sensory blocks are limited in their distribution. In addition, because only local anesthetics are infused in TPV blocks, no opioid-related complications are noted, such as pruritus, urinary retention, sedation, respiratory depression or nausea and vomiting other than the opioid-related side effects of requiring intravenous opioids as an adjunct to TPV analgesia.

Complications of TPV analgesia include failure of the block, both due to inability to place catheter correctly in TPV space or due to suboptimal spread of local anesthetic. Vascular punctures and intravascular placement may occur, but the consequences of bleeding are not as catastrophic as bleeding in the epidural space. Isolated puncture of parietal pleura may result in pneumothorax, either from the needle or from catheter advancement, but usually is Insignificand and does not require treatment. However, puncture of the visceral pleura and subsequent use of positive pressure mechanical ventilation may result in a tension pneumothorax with hemodynamic and respiratory compromise that will increase the need for chest tube placement. Visceral injury can be detected by aspiration of air through the needle or through the catheter.

A benefit of paravertebral nerve block is unilateral block. However, epidural and contralateral spread may occur with high volume dosing and pressurized dosing (such as with bolus injection). In a study halted early because of high rate of epidural spread, half (5/10) of patients who received high-pressure (>20 psi) lumbar paravertebral injection had evidence of neuraxial spread with a level at or above T11 although none (0/10) of the patients who received low-pressure (<15 psi) injection did. Additionally, 6/10 patients in the high-pressure group had bilateral femoral nerve sensory block and none in the low-pressure group had bilateral block [30]. While the study is performed in lumbar paravertebral blocks, these results can be extrapolated to thoracic paravertebral blocks. At the author's institution, greater reductions in blood pressure have been noted with bolus dosing as compared to basal infusions alone.

As demonstrated in the diagram (Figure 9), inadvertent dural puncture is possible since the dural sleeve may extend beyond the neuraxial space, resulting in total spinal anesthesia. The use of small gauge needles is not recommended because CSF leakage with dural puncture may not be easily detected or aspirated. The same is true for puncture of a blood vessel. Intravascular needle placement is less detectable and not easily aspirated. The inability to detect an intrathecal or intravascular needle placement can potentially lead to catastrophic complications with local anesthetic dosing. Use of sharp needles is also discouraged since resistance as the needle traverses the ligaments is less notable and identification of the thoracic paravertebral space more subtle. Medial angulation of the needle should be avoided so that you do not introduce a catheter into the neuraxial space, resulting in a transforaminal epidural catheter. Despite strict parasaggital needle manipulation, extension of a dural sleeve or a Tarlov cyst can still result in intrathecal needle or catheter placement and observation for CSF flow through the needle and test dose is recommended.

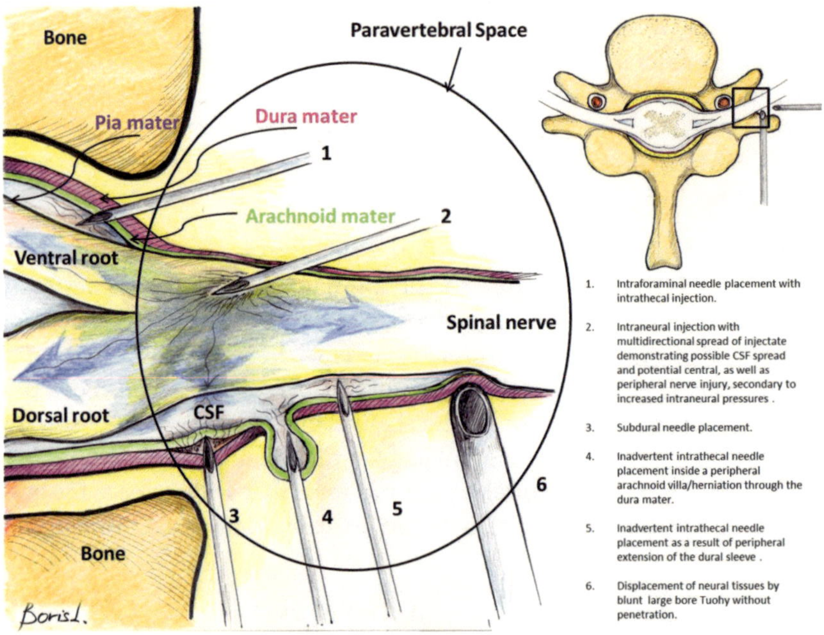

Figure 9. A possible mechanism for catastrophic outcomes from paravertebral block is inadvertent dural puncture. The above diagram demonstrates the potential extension of the dural sleeve in the cervical spine. This diagram can also be extrapolated to the thoracic spine. Catastrophic total spinal anesthesia has occurred with attempted thoracic paravertebral block placements.

17. Transversus Abdominis Plane (TAP) block

The Transversus Abdomins Plane (TAP) block was initially introduced by Rafi in 2001 [31]. Rafi described an anterior approach to the lumbar triangle of Petit in which he used a "pop" technique to reach the plane between the internal oblique and transversus abdominis muscles. Injection and spread of local anesthetic within this neurovascular plane can reach the anterior divisions of the thoracolumbar nerves, T6-L1, providing analgesia to the abdominal wall. With the traditional approach, however, sensory testing and cadaver studies have shown that dermatomes of T11-12 are most readily blocked, with spread to T9 and L1 much less often and usually requiring larger volumes of local anesthetic [32]. A block at this level provides analgesia of the abdominal wall in surgery of the lower abdomen, such as cesarean section, hysterectomy, inguinal hernia repair, and appendectomy.

Hebbard initially introduced standard posterior US-guided TAP block where local anesthetic was deposited between the internal oblique and transversus abdominis muscle above the iliac crest for analgesia of the lower abdomen. Then, in 2008, Hebbard introduced the oblique subcostal TAP block, in which local anesthetic is deposited along the costal margin between the transversus abdominis and rectus abdominis muscle medially, and the transversus abdominis and internal oblique muscle laterally, thus providing analgesia of the abdominal wall above the umbilicus [33].

It is important to emphasize that TAP blocks target peripheral nerves, and their effect is limited to blockade of afferent sensory nerves of the abdominal wall and not viscerally derived pain [34]. Therefore, the role of TAP blocks in major abdominal surgery is limited and should be used as an alternative if neuraxial or paravertebral analgesia is contraindicated or difficult.

17.1. Benefits and indications

When compared to neuraxial blockade, TAP blocks do not result in a sympathectomy and resultant hypotension. Sensory and motor blockade is limited to the abdominal wall musculature and lower extremity weakness is rare, only occurring with the TAP block performed at the level of the iliac crest and not the subcostal TAP approach. Lower extremity weakness is likely due to spread of local anesthetic to the femoral nerve. Side effects such as urinary retention, pruritus, nausea and vomiting, and sedation do not occur with TAP blocks.

In addition, TAP blocks provide an alternative to epidurals for patients receiving potent anticoagulation due to the minimal risk of epidural hematoma. Placement under general anesthesia is not considered unsafe because the target for local anesthetic infiltration is along a muscle plane and not a nerve root or outside the spinal cord. Furthermore, the procedure may be performed with the patient in the supine position.

Single injection TAP blocks have an analgesic duration of no greater than 24 hours despite use of long-acting local anesthetics such as bupivacaine or ropivacaine. The use of continuous TAP blocks will result in prolonged duration of analgesia. However, continuous TAP blocks, as compared to continuous neuraxial or paravertebral analgesia, will result in catheters that are located near the surgical site and may be dislodged or interfere with surgical field when placed prior to surgery.

17.2. Risks and complications

Although generally considered safe, potential adverse effects of TAP blocks include intraperitoneal injection, neural or muscle ischemia, and femoral nerve palsy. Failed block analgesia can stem from incomplete local anesthetic spread within the TAP plane, or a superior block on one side compared to the other in bilateral TAP blocks. Liver trauma is possible, particularly when employing a subcostal approach. Most of these adverse outcomes are relatively minor and self-limited when compared to that of epidurals.

Ultrasound guidance has gained acceptance as a standard over the traditional landmark "double pop" technique. One study looking at needle placement by blind TAP block showed correct needle placement in 23.6% of attempts, and incorrect needle placement included 18% in the peritoneum. The risk of visceral injury has led most proceduralists to employ the use of ultrasound and abandon the landmark approach alone [35]. Furthermore, ultrasound guidance has proven beneficial for ease of block performance because the Triangle of Petit can be difficult to identify, particularly in obese and peripartum patients [36].

Another risk of TAP blocks is systemic local anesthetic toxicity. As this block requires injection of local anesthetic within an intermuscular plane, a larger volume is required for wider dermatomal spread. The usual dose in adults is 15-30 mL of local anesthetic, which is doubled when bilateral injections are used. In particular, pediatric patients and post-caesarean section patients would be more susceptible to this systemic toxicity [37].

17.3. Clinical pearls

The lateral decubitus position for TAP blocks of the lower abdomen, especially in obese patients, will allow displacement of fat and excess soft tissue anteriorly and improved ease of access to the space (Figure 10). Two-inch silk tape can be used to deflect breast tissue cephalad and tissue surrounding the hip caudally. A pillow placed underneath the dependent side further opens the space between the 12th rib and iliac crest. An added benefit is that by placing the entry point on the side and tunneling posteriorly, the catheter can in most, but not all instances, be located away from the surgical field. In the cases of chevron and long subcostal incisions, this may not be possible. The use of multiple ports along the catheter may afford some benefit because analgesia is dependent on the spread of local anesthetic to all terminal nerves innervating the abdominal wall. For incisions crossing midline, bilateral catheters will be needed.

Subcostal catheters for upper abdominal surgery placed along the subcostal margin anteriorly will anesthetize the sensory nerves of the upper abdominal wall [38]. These catheters can be performed in the supine position in a medial-to-lateral direction along the costal margin. The proceduralist stands on the contralateral side with the ultrasound machine on the ipsilateral side. This allows ease of in-plane needle placement and catheter advancement. The drawback of this approach is that the catheter entry points (or the catheter itself) may be located in the surgical field. Therefore, catheter placement may be done under direct visualization or ultrasound guidance by the surgeon prior to fascial closure or at the conclusion of surgery prior to emergence.

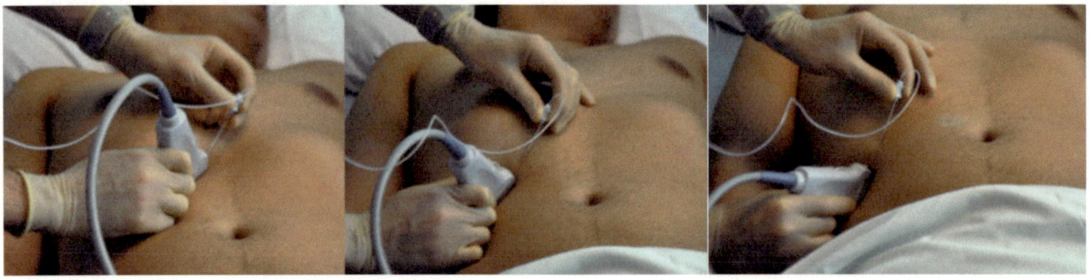

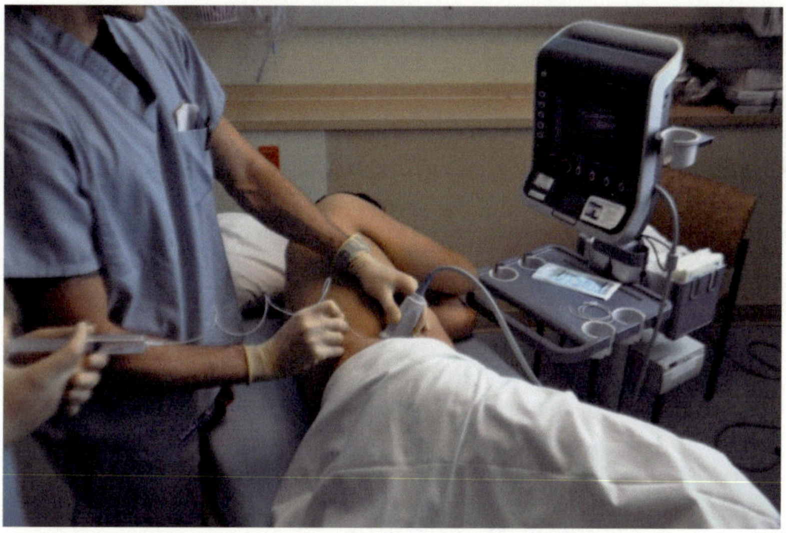

Figure 10. Lateral position for TAP blocks allow tissue deflection away from site of block placement.

Figure 11. Subcostal TAP block single injection performed. Due to the spread of nerves of the upper abdominal wall, when single injections are performed, usually the needle is reintroduced multiple times along the subcostal margin in order to achieve optimal spread of LA.

Local anesthetic infusions can be initiated at higher rates (8 ml per hour per catheter). As with TPV block, large boluses may be necessary to improve spread of local anesthetic. Systemic absorption is notable with this block [39] and use of epinephrine with local anesthetic may reduce absorption and increase duration of analgesia. Total dose in milligrams of local anesthesia should be assessed periodically and patients observed for signs of LAST.

18. Utility of TAP blocks

Overall, TAP blocks are most often considered as part of a multimodal analgesia approach to major abdominal surgery. There is some evidence that TAP blocks are opioid-sparing or delay the use of opioids, making them helpful as adjuncts to systemic analgesics. However, they should not be considered as first-line when superior analgesic modalities such as thoracic epidural or thoracic paravertebral blockade are available.

19. Conclusion

Regional anesthesia provides an superior analgesic modality. Thoracic epidural analgesia, thoracic paravertebral analgesia and continuous transversus abdominis plane blocks have all been utilized as part of a multimodal analgesic approach with success. TEA provides the most complete analgesia, but may be limited due to its side effect profile. TPV and TAP blocks may be less effective, but still substantial analgesic modalities. In order to provide optimal analgesia, knowledge of the benefits and limitations of each is imperative.

Author details

Linda Le-Wendling[1], Julia DeLoach[2], Allison Haller[1] and Barys Ihnatsenka[1]

1 University of Florida College of Medicine, Department of Anesthesiology, Division of Regional Anesthesiology and Perioperative Pain Medicine, Gainesville, Florida, USA

2 Regional Anesthesiology and Perioperative Pain Medicine, University of Florida, College of Medicine, Department of Anesthesiology, Gainesville, Florida, USA

References

[1] Marandola M, Cilli T, Alessandri F, Tellan G, Caronna R, Chirletti P, Delogu G. Perioperative management in patients undergoing pancreatic surgery: the anesthesiologist's point of view. Transplantation Proceedings 2008;40:1195-1199.

[2] Rorarius MG, Kujansuu E, Baer GA, Suominen P, Teisala K, Miettinen A, YlItalo P, Laippala P. Laparoscopically assisted vaginal and abdominal hysterectomy: comparison of postoperative pain, fatigue and systemic response. A case-controlled study. European Journal of Anesthesiology 2001;18:530-539.

[3] Bjerregaard N, Nikolajsen L, Bendtsen TF, Rasmussen BS. Transversus abdominis plane catheter bolus analgesia after major abdominal surgery. Anesthesiology Research and Practice 2012; 2012:1-5. doi: 10.1155/2012/596536.

[4] Bouman EA, Theunissen M, Bons SA, van Mook WN, Gramke HF, van Kleef M, Marcus MA. Reduced incidence of chronic postsurgical pain after epidural analgesia for abdominal surgery. Pain Practice 2013 doi: 10.1111/papr.12091.

[5] Thompson TK, Hutchison RW, Wegmann DJ, Shires GT 3rd, Beecherl E. Pancreatic resection pain management: is combining PCA therapy and a continuous local infusion of 0.5% ropivacaine beneficial? Pancreas 2008;37(1):103-104.

[6] Habib AS, Wahl K, Gu J, Gan TJ, Adenosine Study Group. Comparison of postoperative pain outcomes after vertical or Pfannenstiel incision for major gynecologic surgery. Current Medical Research and Opinions 2009;25(6):1529-34.

[7] Derrode N, Lebrun F, Levron JC, Chauvin M, Debaene B. Influence of preoperative opioid on postoperative pain after major abdominal surgery: sufentanil TCI versus remifentanil TCI. A randomized, controlled study. British Journal of Anesthesia 2003;91(6):842-9.

[8] Sun Y, Li T, Wang N, Yun Y, Gan TJ. Perioperative systemic lidocaine for postoperative analgesia and recovery after abdominal surgery: a meta-analysis of randomized controlled trials. Diseases of the Colon & Rectum

[9] Nguyen NT, Lee SL, Goldman C, Fleming N, Arango A, McFall R, Wolfe BM. Comparison of pulmonary function and postoperative pain after laparoscopic versus open gastric bypass: a randomized trial. Journal of the American College of Surgeons 2001;192:469-477.

[10] Minkowitz HS, Rathmell JP, Vallow S, Gargiulo K, Damaraju CV, Hewitt DJ. Efficacy and safety of the fentanyl iontophoretic transdermal system (ITS) and intravenous patient-controlled analgesia (IV PCA) with morphine for pain management following abdominal or pelvic surgery. Pain Medicine 2007;8(8):657-668.

[11] Fyneface-Ogan S. Anatomy and Clinical Importance of th e Epidural Space. Epidural Analgesia – Current Views and Approaches, 2012. ISBN: 978-953-51-0332-5, In Tech. http://cdn.intechopen.com/pdfs/32648/InTech-Anatomy_and_clinical_importance_of_the_epidural_space.pdf. Accessed August 30, 2012.

[12] Lirk P, Colvin J, Steger B, Colvin HP, Keller C, Rieder J, Kolbitsch C, Moriggi B. Incidence of lower thoracic ligamentum flavum midline gaps. British Journal of Anaesthesia 2005;94:852-855.

[13] Nishimori M, Low JH, Zheng H, Ballantyne JC. Epidural pain relief versus systemic opioid-based pain relief for abdominal arotic surgery. Cochrane Database System Reviews 2012 doi: 10.1002/14651858.CD005059.

[14] O'connor CJ. Thoracic epidural analgesia: physiologic effects and clinical applications. Journal of Cardiothoracic and Vascular Anesthesia 1993;7(5):595-609.

[15] Lubawski J, Saclarides T. Postoperative ileus: strategies for reduction. Therapeutics and Clinical Risk Management 2008;4(5)913-917.

[16] Bonnet MP, Migon A, Mazoit JX, Ozier Y, Marret E. Analgesic efficacy and adverse effects of epidural morphine compared to parenteral opioids after elective caesarean section: a systematic review. European Journal of Pain 2010;894.e1-894.e899.

[17] Bujedo BM, Santos SG, Azpiazu AU. A review of epidural and intrathecal opioids used in the management of postoperative pain. Journal of Opioid Management 2012;8(3)177-192.

[18] Sultan P, Gutierrez MC, Carvalho B. Neuraxial morphine and respiratory depression: finding the right balance. Drugs 2011;71(14):1807-1819.

[19] Wuethrich PY, Metzger T, Mordasini L, Kessler TM, Curatolo M, Burkhard FC. Influence of epidural mixture and surgery on bladder function after open renal surgery: a randomized clinical trial. Anesthesiology 2013;118(1):70-77.

[20] Zaouter C, Kaneva P, Carli F. Less urinary tract infection by earlier removal of bladder catheter in surgical patients receiving thoracic epidural analgesia. Regional Anesthesia and Pain Medicine 2009;34(6):542-548.

[21] Webb CA, Weyker PD, Zhang L, Stanley S, Coyle DT, Tang T, Smiley RM, Flood P. Unintentional dural puncture with a Tuohy needle increases risk of chronic headache. Anesthesia and Analgesia 2012;115(1):124-132.

[22] Neal JM, Bernards CM, Hadzic A, Hebl J, Hogan Q, Horlocker TT, Lee LA, Rathmell JP, Sorenson EJ, Suresh S, Wedel DJ. ASRA practice advisory on neurologic complications in regional anesthesia and pain medicine. Regional Anesthesia and Pain Medicine 2008;33(5):404-415.

[23] Horlocker TT, Wedel DJ, Rowlingson JC, Enneking FK, Kopp SL, Benzon HT, Brown DL, Heit JA, Mulroy MF, Rosenquist RW, Tryba M, Yuan CS. Regional anesthesia in the patient receiving antithrombotic or thrombolytic therapy: American Society of Regional Anesthesia and Pain Medicine Evidence-Based Buidelines (Third Edition). Regional Anesthesia and Pain Medicine 2010;35(1):64-101].

[24] Wang LP, Hauerberg JM, Schmidt FJ. Incidence of spinal epidural abscess after epidural analgesia: a national 1-year survey. Anesthesiology 1999;91(6):1928-1936.

[25] Dodd M, Hunsley J. Thoracic paravertebral block: landmark techniques. Anaesthesia Tutorial of the week 224. 2011. http://www.frca.co.uk/Documents/224%20Paravertebral%20block, %20Landmark%20techniques.pdf. Assessed August 30, 2013.

[26] Marhofer D, Marhofer P, Kettner SC, Fleischmann E, Prayer D, Schernthaner M, Lackner E, Willschke H, Schwetz P, Zeitlinger M. Magnetic resonance imaging analysis of the spread of local anesthetic solution after ultrasound-guided lateral thoracic paravertebral blockade: a volunteer study. Anesthesiology 2013;118(5):1106-1112.

[27] Pintaric TS, Potocnik I, Hadzic A, Stupnik T, Pintaric M, Jankovic VN. Comparison of continuous thoracic epidural with paravertebral block on perioperative analgesia and hemodynamic stability in patients having open lung surgery. Regional Anesthesia and Pain Medicine 2011;36(3):256-260.

[28] Melnikov AL, Bjoergo S, Kongsgarrd UE. Thoracic paravertebral block versus transversus abdominis plane block in major gynecological surgery: a prospective randomized, controlled, observer-blinded study. Local and Regional Anesthesia 2012;5:55-61.

[29] Joshi GP, Bonnet F, Shah R, Wilkinson TC, Camu F, Fischer B, Neugebauer EAM, Rawal N, Schug SA, Simanski C, Kehlet H. A systematic review of randomized trials evaluating regional techniques for postthoracotomy analgesia. Anesthesia and Analgesia 2008;107(3):1026-1040.

[30] Gadsden JC, Lindenmuth DM, Hadzic A, Xu D, Somasundarum L, Flisinski KA. Lumbar plexus block using high-pressure injection leads to contralateral and epidural spread. Anesthesiology 2008;109(4):683-688.

[31] Rafi AN. Abdominal field block: a new approach via the lumbar triangle. Anaesthesia 2001;56:1024-1026.

[32] Taylor R Jr, Pergolizzi JV, Sinclair A, Raffa RB, Aldington D, Plavin S, Apfel CC. Transversus abdominis block: clinical uses, side effects, and future perspectives. Pain Practice 2013;12(4):332-344.

[33] Hebbard P. Subcostal transversus abdominis plane block under ultrasound guidance. Anesthesia and Analgesia 2008;106(2):674-675.

[34] Niraj G, Kelkar A, Jeyapalan I, Graff-Baker P, Williams O, Darbar A, Maheshwaran A, Powell R. Comparison of analgesic efficacy of subcostal transversus abdominis plane blocks with epidural analgesia following upper abdominal surgery. Anaesthesia 2011;66(6):465-471.

[35] McDermott G, Korba E, Mata U, Jaigirdar M, Narayanan N, Boylan J, Conlon N. Should we stop using blind transversus abdominis plane blocks? British Journal of Anaesthesia 2012;108(3)499-502.

[36] Finnerty O, McDonnel JG. Transversus abdominis plane block. Current Opinion in Anesthesiology 2012;25(5):610-614.

[37] Griffiths JD, Le NV, Grant S, Bjorksten A, Hebbard P, Royse C. Symptomatic local anaesthetic toxicity and plasma ropivacaine concentrations after transversus abdominis plane block for Caesarean section. British Journal of Anaesthesia 2013;110(6): 996-1000.

[38] Hebbard PD, Barrington MJ, Vasey C. Ultrasound-guided continuous oblique subcostal transversus abdominis plane blockade: description of anatomy and clinical technique. Regional Anesthesia and Pain Medicine 2010;35(5):436-441.

[39] Hessian EC, Evans BE, Woods JA, Taylor, Kinkel E, Bjorksten AR. Plasma ropivacaine concentrations during bilateral transversus abdominis plane infusions. British Journal of Anaesthesia 2013;111(3):488-495.

Chapter 9

The Navigable Percutaneous Disc Decompression Device (L'DISQ & L'DISQ-C) in Patients with Herniated Nucleus Pulposus Related to Radicular Pain

Sang Chul Lee and Sang Heon Lee

Additional information is available at the end of the chapter

http://dx.doi.org/10.5772/57600

1. Introduction

Minimally-invasive disc decompression procedures have been developed over the last circa twenty years to treat radicular pain caused by disc herniations as an alternative treatment to open disc surgery. [1] Various interventional techniques include chemonucleolysis, ozone, automated percutaneous lumbar discectomy, intradiscal laser discectomy, intradiscal electrothermal therapy, and percutaneous nucleoplasty. [2-7] Even injectable liquids and gasses may reach the herniated nucleus, most devices are designed to decompress the center of the nucleus instead of the herniated disc. Although partial nuclear decompression by various minimally invasive techniques is generally safe and less invasive than open surgery, studies report inconsistent axial pain relief and most studies report a lower success rate than open and microdiscectomy for relieving radicular pain. [8] One reason for these inconsistent results may be the device design does not easily allow direct decompression of herniated disc material.

Introduced in 1999 and promoted to cause minimal collateral thermal damage, [9] Nucleoplasty (ArthroCare Co., Sunnyvale, CA) is representative of nuclear decompression devises that remove nuclear tissue through introducer needles that is typically inserted into a lumbar disc using a posterior lateral approach. Although different devises use various methods to remove nuclear tissue, the Nucleoplasty wand vaporizes nuclear tissue using a bipolar radiofrequency technology applied to a saline conducting medium. The disadvantage of the Nucleoplasty device, and indeed the disadvantage of most other minimally invasive devices and techniques, is the inability to easily reach the herniated nucleus. Direct removal of herniated disc tissue is, therefore, limited and removal of disc extrusions is impossible. Instead, nuclear decompression relies on pressure reduction and "implosion" of a disc protrusion to

INTECH
open science | open minds

© 2015 The Author(s). Licensee InTech. This chapter is distributed under the terms of the Creative Commons Attribution License (http://creativecommons.org/licenses/by/3.0), which permits unrestricted use, distribution, and reproduction in any medium, provided the original work is properly cited.

reduce pressure on the traversing or exiting nerve roots. While studies show reduced disc pressure in hydrated discs, [10] implosion of nuclear material has not been validated. [11]

2. Navigable percutaneous disc decompression device (L'DISQ) for lumbar spine

A new navigable percutaneous disc decompressor (L'DISQ, U&I Co., Uijeongbu, Korea) is designed to allow direct access to herniated disc material. The device vaporizes herniated nucleus using bipolar radiofrequency current similar to Nucleoplasty. (Figure 1) Unlike the Nucleoplasty device, the L'DISQ wand can be curved by rotating a control wheel and directed into a disc herniation.

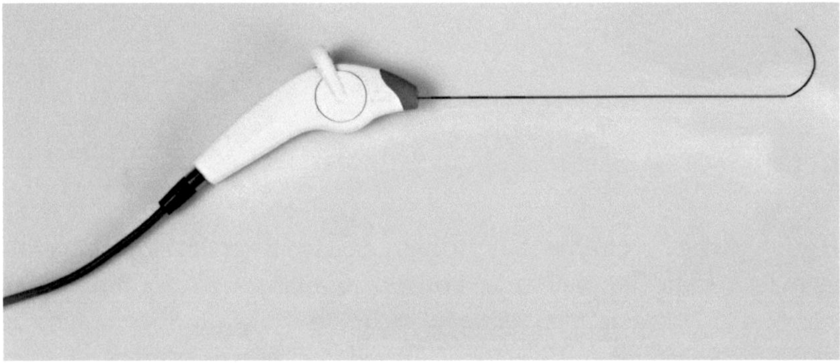

Figure 1. The wand and navigable tip of the L'DISQ is illustrated. The tip of the wand is curved to the desired angle by rotating the control wheel.

Unlike most percutaneous nuclectomy devices that use a rigid and uncontrolled tip, L' DISQ has a navigable tip that can be curved to the desired angles by rotation of the control wheel. Direct removal of the herniated tissue by the L'DISQ allows access to larger herniations and extruded fragments which are currently considered a contraindication for most percutaneous devices. [12-14] In addition, compared to open surgical discectomy, percutaneous removal through a relatively small bore introducer cannulae placed directly into the herniation or though the posterior-lateral annulus will theoretically better preserve the integrity of the outer annulus and potentially reduce the re-herniation rate following open discectomy. [15]

3. Safety of the procedure

Although the L'DISQ uses bipolar radio-frequency current to ablate tissue and therefore has the potential to injure unintended tissue due to high temperature caused by electric current and plasma energy, a previous study reported the thermal safety of this procedure. [16] The temperature did not exceed 13ºC above the initial temperature at any location and no denaturation of the adjacent neural tissue was observed. The histopathology examination demonstrated decompression of the nucleus pulposus without thermal damage to the surrounding neural tissues. [16]

Furthermore, as the distance between the two electrodes on L'DISQ tip is 1 mm, a nerve root greater than 1 mm from the tip is theoretically safe from electric injury. Indeed, the electric currents should pass to the other electrode instead of the nerve root rather than passing to the nerve root. In addition, the thin outer annulus membrane is at best a poor conductor of electrical current which should theoretically reduce neural damage due to the bipolar electrical current. Closely monitoring for the occurrence of leg pain should prevent injury due to heat. In addition, the wand tip should obviously be moved if electric stimulation causes lower extremity contraction.

4. Procedure technique

Patient preparation. Prophylactic intravenous antibiotics must be administered 30 minutes before the procedure and monitor patients with electrocardiogram, pulse oximetry, and automated blood pressures. The patients are positioned prone on the surgical table and fluoroscopic examination of the spine is performed to confirm segmentation and determine the appropriate level of needle. Sedation is limited to 20 mg of propofol administered as necessary during anesthetization of the skin and subcutaneous fascia onto the superior articular process contralateral to the herniated disc.

Standard procedure. Use a standard posterior lateral approach to the disc as previously described, [17] but modified technique is to approach the disc further lateral so that the introducer needle would contact the disc margin at a line drawn between the medial border of adjacent pedicles rather than the midline. Slightly curve the distal end of the introducer needle to facilitate directing the introduced wand medial across the posterior annulus either slightly within or in some cases outside the posterior disc annulus.

A 25 gauge needle is first inserted into the target disc nucleus and 0.5 to 1 ml of contrast can be injected to outline the disc herniation. Next, mark the skin 12 to 15 cm from the midline to provide the approximate site of needle entry. The endplates of the target disc space are aligned and the C-arm rotated ipsilateral to position the lateral margin of the ipsilateral superior articular process approximately 3/5 distance across the vertebral body as visualized in the oblique position. This typically required rotating the C-Arm 20 degrees from a zero degree lateral projection (70°oblique view). After anesthetizing the skin and subcutaneous fascia to the superior articular process, manually curve the 15 gauge introducer needle approximately 15 degrees in the distal ~ 1cm from the distal tip. The introducer needle is directed toward the lateral edge of the superior articular process following the local anesthesia tract and guided by intermittent fluoroscopic "down the beam" projection using a "corkscrew" rotation of the slightly curved distal tip. Once the lateral edge is touched, the needle tip is directed laterally over the process and once the tip is over the SAP, the tip is rotated back toward the midline.

Prior to advancing the introducer needle across the midline the AP projection need to be checked. A lateral projection is used to slowly advance the needle across the foramen toward the disc margin. As the needle tip is directed toward the midline, the AP projection is intermittently checked to assure that the needle tip is always lateral the medial border of the pedicle. Be careful not to penetrate the neural tissues and the patient need to be asked to report any buttock or leg pain. Ideal technique is to avoid puncturing a normal posterior annulus if doctor feet that he could safely pass the introducer needle directly into central protrusions, or pass the wand posterior to the disc annulus in cases of contra-lateral disc extrusions. (Figure 2)

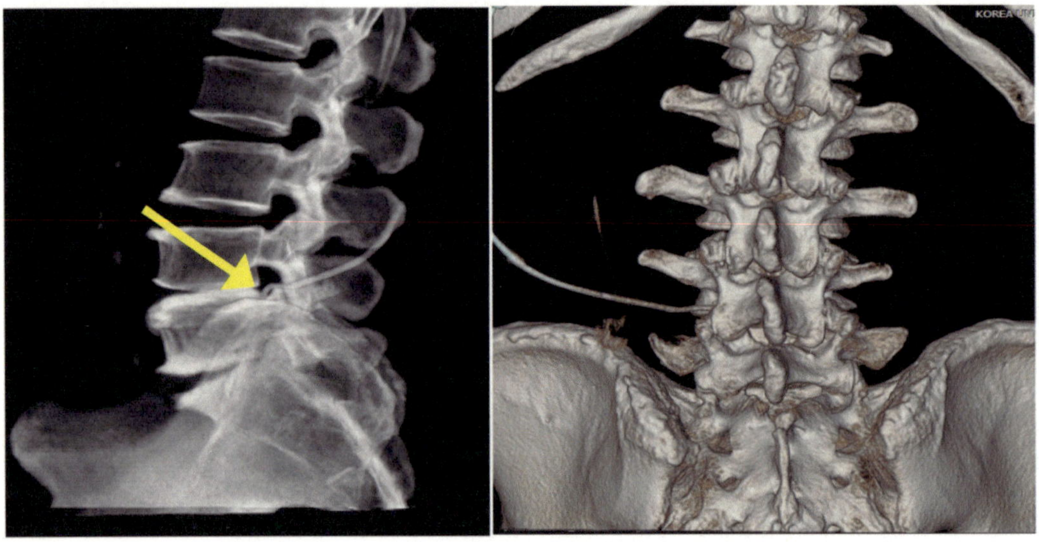

Figure 2. A three-dimension computed tomographic reconstruction image of the pathway of the L'DISQ wand is shown. In this case, the introducer needle was advanced posterior to the annulus into the annular extrusion. The tip of the L'DISQ wand (yellow arrow) is seen within the extrusion disc. The computed tomography scan was obtained with the patient's permission to evaluate immediate post procedure changes.

The advancement of the needle is precisely controlled by rotating the direction of the needle tip bend. Entering the herniation is identified by a sudden loss of resistance. After confirming the introducer needle position with the lateral and AP view, the stylet is removed and the through the introducer needle the wand is advanced to the center of the herniated disc using fluoroscopic monitoring of the AP and lateral views. Before ablation, negative motor nerve stimulation confirmed the needle is not close to the traversing or exiting nerve root. During the ablation, the tip of the wand the tip is continuously rotated and moved back and forth to increase the ablated volume. We also strived to remove disc material within the annular tears with either the same wand position or in some cases after repositioning of the wand.(Figure 3) The entire procedure need to be monitored, recorded and evaluated by C-arm fluoroscopy.

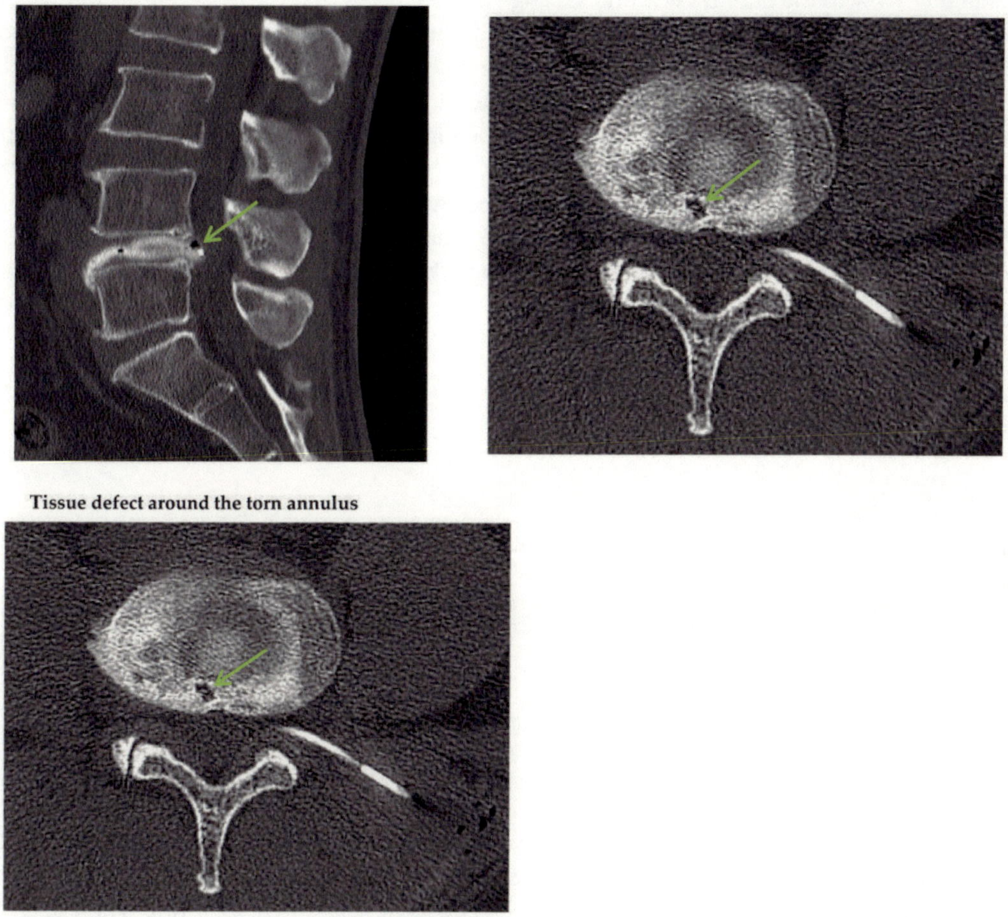

Figure 3. A computed tomographic scan performed just after the procedure illustrates the probable results of radiofrequency ablation as indicated by opacity (arrow) around the treated disc herniation.

5. Trans-annulus approach technique by directly inserting the wand into the herniated disc

For this technique, 70°oblique view is recommended. Trocar needle pass through the skin, fat, and muscle, so it is easy to correct the needle position or pathway up to 1cm before reaching the disc. With the guide needle continuing toward the target as a single spot in the C-arm image, check the position every 1-2cm until the guide needle reaches the disc. Although the needle tip continues in toward the target, because the tip of the needle is bent, pushing straight will cause the needle to rotate posteriorly. In a 70°oblique view, needle is seen as slightly bent posteriorly, rather than a single spot. Once the needle tip reaches the disc, change from the 70°oblique view to the lateral view and arrange the needle so that the distal end is in-line as a spot with the C-arm image. Push the guide needle in between the rear portion of the disc's vertebral pulp to the herniated disc. At this time, inject small amounts of contrast dye in the herniated disc. If the contrast dye does not visualize clearly in the image, inject saline solution and then reposition the needle into the desired location. When entering the annulus fibrosus, saline solution is not injected, but once the needle tip enters the herniated portion of the intervertebral disc, saline solution is easily injected. Also, the herniated position from the MRI image and the C-arm's AP & lateral views should match to indicate the correct location. The location of the guide needle tip is confirmed through the image of the A-P view and the contrast dye.(figure4)

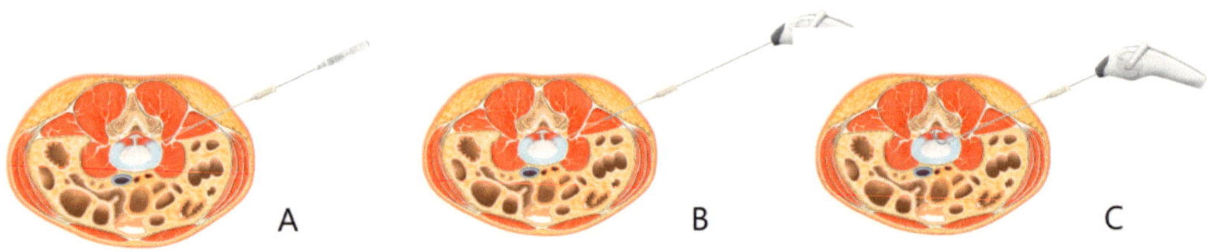

Figure 4. Trocar needle pass through the skin, fat, and muscle, so it is easy to correct the needle position or pathway up to 1cm before reaching the disc.(A) Push the guide needle in between the rear portion of the disc's vertebral pulp to the herniated disc.(B). The needle tip enters the herniated portion of the intervertebral disc.(C)

After the removal of the stylet, the L'DISQ wand is inserted into the guide polymer needle. After inserting the wand tip into the lesion, carry out a nerve impulse test with a test ablation. If the patient does feel anything, then the wand is in a safe position to continue with the high-frequency ablation. Using the control wheel for the wand tip, pull the wand while rotating it in a bent position. This method will allow the wand to contact the largest area and remove the most vertebral pulp. Inject 0.5-1cc saline solution, as needed, for improved plasma effect.

6. 30° rotation technique for L5/S1 disc

The best view to avoid getting caught on the pelvic bone is the 30°rotation view (60°oblique view).

However, it is difficult to approach a large herniated disc with the guide needle at this position because of the angle and the anatomical structure. The target region using the 60°oblique view is the center or rear 2/5 of the disc. This region of the L5/S1 is where the intervertebral foramen or neural foramen is located. Since the pelvic bone is blocking the target, the start position should be 1cm above the pelvic bone. For the Lumbar 4/5 (L4/5) disc, position the needle so that the tip creates a spot and advancement into the annulus fibrosus should be easy. For the lumbosacral joint (L5/S1), after passing the pelvic bone, guide the bent tip of the needle like a car by pointing the bent portion down toward the disc before pushing the tip in. Advance forward into the neural foramen, particularly at the S1 vertebral body, until you reach the superior articular process. Once the superior articular process of the S1 vertebral body is reached, rotate to the lateral view and proceed. Using the oblique 60° lateral view make visualization of the needle easier. Once the needle reached the vertebral pulp and the feeling of the hard vertebral pulp disappears, use the AP & lateral views to check location while injecting saline solution. Position the guide needle in the disc and remove the stylet. Then replace the stylet with the wand tip and begin high frequency ablation.(figure5)

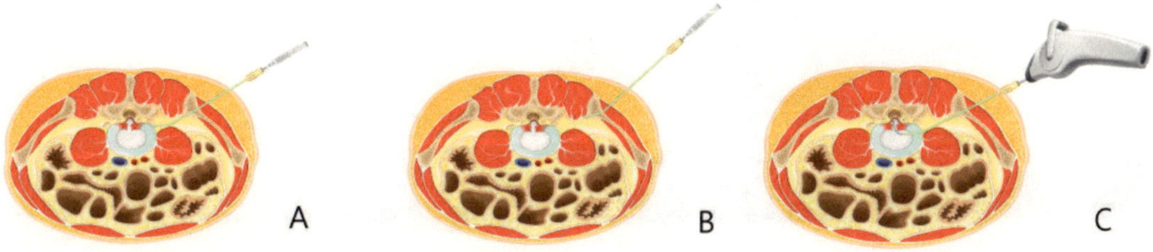

Figure 5. For the lumbosacral joint (L5/S1), after passing the pelvic bone, guide the bent tip of the needle like a car by pointing the bent portion down toward the disc before pushing the tip in.(A) Once the needle reached the vertebral pulp and the feeling of the hard vertebral pulp disappears, use the AP & lateral views to check location while injecting saline solution.(B) Place the stylet with the wand tip and begin high frequency ablation(C)

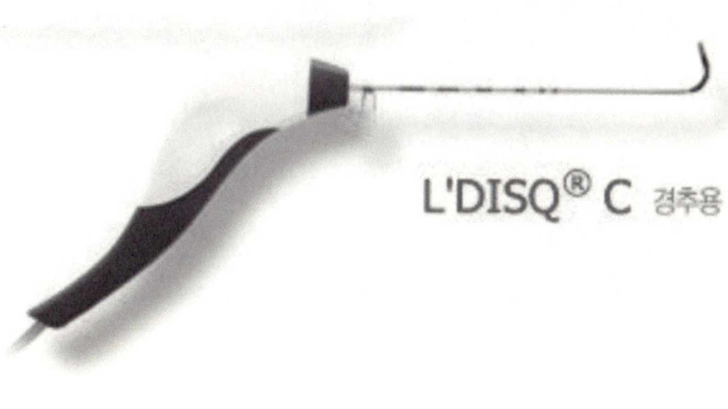

Figure 6. The wand and navigable tip of the L'DISQ-C is shown. The tip of the wand can be curved to the desired angle by rotating the control wheel. After placing the tip into the posterior annulus, plasma energy induced by radio-frequency is used to ablate and decompress the disc herniation.

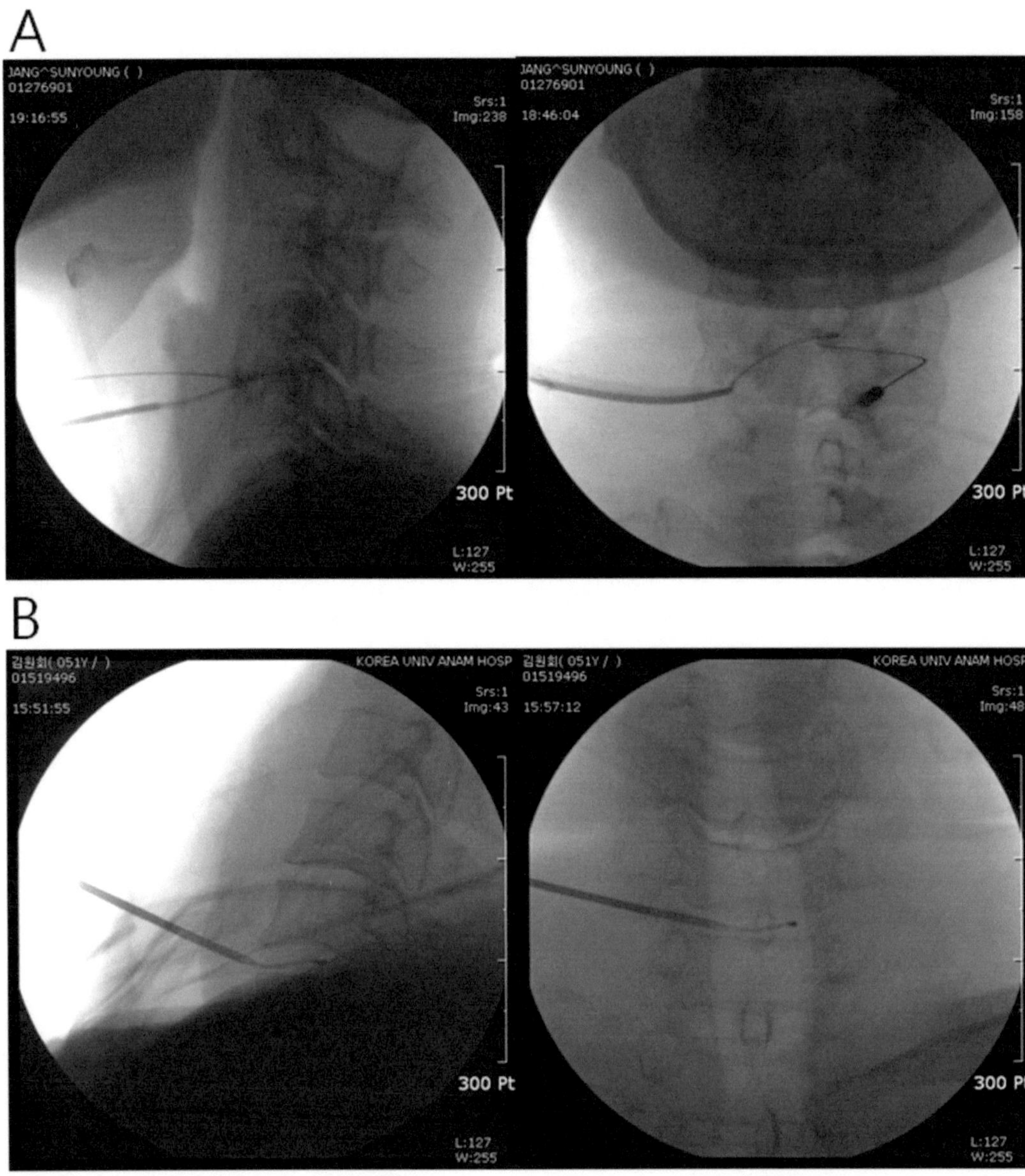

Figure 7. Exact positions of the L'DISQ-C wand tip (arrow) placed in the center of herniation. C-arm fluoroscopy was used in anteroposterior and lateral planes to confirm the correct placement with reference to MRI studies. (A) Placing the tip of the L-DISQ catheter into the herniated disc. (B) Cervical disc decompressions were performed using L-DISQ catheter with fluoroscopic guidance

http://dx.doi.org/10.5772/57600

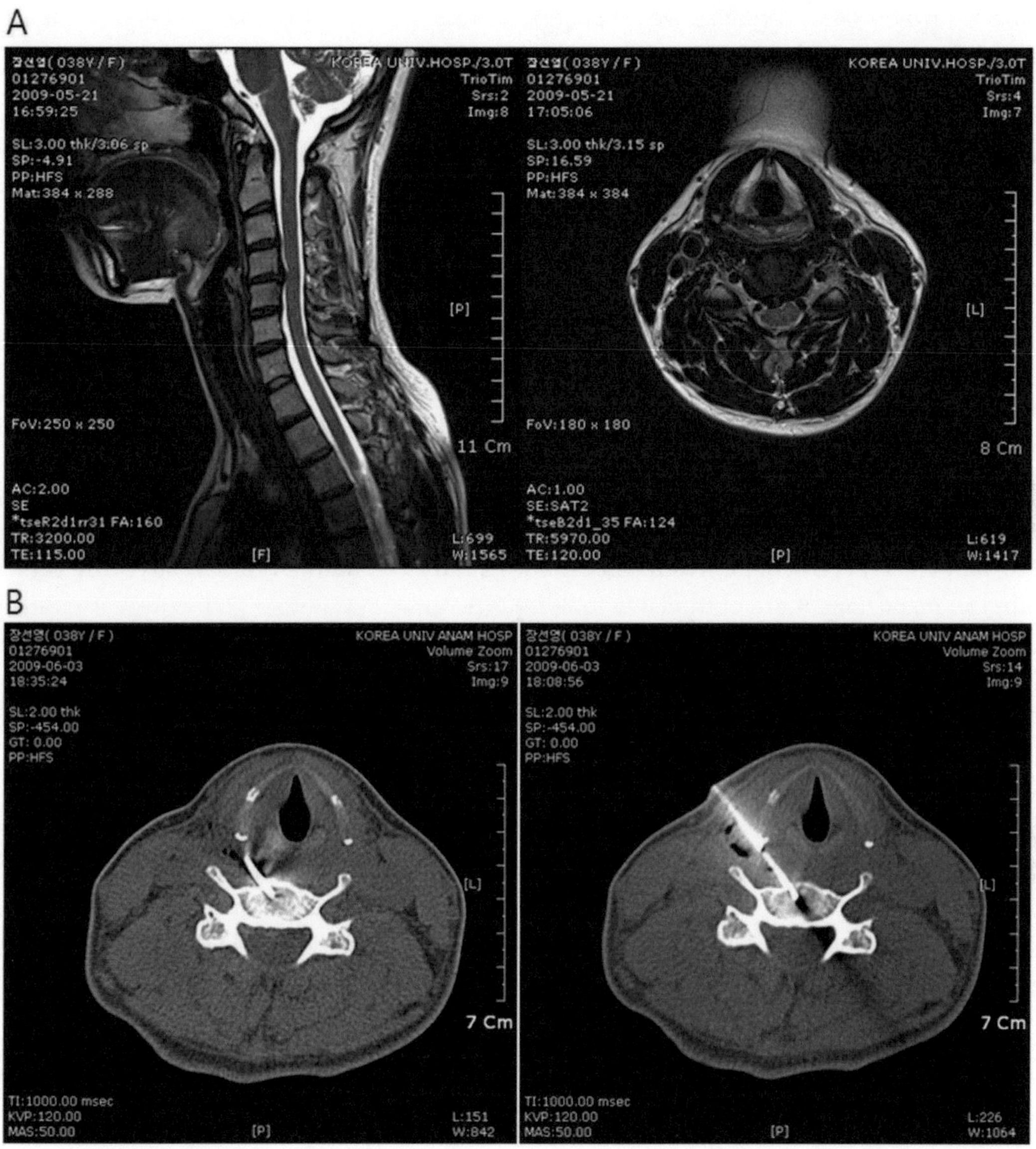

Figure 8. (A) Pre-procedure MRI noted a central disc extrusion at C4/5.(B) Placing the tip of the L-DISQ catheter into the herniated disc with computed tomography guidance of the standard midline approach

7. Outcomes

Recently, Lee et al. [18] reported the outcomes of this procedure. Results were shown that the VAS fell from 7.08 to 1.84 at 24 weeks post-procedure. At 6 months, the success rate, defined as a reduction of VAS more than 50%, was reported 88%. [18]

The L'DISQ device is specifically designed to remove herniated disc using a wand that can be navigated into a disc protrusion or extrusion. [18] Following decompression, we measured clinically significant pain improvement and decreased disability for patients with both radicular and axial pain caused by protruded and extruded discs. [18]

8. Navigable percutaneous disc decompression device (L'DISQ-C) for cervical spine

Neck pain is the second most common problem following back pain [19]. Although typically self-limiting, cervical disc herniation (CDH) with an annual incidence of 83.2/100,000 persons [20] may cause persistent pain refractory to conservative. Continued conservative care versus surgical management are both viable long term treatment strategies [21], however patients suffering more extreme pain, neurological compromise, or both are more likely to be offered a variety of disc decompression techniques [6, 7, 22, 23]. Although the efficacy and safety of the disc ablation with radiofrequency energy has been previously demonstrated[9, 24], focal direct removal of the herniated disc is restricted by the inability to navigate the catheter within the herniation. To overcome this liability, a navigable decompression device named L'DISQ-C was developed that is designed to allow direct access to the herniated disc material by rotating a control wheel directed into the disc herniation. In addition to direct mechanical decompression, the plasma energy applied within the disc herniation would theoretically destroy nociceptive nerve endings and disrupt inflammatory cytokines in the periphery of the annulus [25-28].

The perceived benefits of percutaneous disc decompression compared to open surgical decompression initiated the development and use of minimally invasive percutaneous devices to ablate nuclear tissue. The effectiveness versus risk of cartilaginous end plate damage, bleedings, osteonecrosis of the vertebral body, and end plate damage [29, 30] are ongoing debate.

It is crucial that interventionalists are careful when manipulating the device and before each ablation, one should perform a brief test electrical stimulation. If stimulation or limb movement is detected, the wand must be repositioned. Movement of the wand forward during ablation must be prevented.

9. Procedure technique

Patient preparation. First, inject antibiotics intravenously 30 minutes prior the procedure and monitor blood pressure, heart rate, electrocardiogram, oxygen saturation, and respiration rate during the procedure. Patients are placed in the supine position with the neck extended by placing a cushion beneath the shoulder. A soft strap is placed over the forehead for stabilization. Patients are asked to gently distract both shoulders downward the operation table. The neck is prepped and draped in a sterile fashion. An aseptic technique must be used throughout the procedure. Deep sedation should be avoided so that complete neurological monitoring of the patient is possible during the whole procedure.

Standard procedure. The procedure is performed under fluoroscopic guidance using a standard midline approach [31]. During the initiatory stage, fluoroscopic examination identifies the target disc and appropriate skin site to needle trajectory. Displace the trachea medially and vessels laterally using two digits applied with firm pressure to the space between the trachea and the medial border of the sternocleidomastoid muscle. After encounter with the anterior cervical spine, a 25 gauge needle is inserted into the disc ipsilateral to the herniation and the 16 gauge introducer needle(Fig. 2) passed contralateral to the herniation. After confirming needle placement with AP and lateral fluoroscopic views, Outline the herniation with 0.2 mL contrast injected through the 25 gauge needle. The stylet of the introducer needle is withdrawn from the introducer cannula and the L'DISQ-C wand with 17mm flexible tip is replaced. By manipulating the L'DISQ-C control wheel with or without force of the wand into the introducer needle, advance the tip of the wand to the center of the herniation. After connecting the L'DISQ-C wand to the power generator and testing with a brief test electrical stimulation before each ablation and any complaint of radiating pain or muscular contraction prompted withdrawal of the tip by 1 mm and retesting. Use brief bursts of 50W-75W for 2~5 seconds to ablate disc tissue. After each ablation the wand slightly repositioned and after test stimulation, ablation is repeated to a total of 100~150 seconds. In the intervals of ablation a small amount of saline can be injected through the 25 gauge needle to support the plasma well-evoking.

10. Outcomes

Recently, Lee et al. [32] reported the outcomes of this procedure in the patients with cervical herniated nucleus pulposus. Results were shown that the average VAS fell from 7.29 to 1.14 scores at 1 year post procedure. [32] All seven patients reported successful outcomes with a reduction of VAS more than 50%. However, the lack of a control group and a few patients are limitations. Following decompression with L'DISQ-C patients reported clinically significant pain improvement and decreased disability for patients with both cervical radicular and axial pain caused by protruded and extruded discs. [32]

Author details

Sang Chul Lee[1] and Sang Heon Lee[2,3,4]

1 Department of Anesthesiology and Pain, Seoul National University Medical Center, Seoul National University, Seoul, South Korea

2 Department of Physical Medicine & Rehabilitation, Korea University Medical Center, Seoul, South Korea

3 Spinal Diagnostics & Treatment Center, Daly City, CA, USA

4 Department of Biomedical Science, Korea University Graduate School, South Korea

References

[1] Chen Y, Derby R, Lee SH. Percutaneous disc decompression in the management of chronic low back pain. *Orthop Clin North Am.* Jan 2004;35(1):17-23.

[2] Mirzai H, Tekin I, Yaman O, Bursali A. The results of nucleoplasty in patients with lumbar herniated disc: a prospective clinical study of 52 consecutive patients. *Spine J.* Jan-Feb 2007;7(1):88-92; discussion 92-83.

[3] Erdine S, Ozyalcin NS, Cimen A. [Percutaneous lumber nucleoplasty]. *Agri.* Apr 2005;17(2):17-22.

[4] Andreula C, Muto M, Leonardi M. Interventional spinal procedures. *European journal of radiology.* May 2004;50(2):112-119.

[5] Kambin P, Schaffer JL. Percutaneous lumbar discectomy. Review of 100 patients and current practice. *Clinical orthopaedics and related research.* Jan 1989(238):24-34.

[6] Karasek M, Bogduk N. Twelve-month follow-up of a controlled trial of intradiscal thermal anuloplasty for back pain due to internal disc disruption. *Spine.* Oct 15 2000;25(20):2601-2607.

[7] Nerubay J, Caspi I, Levinkopf M, Tadmor A, Bubis JJ. Percutaneous laser nucleolysis of the intervertebral lumbar disc. An experimental study. *Clinical orthopaedics and related research.* Apr 1997(337):42-44.

[8] Faciszewski T, Winter RB, Lonstein JE, Denis F, Johnson L. The surgical and medical perioperative complications of anterior spinal fusion surgery in the thoracic and lumbar spine in adults. A review of 1223 procedures. *Spine.* Jul 15 1995;20(14):1592-1599.

[9] Chen YC, Lee SH, Saenz Y, Lehman NL. Histologic findings of disc, end plate and neural elements after coblation of nucleus pulposus: an experimental nucleoplasty study. *Spine J.* Nov-Dec 2003;3(6):466-470.

[10] Chen YC, Lee SH, Chen D. Intradiscal pressure study of percutaneous disc decompression with nucleoplasty in human cadavers. *Spine (Phila Pa 1976).* Apr 1 2003;28(7):661-665.

[11] Delamarter RB, Howard MW, Goldstein T, Deutsch AL, Mink JH, Dawson EG. Percutaneous lumbar discectomy. Preoperative and postoperative magnetic resonance imaging. *J Bone Joint Surg Am.* Apr 1995;77(4):578-584.

[12] Hirsch JA, Singh V, Falco FJ, Benyamin RM, Manchikanti L. Automated percutaneous lumbar discectomy for the contained herniated lumbar disc: a systematic assessment of evidence. *Pain Physician.* May-Jun 2009;12(3):601-620.

[13] Ohnmeiss DD, Guyer RD, Hochschuler SH. Laser disc decompression. The importance of proper patient selection. *Spine (Phila Pa 1976).* Sep 15 1994;19(18):2054-2058; discussion 2059.

[14] Philip SK. Nucleoplasty. *Techniques in Regional Anesthesia and Pain Management.* 2004;8(1):46-52.

[15] Carragee EJ, Spinnickie AO, Alamin TF, Paragioudakis S. A prospective controlled study of limited versus subtotal posterior discectomy: short-term outcomes in patients with herniated lumbar intervertebral discs and large posterior anular defect. *Spine.* Mar 15 2006;31(6):653-657.

[16] Kang CH, Kim YH, Lee SH, et al. Can magnetic resonance imaging accurately predict concordant pain provocation during provocative disc injection? *Skeletal radiology.* Sep 2009;38(9):877-885.

[17] Derby R, Lee SH, Kim BJ. Discography. In: Slipman CW, Derby R, Simeone FA, Mayer TG, eds. *Interventional Spine: an algorithmic approach*: Elsevier; 2008:291-302.

[18] Lee SH, Derby R, Sul D, et al. Efficacy of a new navigable percutaneous disc decompression device (L'DISQ) in patients with herniated nucleus pulposus related to radicular pain. *Pain Med.* Mar 2011;12(3):370-376.

[19] Nachemson A, Waddell G, Norlund A. Epidemiology of neck and neck pain. In: Nachemson AL, Jonsson E, editors. Neck and back pain: the scientific evidence of causes,diagnosis and treatment. Philadelphia (PA): Lippincott Williams and Wilkins; 2000. 164-87.

[20] Radhakrishnan K, Litchy WJ, O'Fallon WM, Kurland LT. Epidemiology of cervical radiculopathy. A population-based study from Rochester, Minnesota, 1976 through 1990. *Brain : a journal of neurology.* Apr 1994;117 (Pt 2):325-335.

[21] Persson LC, Carlsson CA, Carlsson JY. Long-lasting cervical radicular pain managed with surgery, physiotherapy, or a cervical collar. A prospective, randomized study. *Spine (Phila Pa 1976).* Apr 1 1997;22(7):751-758.

[22] Smith L. Enzyme Dissolution of the Nucleus Pulposus in Humans. *JAMA.* Jan 11 1964;187:137-140.

[23] Hijikata S. Percutaneous nucleotomy. A new concept technique and 12 years' experience. *Clin Orthop Relat Res.* Jan 1989(238):9-23.

[24] Lee MS, Cooper G, Lutz GE, Doty SB. Histologic characterization of coblation nucleoplasty performed on sheep intervertebral discs. *Pain physician.* Oct 2003;6(4):439-442.

[25] Bogduk N, Tynan W, Wilson AS. The nerve supply to the human lumbar intervertebral discs. *J Anat.* Jan 1981;132(Pt 1):39-56.

[26] Konttinen YT, Gronblad M, Antti-Poika I, et al. Neuroimmunohistochemical analysis of peridiscal nociceptive neural elements. *Spine (Phila Pa 1976).* May 1990;15(5): 383-386.

[27] Ashton IK, Roberts S, Jaffray DC, Polak JM, Eisenstein SM. Neuropeptides in the human intervertebral disc. *J Orthop Res.* Mar 1994;12(2):186-192.

[28] Freemont AJ, Peacock TE, Goupille P, Hoyland JA, O'Brien J, Jayson MI. Nerve ingrowth into diseased intervertebral disc in chronic back pain. *Lancet.* Jul 19 1997;350(9072):178-181.

[29] Melrose J, Taylor TK, Ghosh P, Holbert C, Macpherson C, Bellenger CR. Intervertebral disc reconstitution after chemonucleolysis with chymopapain is dependent on dosage. *Spine.* Jan 1 1996;21(1):9-17.

[30] Tonami H, Kuginuki M, Kuginuki Y, et al. MR imaging of subchondral osteonecrosis of the vertebral body after percutaneous laser diskectomy. *AJR. American journal of roentgenology.* Nov 1999;173(5):1383-1386.

[31] Slipman CW. *Interventional spine : an algorithmic approach.* Philadelphia, PA: Saunders Elsevier; 2008.

[32] Lee SH, Derby R, Sul D, et al. Efficacy of the Navigable Percutaneous Disc Decompression Device (L'DISQ-C) in Patients with the Cervical Herniated Nucleus Pulposus: prospective outcome study with a minimum 1-year follow-up. Pain Med. 2013;on submission.

Chapter 10

Epidural Lysis of Adhesions and Percutaneous Neuroplasty

Gabor B. Racz, James E. Heavner, Jeffrey P. Smith, Carl E. Noe, Adnan Al-Kaisy, Tomikichi Matsumoto, Sang Chul Lee and Laszlo Nagy

Additional information is available at the end of the chapter

http://dx.doi.org/10.5772/58753

1. Introduction

Chances are relatively high that each of us will experience low back pain at some point in our lives. The usual course is rapid improvement with 5% to 10% developing persistent symptoms [1]. In the 1990s the estimated cost of low back pain to the health industry was in the billions of dollars, and with a larger proportion of our population now reported to be older, this number can only be expected to increase [2,3]. Treatment typically begins with conservative measures such as medication and physical therapy and may even include minimally and highly invasive pain management interventions. Surgery is sometimes required in patients who have progressive neurologic deficits or those who do not respond to conservative treatment sometimes chose surgery. A quandary sometimes arises, following a primary surgery, as to whether repeat surgery should be attempted or another alternative technique should be tried. This is the exact problem that the epidural adhesiolysis procedure was designed to address. Failed back surgery or postlaminectomy syndrome led to the development of the epidural adhesiolysis procedure. It was shown to be effective in many patients with chronic pain after back surgery presumably by freeing up nerves and breaking down scar formation, delivering site-specific corticosteroids and local anesthetics, and reducing edema with the use of hyaluronidase and hypertonic saline. Epidural adhesiolysis has afforded patients a reduction in pain and neurologic symptoms without the expense and occasional long recovery period associated with repeat surgery, and often prevents the need for surgical intervention. Epidural adhesiolysis was given an evidence rating of strong correlating to a 1B or 1C evidence level for post–lumbar surgery syndrome in the most recent American Society of Interventional Pain Physicians evidence-based guidelines. The therapy is supported by observational studies and case series along with randomized-control trials. The recommendation was also made that this therapy could apply to most patients with post laminectomy syndrome or failed back syn-

INTECH
open science | open minds

© 2015 The Author(s). Licensee InTech. This chapter is distributed under the terms of the Creative Commons Attribution License (http://creativecommons.org/licenses/by/3.0), which permits unrestricted use, distribution, and reproduction in any medium, provided the original work is properly cited.

drome in many circumstances with informed consent [4]. Additionally, current procedural terminology (CPT) codes have been assigned to the two different kinds of adhesiolysis: CPT 62263 for the three-times injections over 2 to 3 days, which has recently changed to 3 injections 6- 8 hours apart within 24 hours, usually done in an inpatient hospital setting, and CPT 62264 for the one-time injection series surgery-center model that may need to be repeated 3 to 3.5 times in a 12-month period.

2. Pathophysiology of epidural fibrosis (scar tissue) as a cause of low back pain with radiculopathy

The etiology of chronic low back pain with radiculopathy after appropriate surgery is not well understood. Kuslich et al [5] addressed this issue when they studied 193 patients who had undergone lumbar spine operations given local anesthesic into the epidural space. It was postulated that sciatica could only be produced by stimulation of a swollen, stretched, restricted (i.e., scarred) or compressed nerve root [5]. Back pain could be produced by stimulation of several tissues, but the most common tissue of origin was the outer layer of the annulus fibrosus and the posterior longitudinal ligament. Stimulation for pain generation of the facet joint capsule rarely generated low back pain, and facet synovium and cartilage surfaces of the facet or muscles were never tender [6].

The contribution of fibrosis to the etiology of low back pain has been debated [7–9]. There are many possible etiologies of epidural fibrosis, including surgical trauma, an annular tear, infection, hematoma, or intrathecal contrast material [10]. These etiologies have been well documented in the literature. LaRocca and Macnab [11] demonstrated the invasion of fibrous connective tissue into postoperative hematoma as a cause of epidural fibrosis, and Cooper et al [12] reported periradicular fibrosis and vascular abnormalities occurring with herniated intervertebral disks. McCarron et al [13] investigated the irritative effect of nucleus pulposus on the dural sac, adjacent nerve roots, and nerve root sleeves independent of the influence of direct compression on these structures. Evidence of an inflammatory reaction was identified by gross inspection and microscopic analysis of spinal cord sections after homogenized autogenous nucleus pulposus was injected into the lumbar epidural space of four dogs. In the control group consisting of four dogs injected with normal saline, the spinal cord sections were grossly normal. Parke and Watanabe [14] showed significant evidence of adhesions in cadavers with lumbar disk herniation.

It is widely accepted that postoperative scar renders the nerve susceptible to injury by a compressive phenomena [9]. It is natural for connective tissue or any kind of scar tissue to form fibrous layers (scar tissue) as a part of the process that transpires after disruption of the intact milieu [15]. Scar tissue is generally found in three components of the epidural space. Dorsal epidural scar tissue is formed by reabsorption of surgical hematoma and may be involved in pain generation [16]. In the ventral epidural space, dense scar tissue is formed by ventral defects in the disk, which may persist despite surgical treatment and continue to produce low back pain and radiculopathy past the surgical healing phase [17]. The lateral epidural space includes the epiradicular structures outside the root canals, known as the lateral recesses or "sleeves," which are susceptible to lateral disk defects, facet hypertrophy, and neuroforaminal stenosis [18].

Although scar tissue itself is not tender, an entrapped nerve root is. Kuslich et al [5] surmised that the presence of scar tissue compounded the pain associated with the nerve root by fixing it in one position and thus increasing the susceptibility of the nerve root to tension or compression. They also concluded that no other tissues in the spine are capable of producing leg pain. In a study of the relationship between peridural scar evaluated by magnetic resonance imaging (MRI) and radicular pain after lumbar diskectomy, Ross et al [19] demonstrated that subjects with extensive peridural scarring were 3.2 times more likely to experience recurrent radicular pain.

This evidence also parallels a new study by Gilbert et al [20] in which lumbosacral nerve roots were identified as undergoing less strain than previously published during straight leg raise and in which hip motion greater than 60 degrees was determined to cause displacement of the nerve root in the lateral recess.

3. Fluid foraminotomy: Foraminal adhesiolysis or disentrapment

Relative or functional foraminal root entrapment syndrome secondary to epidural fibrosis with corresponding nerve root entrapment is frequently evident after an epidurogram and signified by lack of epidural contrast flow into epidural finger projections at those levels. The lysis procedure effectively serves as a fluid foraminotomy reducing foraminal stenosis caused by epidural fibrosis. In addition to increasing foraminal cross-sectional area, adhesiolysis serves to decompress distended epidural venous structures that may exert compression at nearby spinal levels (Figures 1 and 2) and inevitably cause needle stick related epidural hematomas. Adhesiolysis has led to the development of flexible epiduroscopy that is being pioneered by, primarily initiated, pursued and to this day supported by Dr. James Heavner [21,22].

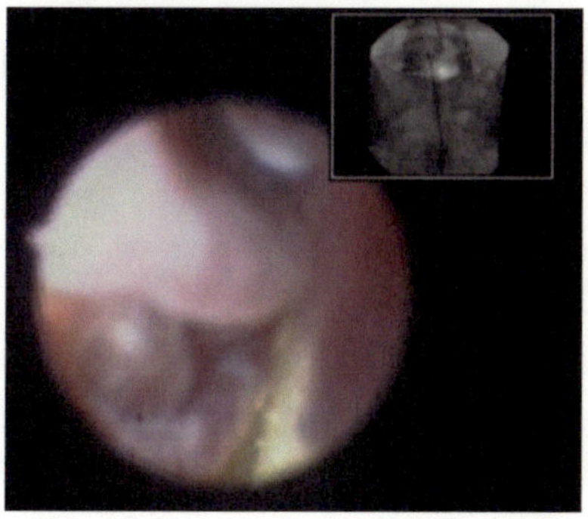

Figure 1. Engorged blood vessels in the epidural cavity as observed during epiduroscopy. Insert in upper right corner is fluoroscopy showing location for epiduroscopy tip (left anterior border of L5).

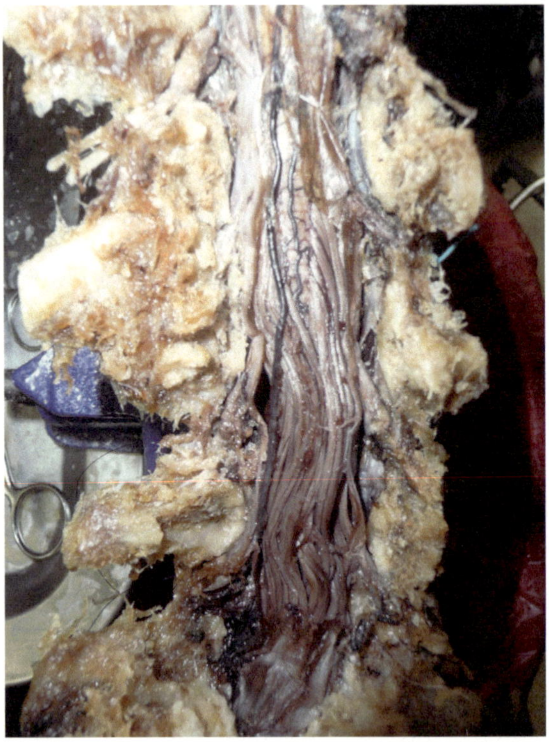

Figure 2. Engorged blood vessels in the epidural cavity in cadaver. See vein on right side next to the nerve root target site for fluid foraminotomy and opening venous run off and decompression.

4. Diagnosis and radiologic diagnosis of epidural fibrosis

As with any patient, a thorough musculoskeletal and neurologic examination should be performed. In addition to standard dural tension provocative tests, we recommend a provocative test called 'dural tug.' To perform the test, the patient should be instructed to sit up with a straight leg, bend forward flexing the lumbar spine until their back pain starts to become evident, and the head and neck flexed rapidly forward. During this maneuver, the dura is stretched cephalad and if adhered to structures such as the posterior longitudinal ligament, the most heavily innervated spinal canal structure, the movement of the dura will elicit back pain that is localized to the pain generator. A positive dural tug maneuver has been observed to resolve after percutaneous neuroplasty. (Figures 3-7).

http://dx.doi.org/10.5772/58753

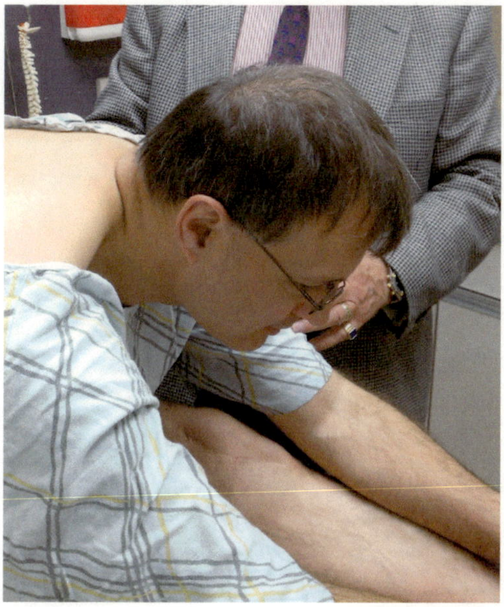

Figure 3. The 'dural tug' maneuver being performed prior to percutaneous neuroplasty.

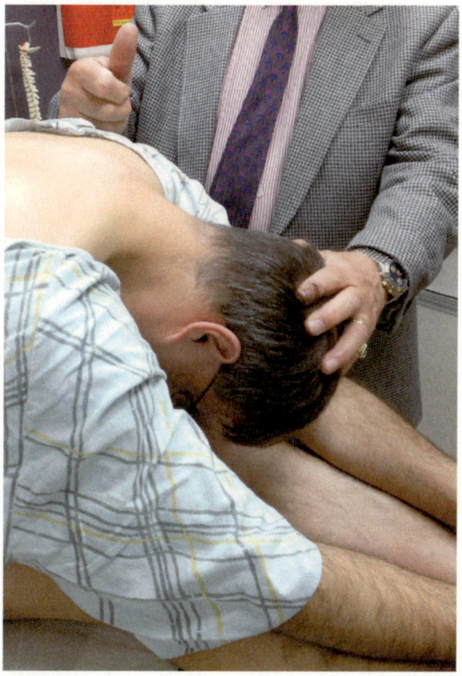

Figure 4. Note pain reproduction prior to full neck flexion secondary to dural adhesions.

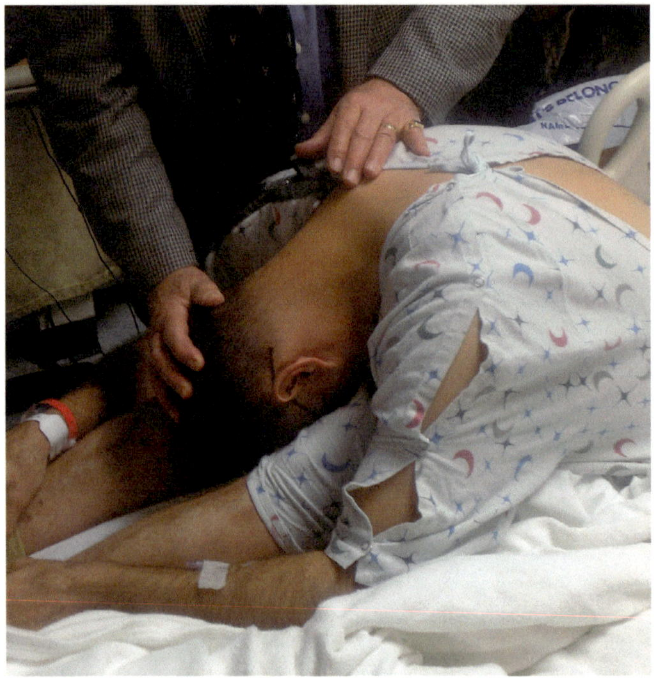

Figure 5. Patient after percutaneous neuroplasty with pain free neck and back flexion due to treatment of dural adhesions.

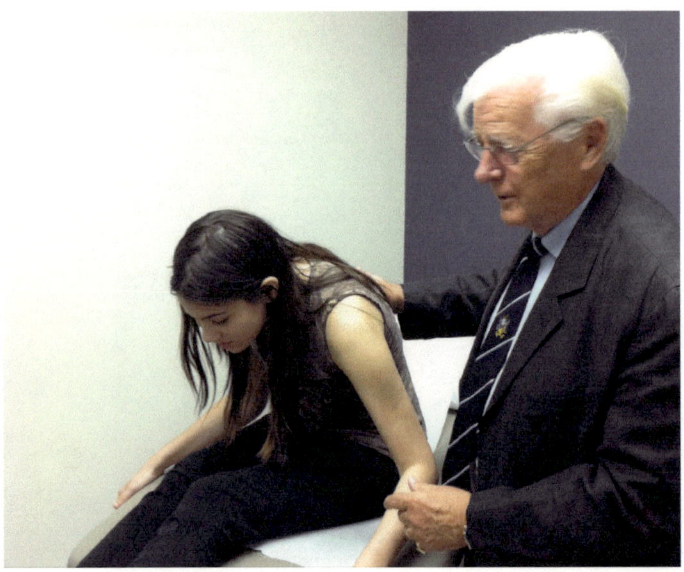

Figure 6. There is decreased spine flexion prior to treatment secondary to dural adhesions. The pain generator was subsequently documented to be T9-T10 dural adhesion from an annular tear.

http://dx.doi.org/10.5772/58753

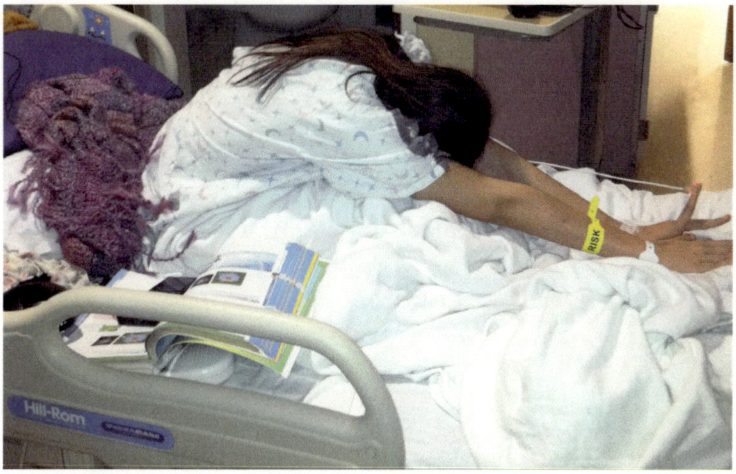

Figure 7. After treatment, the same patient demonstrates increased painless flexion of the spine.

MRI and computed tomography (CT) are diagnostic tools; sensitivity and specificity are 50% and 70%, respectively [15]. CT myelography may also be helpful, although none of the aforementioned modalities can identify epidural fibrosis with 100% reliability. In contrast, epidurography is a technique used with considerable success and it is believed that epidural fibrosis is best diagnosed by performing an epidurogram [23–26]. It can detect filling defects in good correlation with a patient's symptoms in real time [26]. A combination of several of these techniques would undoubtedly increase the ability to identify epidural fibrosis.

4.1. current procedural terminology or CPT codes

The American Medical Association has developed Current Procedural Terminology codes for epidural adhesiolysis, which include 62264 for a single infusion and 62263 for a staged three-series infusion.

4.2. Indications for epidural adhesiolysis

Although originally designed to treat radiculopathy secondary to epidural fibrosis following surgery, the use of epidural adhesiolysis has been expanded to treat a multitude of pain etiologies. These include the following [27]:

1. Failed back surgery syndrome
2. Postlaminectomy syndrome of the neck and back after surgery
3. Disk disruption
4. Metastatic carcinoma of the spine leading to compression fracture
5. Multilevel degenerative arthritis
6. Facet pain

7. Spinal stenosis
8. Pain unresponsive to spinal cord stimulation and spinal opioids
9. Thoracic disk related chest wall and abdominal pain (after mapping)

4.3. Contraindications

The following are absolute contraindications for performing epidural adhesiolysis:

1. Sepsis
2. Chronic infection
3. Coagulopathy
4. Local infection at the procedure site
5. Patient refusal
6. Syrinx formation

A relative contraindication is the presence of arachnoiditis. With arachnoiditis, the tissue planes may be adherent to one another, increasing the chance of loculation of contrast or medication. It may also increase the chance of spread of the medications to the subdural or subarachnoid space, which can increase the chance of complications. Practitioners with limited experience with epidural adhesiolysis should consider referring these patients to a clinician with more training and experience.

5. Patient preparation

When epidural adhesiolysis has been deemed an appropriate treatment modality, the risks and benefits of the procedure should be discussed with the patient and informed consent obtained. The benefits are pain relief, improved physical function, and possible reversal of neurologic symptoms. Risks include, but are not limited to, bruising, bleeding, infection, reaction to medications used (i.e., hyaluronidase, local anesthetic, corticosteroids, hypertonic saline), damage to nerves or blood vessels, no or little pain relief, bowel/bladder incontinence, worsening of pain, and paralysis. Patients with a history of urinary incontinence should have an urodynamic evaluation by a urologist before the procedure to document the preexisting urodynamic etiology and pathology.

6. Anticoagulant medication

Medications that prolong bleeding and clotting parameters should be withheld before performing epidural adhesiolysis. The length of time varies depending on the medication taken. A consultation with the patient's primary physician should be obtained before stopping

http://dx.doi.org/10.5772/58753

any of these medications, particularly in patients who require chronic anticoagulation such as those with drug-eluting heart stents or prosthetic heart valves. Nonsteroidal anti-inflammatory drugs and aspirin, respectively, should be withheld 4 days and 7 to 10 days before the procedure. Although there is much debate regarding these medications and neuraxial procedures, we tend to be on the conservative side. Clopidogrel (Plavix) should be stopped 7 days before, whereas ticlopidine (Ticlid) is withheld 10 to 14 days before the adhesiolysis [28]. Warfarin (Coumadin) stoppage is variable but 5 days is usually adequate [27]. Patients on subcutaneous heparin should have it withheld a minimum of 12 hours before the procedure, whereas those on low-molecular-weight heparin require a minimum of 24 hours [28]. Over-the-counter homeopathic medications that prolong bleeding parameters should also be withheld. These include fish oil, vitamin E, gingko biloba, garlic, ginseng, and St. John's Wort. Adequate coagulation status can be confirmed by the history, INR, prothrombin time, partial thromboplastin time, and a platelet function assay or bleeding time. The tests should be performed as close to the day of the procedure as possible. Tests performed only a few days after stopping the anticoagulant medication may come back elevated because not enough time has elapsed to allow the anticoagulant effects of the medication to resolve. The benefits of the procedure must be weighed against the potential sequelae of stopping the anticoagulant medication and this should be discussed thoroughly with the patient.

7. Preoperative laboratory

Before the procedure, a complete blood count and a clean-catch urinalysis are obtained to check for any undiagnosed infections. An elevated white count and/or a positive urinalysis should prompt the physician to postpone the procedure and refer the patient to the primary care physician for further workup and treatment. In addition, history of bleeding, abnormalities a prothrombin time, partial thromboplastin time, and platelet function assay or bleeding time, are obtained to check for coagulation abnormalities. Any elevated value warrants further investigation and postponement of the procedure until those studies are complete.

8. Technique

This procedure can be performed in the cervical, thoracic, lumbar, and caudal regions of the spine. The caudal and transforaminal placement of catheters will be described in detail, whereas highlights and slight changes in protocol will be provided for cervical and thoracic catheters. Our policy is to perform this procedure under strict sterile conditions in the operating room. Prophylactic antibiotics with broad neuraxial coverage are given before the procedure. Patients will receive either ceftriaxone 1 g intravenously or Levaquin 500 mg orally in those allergic to penicillin. The same dose is also given on day 2. An anesthesiologist or nurse anesthetist provides monitored anesthesia care.

9. Caudal approach

The patient is placed in the prone position with a pillow placed under the abdomen to correct the lumbar lordosis and a pillow under the ankles for patient comfort. The patient is asked to put his or her toes together and heels apart. This relaxes the gluteal muscles and facilitates identification of the sacral hiatus. After sterile preparation and draping, the sacral hiatus is identified via palpation just caudal to the sacral cornu or with fluoroscopic guidance. A skin wheal is raised with local anesthetic 1-inch lateral and 2 inches caudal to the sacral hiatus on the side opposite the documented radiculopathy. A distal subcutaneous approach theoretically provides some protection from meningitis, as a local skin infection would be much preferred over infection closer to the caudal epidural space. The skin is nicked with an 18-gauge cutting needle, and a 15-or 16-gauge RX Coudé (Epimed International) epidural needle is inserted through the nick at a 45-degree angle and guided fluoroscopically or by palpation to the sacral hiatus (Figures 8 and 9).

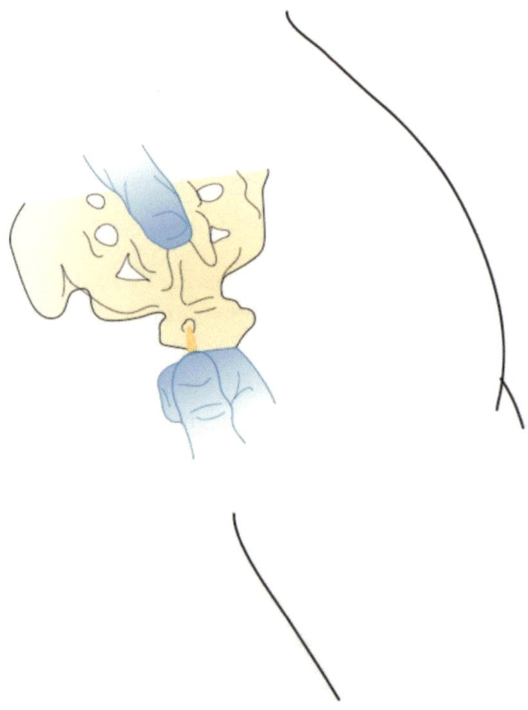

Figure 8. Caudal lysis sequence—first find sacral hiatus and tip of coccyx.

When the needle is through the hiatus, the angle of the needle is dropped to approximately 30 degrees and advanced. The advantages of the RX Coudé needle over other needles are the angled tip, which enables easier direction of the catheter, and the tip of the needle is less sharp. The back edge of the distal opening of the needle is designed to be a noncutting surface that allows manipulation of the catheter in and out of the needle. A Touhy needle has the back edge

http://dx.doi.org/10.5772/58753

of the distal opening, which is a cutting surface and can more easily shear a catheter. A properly placed needle will be inside the caudal canal below the level of the S3 foramen on anteroposterior (AP) and later fluoroscopic images. A needle placed above the level of the S3 foramen could potentially puncture a low-lying dura. The needle tip should cross the midline of the sacrum toward the side of the radiculopathy.

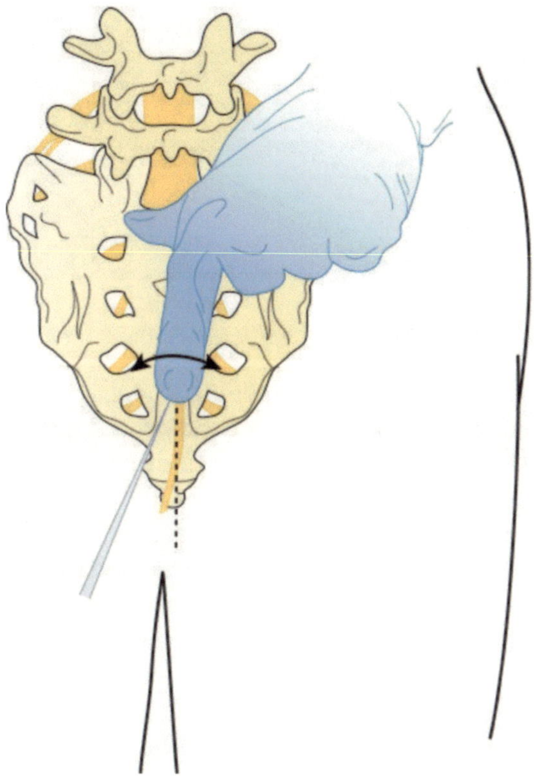

Figure 9. Roll palpating index finger to identify the sacral cornu and thus the target sacral hiatus.

An epidurogram is performed using 10 mL of a non-ionic, water-soluble contrast agent. Confirm a negative aspiration for blood or cerebrospinal fluid before any injection of the contrast or medication. Omnipaque and Isovue are the two agents most frequently used and are suitable for myelography [29, 30]. Do not use ionic, water-insoluble agents such as Hypopaque or Renografin or ionic, water-soluble agents such as Conray [31,32]. These agents are not indicated for myelography. Accidental subarachnoid injections can lead to serious untoward events such as seizure and possibly death. Slowly inject the contrast agent and observe for filling defects. A normal epidurogram will have a "Christmas tree" pattern with the central canal being the trunk and the outline of the nerve roots making up the branches. An abnormal epidurogram will have areas where the contrast does not fill (Figure 10). These are the areas of presumed scarring and typically correspond to the patient's radicular complaints. If vascular uptake is observed, the needle needs to be redirected.

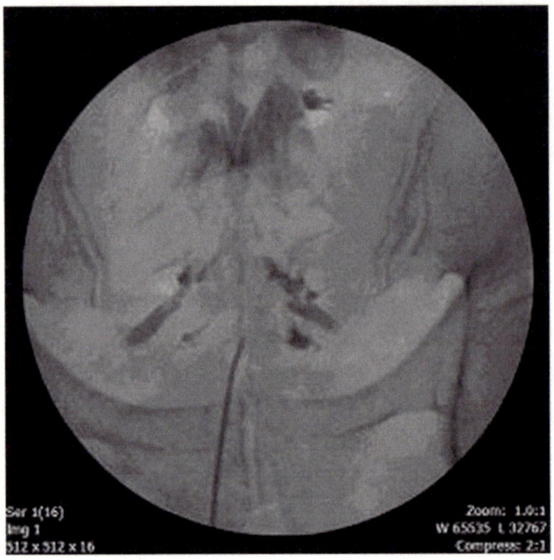

Figure 10. Initial dye injection Omnipaque 240 (10 mL) showing sacral S3 runoff and filling defects at S2, S1, and right L5.

After turning the distal opening of the needle ventral lateral, insert a TunL Kath or TunL-XL (stiffer) catheter (Epimed International) with a bend on the distal tip through the needle (Figures 11 and 12). The bend should be 2.5 cm from the tip of the catheter and at a 30-degree angle. The bend will enable the catheter to be steered to the target level (Figure 13). Under continuous AP fluoroscopic guidance, advance the tip of the catheter toward the ventral-lateral epidural space of the desired level. The catheter can be steered by gently twisting the catheter in a clockwise or counterclockwise direction. Avoid "propellering" the tip (i.e., twisting the tip in circles) because this makes it more difficult to direct the catheter. Do not advance the catheter up the middle of the sacrum because this makes guiding the catheter to the ventral-lateral epidural space more difficult. Ideal location of the tip of the catheter in the AP projection is in the foramen just below the midportion of the pedicle shadow (Figures 14 and 15). Check a lateral projection to confirm that the catheter tip is in the ventral epidural space.

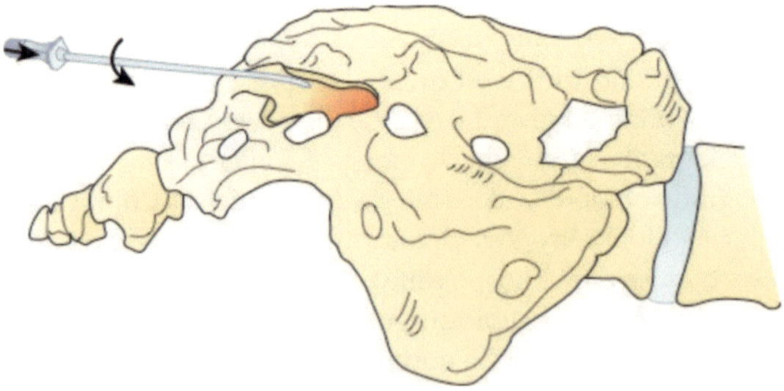

Figure 11. The needle is placed through the sacral hiatus into the sacral canal and rotated in the direction of the target. Do not advance beyond the S3 foramen.

http://dx.doi.org/10.5772/58753

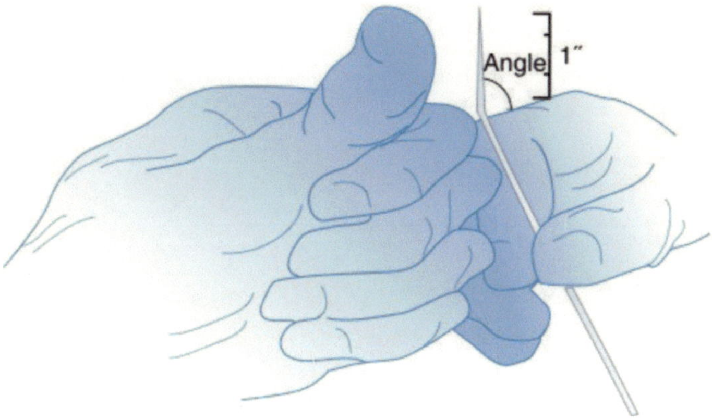

Figure 12. The Epimed Racz catheter is marked for the location of the bend, or use the thumb as reference for the 15-degree angle bend.

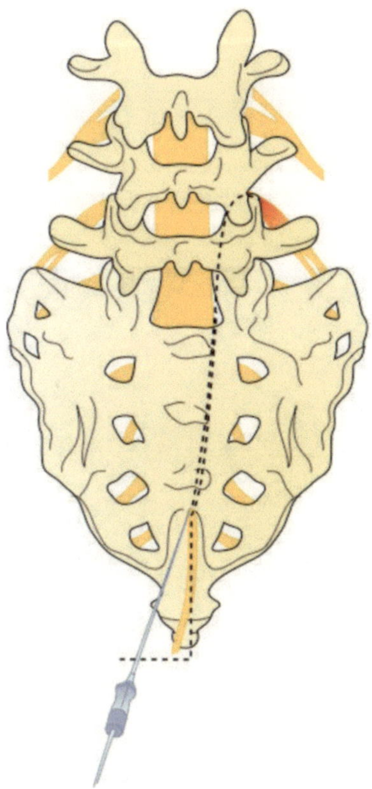

Figure 13. The direction of the catheter is just near the midline; direct the curve under continuous fluoroscopic guidance to the ventral lateral target site. The needle rotation, as well as the catheter navigation, may need to be used to reach the target.

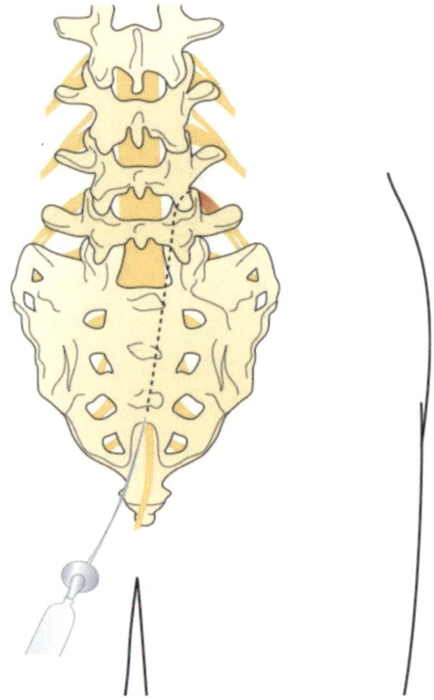

Figure 14. The needle is removed, and the catheter is placed in the ventral lateral epidural space ventral to the nerve root.

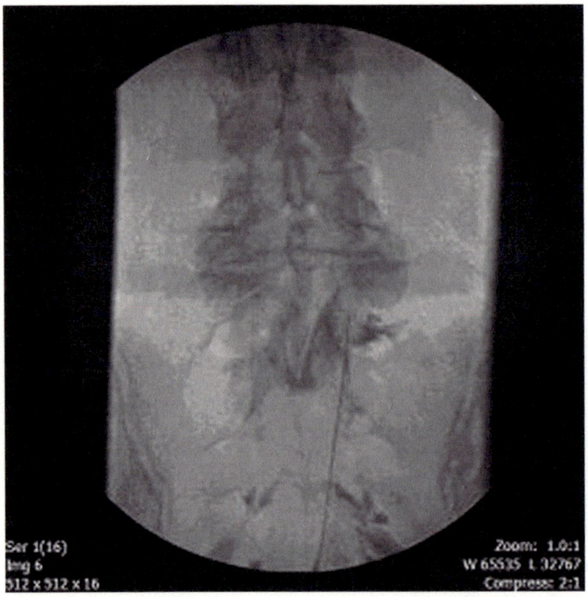

Figure 15. Catheter (24xL) is threaded to lateral L5 neural foramen.

http://dx.doi.org/10.5772/58753

Under real-time fluoroscopy, inject 2 to 3 mL of additional contrast through the catheter in an attempt to outline the "scarred in" nerve root (Figure 16). If vascular uptake is noted, reposition the catheter and reinject contrast. Preferably there should not be vascular runoff, but infrequently secondary to venous congestion, an epidural pattern is seen with a small amount of vascular spread. This is acceptable as long as the vascular uptake is venous in nature and not arterial. Extra caution should be taken when injecting the local anesthetic to prevent local anesthetic toxicity. Toxicity is volume and dose related and so far there has not been any reported complications from small volume venous spread. Any arterial spread of contrast always warrants repositioning of the catheter. We have never observed intra-arterial placement in 25 years of placing soft, spring-tipped catheters.

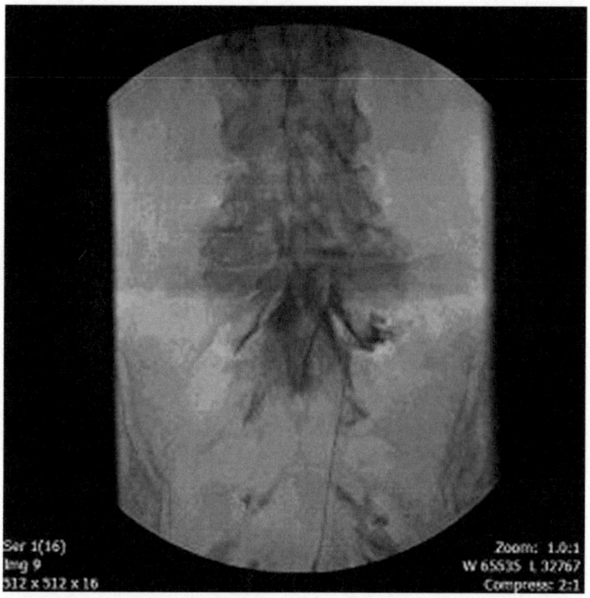

Figure 16. Contrast injection Omnipaque 240, additional 5 mL opening right L5, S1, S2, and S3 perineural spaces; also left L5, S1, S2, and S3 in addition to right L4 spread in cephalad direction.

Inject 1500 U of hyaluronidase dissolved in 10 mL of preservative-free normal saline. A newer development is the use of Hylenex or human-recombinant hyaluronidase, which carries the advantage of a reportedly increased effectiveness at the body's normal pH compared to bovine-recombinant hyaluronidase [33]. This injection may cause some discomfort, so a slow injection is preferable. Observe for "opening up"(i.e. visualization) of the "scarred in" nerve root (Figures 17 and 18 see also Figure 16). A 3 mL test dose of a 10 mL local anesthetic/steroid (LA/S) solution is then given. Our institution used 4 mg of dexamethasone mixed with 9 mL of 0.2% ropivacaine. Ropivacaine is used instead of bupivacaine for two reasons: the former produces a preferential sensory versus a motor block, and it is less cardiotoxic than a racemic bupivacaine. Doses for other corticosteroids commonly used are 40 to 80 mg of methylprednisolone (Depo-Medrol), 25 to 50 mg of triamcinolone diacetate (Aristocort), 40 to 80 mg of triamcinolone acetonide (Kenalog), and 6 to 12 mg of betamethasone (Celestone Solu span). If, after 5 minutes, there is no evidence of intrathecal or intravascular injection of medication, inject the remaining 7 mL of the LA/S solution.

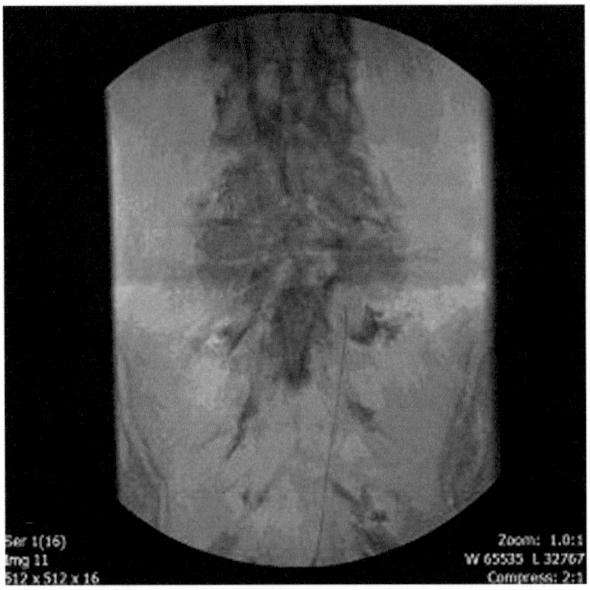

Figure 17. Additional contrast and hyaluronidase injection opens up bilaterally formerly scarred areas. The Christmas tree appearance is obvious.

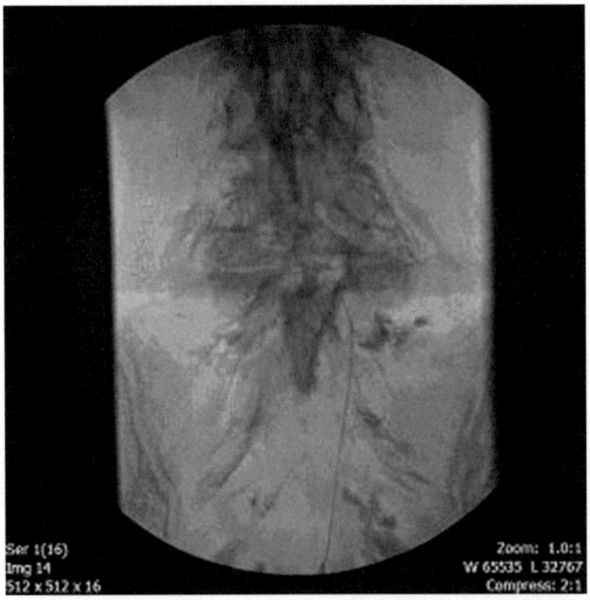

Figure 18. Catheter advances to the desired symptomatic level of right L5 in the ventral lateral epidural space. Injection of contrast followed by 10 mL hyaluronidase 1,500 units opens up bilaterally L3-5, S1, S2, and S3 neural foramina.

http://dx.doi.org/10.5772/58753

Remove the needle under continuous fluoroscopic guidance to ensure the catheter remains at the target level (Figure 19). Secure the catheter to the skin using nonabsorbable suture and coat the skin puncture site with antimicrobial ointment. Apply a sterile dressing and attach a 0.2 μ m filter to the end of the catheter. Affix the exposed portion of the catheter to the patient with tape and transport the patient to the recovery area.

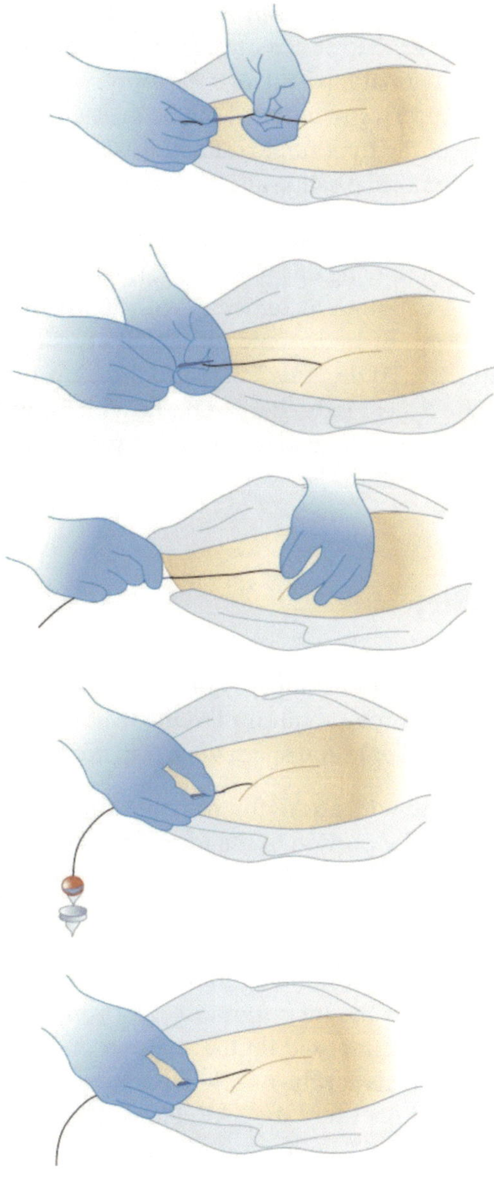

Figure 19. Five picture sequence of removal of the needle to prevent dislodging the catheter from target site before suturing and application of dressing.

A 20-to 30-minute period should elapse between the last injection of the LA/S solution and the start of the hypertonic saline (10%) infusion. This is necessary to ensure that a subdural injection of the LA/S solution has not occurred. A subdural block mimics a subarachnoid block but it takes longer to establish, usually 16 to 18 minutes. Evidence for subdural or subarachnoid spread is the development of motor block. If the patient develops a subarachnoid or subdural block at any point during the procedure, the catheter should be removed and the remainder of the adhesiolysis canceled. The patient needs to be observed to document the resolution of the motor and sensory block and to document that 10 mL of the hypertonic saline is then infused through the catheter over 15 to 30 minutes. If the patient complains of discomfort, the infusion is stopped and an additional 2 to 3 mL of 0.2% ropivacaine is injected and the infusion is restarted. Alternatively, 50 to 75 μ g of fentanyl can be injected epidurally in lieu of the local anesthetic. After completion of the hypertonic saline infusion, the catheter is slowly flushed with 2 mL of preservative-free normal saline and the catheter is capped.

Our policy is to admit the patient for 24-hour observation status and do a second and a third hypertonic saline infusion the following day. On post–catheter insertion day 2, the catheter is twice injected (separated by 4-to 6-hour increments) with 10 mL of 0.2% ropivacaine without steroid and infused with 10 mL of hypertonic saline (10%) using the same technique and precautions as the day 1 infusion. At the end of the third infusion, the catheter is removed and a sterile dressing applied. The patient is discharged home with 5 days of oral cephalexin at 500 mg twice a day or oral levofloxacin (Levaquin) at 500 mg once a day for penicillin-allergic patients. Clinic follow-up is in 30 days.

10. Transforaminal catheters

Patients with an additional level of radiculopathy or those in whom the target level cannot be reached by the caudal approach may require placement of a second catheter. The second catheter is placed into the ventral epidural space via a transforaminal approach.

After the target level is identified with an AP fluoroscopic image, the superior endplate of the vertebra that comprises the caudal portion of the foramina is "squared," that is, the anterior and posterior shadows of the vertebral endplate are superimposed. The angle is typically 15 to 20 degrees in a caudocephalad direction. The fluoroscope is then oblique approximately 15 degrees to the side of the radiculopathy and adjusted until the spinous process is rotated to the opposite side. This fluoroscope positioning allows the best visualization of the superior articular process (SAP) that forms the inferoposterior portion of the targeted foramen. The image of the SAP should be superimposed on the shadow of the disk space on the oblique view. The tip of the SAP is the target for the needle placement (Figure 20). Raise a skin wheal slightly lateral to the shadow of the tip of the SAP. Pierce the skin with an 18-gauge needle and then insert a 15-or 16-gauge RX Coudé needle and advance using gun-barrel technique toward the tip of the SAP. Continue to advance the needle medially toward the SAP until the tip contacts bone. Rotate the tip of the needle 180 degrees laterally and advance about 5 mm (Figure 21). Rotate the needle back medially 180 degrees (Figure 22).

http://dx.doi.org/10.5772/58753

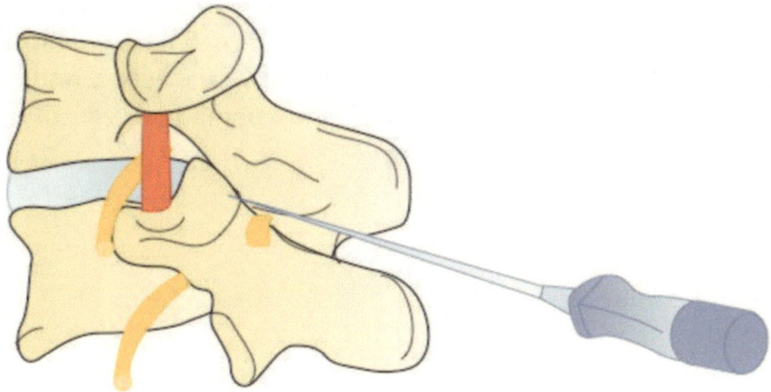

Figure 20. Transforaminal lateral-oblique view. Target the SAP with the advancing RX Coude needle.

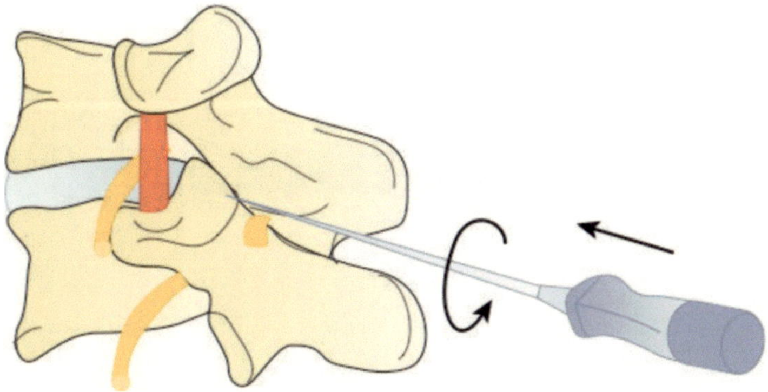

Figure 21. Following bony contact with SAP. Lateral rotation of 180 degrees to allow passage toward the target.

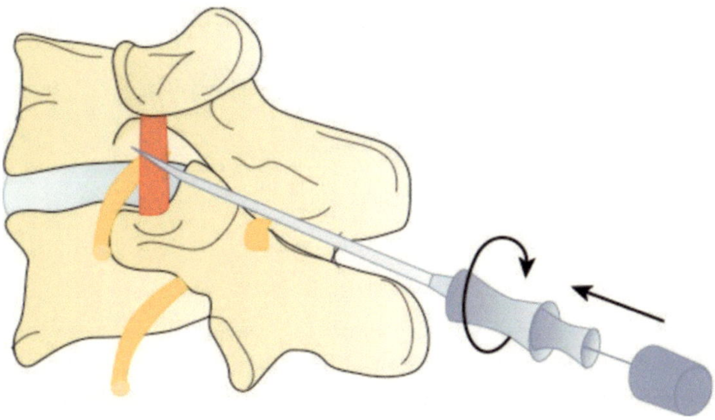

Figure 22. Note the intertransverse ligament. The needle tip with the RX Coude 2 that has 1 mm protruding blunt stylet will pass through the ligament and will be less likely to damage the nerve.

As the needle is advanced slowly, a clear "pop" is felt as the needle penetrates the intertransverse ligament. Obtain a lateral fluoroscopic image. The tip of the needle should be just past the SAP in the posterior foramen. In the AP plane, the tip of the needle under continuous AP fluoroscopy, insert the catheter slowly into the foramen and advance until the tip should be just short of the middle of the spinal canal (Fig 23-25).

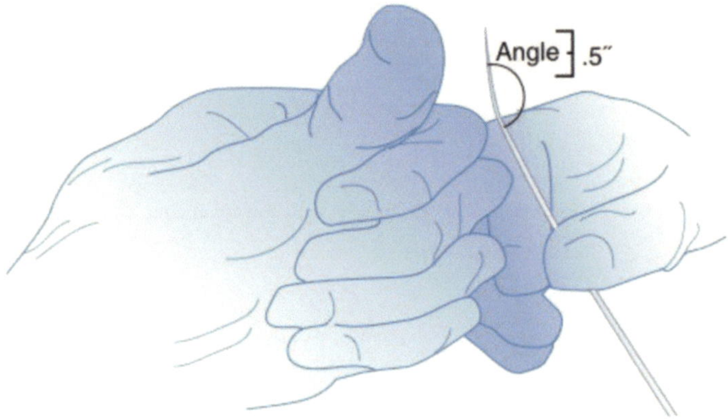

Figure 23. The distal tip of the catheter may be bent 15-degrees, 3/4 inch length.

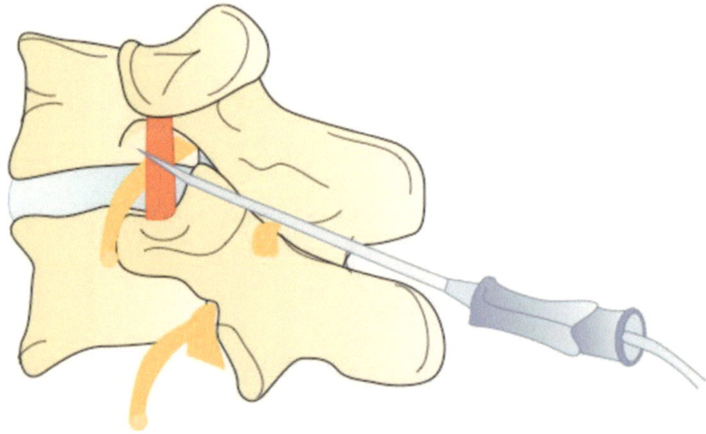

Figure 24. Once the intertransverse ligament is perforated, the catheter is steered to the ventral lateral epidural space (lateral view).

Confirm that the catheter is in the anterior epidural space with a lateral image (Figure 26). Anatomically, the catheter is in the foramen above or below the exiting nerve root (Figure 27). If the catheter cannot be advanced, it usually means the needle is either too posterior or too lateral to the foramen. It can also indicate that the foramen is too stenotic to allow passage of the catheter. The needle can be advanced a few millimeters anteriorly in relation to the foramen, and that will also move it slightly medial into the foramen. If the catheter still will

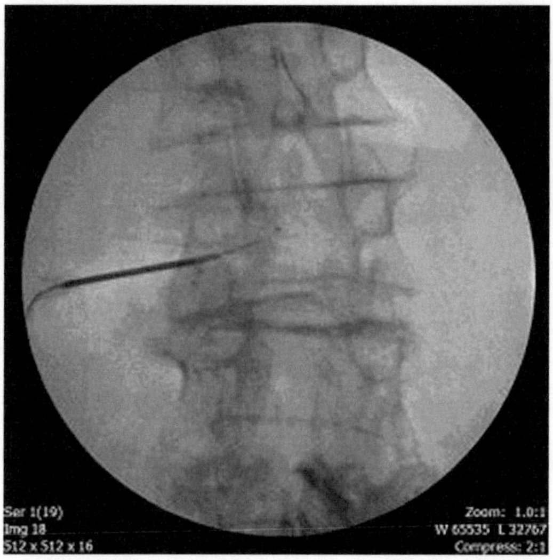

Figure 25. Transforaminal 15-gauge RX-Coude 2 (Epimed International, Johnstown, NY) catheter at left L3-4 threaded almost to near *midcanal* position (anteroposterior view).

not pass, the initial insertion of the needle will need to be more lateral. Therefore the fluoroscope angle will be about 20 degrees instead of 15 degrees. The curve of the needle usually facilitates easy catheter placement. The final position of the catheter tip is just short of the midline.

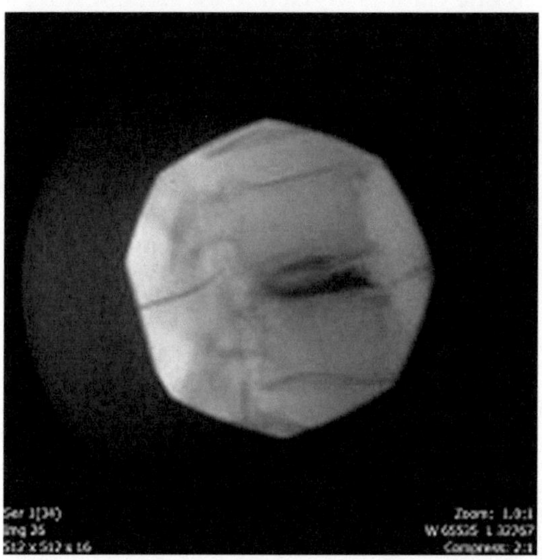

Figure 26. Lateral view of Figure. 16-13. Transforaminal-ventral-anterior catheter dye spread to epidural and L3-4 intradiscal area (through annular tear).

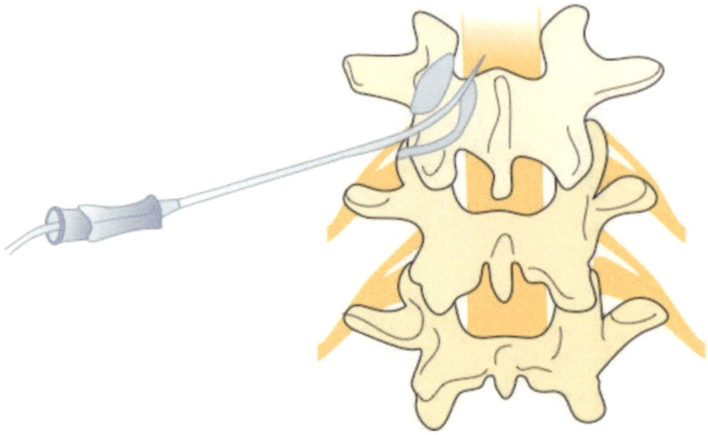

Figure 27. Anteroposterior view. The catheter is in optimal position near midline via the transforaminal placement.

Inject 1 to 2 mL of contrast to confirm epidural spread. When a caudal and a transforaminal catheter are placed, the 1500 U of hyaluronidase are divided evenly between the two catheters (5 mL of the hyaluronidase/saline solution into each). The LA/S solution is also divided evenly, but a volume of 15 mL (1 mL steroid and 14 mL 0.2% ropivacaine; of the total volume, 5 mL is transforaminal and 10 mL is caudal) is used instead of 10 mL. Remove the needle under fluoroscopic guidance to make sure the catheter does not move from the original position in the epidural space. Secure and cover the catheter as described previously. The hypertonic saline solution is infused at a volume of 4 to 5 mL per transforaminal and 8 to 10 mL per caudal catheter over 30 minutes. The hypertonic saline injection volume should always be less than or equal to the local anesthetic volume injected to avoid pain from injection. It behooves the practitioner to check the position of the transforaminal catheter under fluoroscopy before performing the second and third infusions. The catheter may advance across the epidural space into the contralateral foramen or paraspinous muscles or more commonly back out of the epidural space into the ipsilateral paraspinous muscles.

This results in deposition of the medication in the paravertebral tissue rather than in the epidural space. As with the caudal approach, remove the transforaminal catheter after the third infusion. A recent development is the R-X Coude 2 needle in which a second protruding stylet may allow closer needle placement and less chance of nerve injury.

11. 1st sacral foramen approach

The area at the L5S1 anterolateral epidural space is frequently occupied with epidural adhesions which are associated with pain and a lack of contrast filling on epidurography. This volume of this space has been measured to be 1.1 ml anatomically and 0.9 ml surgically [34]. Lysis of adhesions via the caudal approach may be difficult in patients with epidural adhesions at this location and the S1 foraminal approach may be used to achieve lysis and fluid foraminotomy at this level [35].

http://dx.doi.org/10.5772/58753

Matsumoto reported 36 cases with adhesive S-1 radiculopathy. After the procedure, the patients were followed up for 12 months. A marked decrease in VAS and improvement in ADL (improvement in ODI scores) were observed [36].

http://www.paincast.com has video information regarding this procedure [37].

12. Cervical lysis of adhesions

The success of the caudal approach for lysis of adhesions led to the application of the same technique to the cervical epidural space. The indications and preprocedure workup are the same as those for the caudal lysis technique, but there are a few differences in technique and volumes of medication used.

The epidural space should be entered via the upper thoracic interspaces using a paramedian approach on the contralateral side. The most common levels are T1-2 and T2-3. Entry at these levels allows for a sufficient length of the catheter to remain in the epidural space after the target level has been reached. If the target is the lower cervical nerve roots, a more caudal interspace should be selected. We place the patient in the left lateral decubitus position, but use a prone approach in larger patients.

A technique referred to as the "3-D technique" is used to facilitate entry into the epidural space. The "3-D" stands for *direction, depth,* and *direction.* Using an AP fluoroscopic image, the initial *direction* of the 15-or 16-gauge RX Coudé needle is determined. Using a modified paramedian approach with the skin entry one and a half levels below the target interlaminar space, advance and direct the needle toward the midpoint of the chosen interlaminar space with the opening of the needle pointing medial. Once the needle engages the deeper tissue planes (usually at 2 to 3 cm), check the depth of the needle with a lateral image. Advance the needle toward the epidural space and check repeat images to confirm the *depth.* The posterior border of the dorsal epidural space can be visualized by identifying the junction of the base of the spinous process of the vertebra with its lamina. This junction creates a distinct radiopaque "straight line." Once the needle is close to the epidural space, obtain an AP fluoroscopic image to recheck the *direction* of the needle. If the tip of the needle has crossed the midline as defined by the spinous processes of the vertebral bodies, pull the needle back and redirect. The "3-D" process can be repeated as many times as is necessary to get the needle into the perfect position.

Using loss-of-resistance technique, advance the needle into the epidural space with the tip of the RX-Coudé needle, pointed caudally. Once the tip is in the epidural space, rotate the tip cephalad, and inject 1 to 2 mL of contrast to confirm entry. Rotation or movement of any needle in the epidural space can cut the dura. This technique has been improved with the advent of the RX Coudé 2 needle, which has a second interlocking stylet that protrudes slightly beyond the tip of the needle and functions to push the dura away from the needle tip as it is turned 180 degrees cephalad (Figures 28-32).

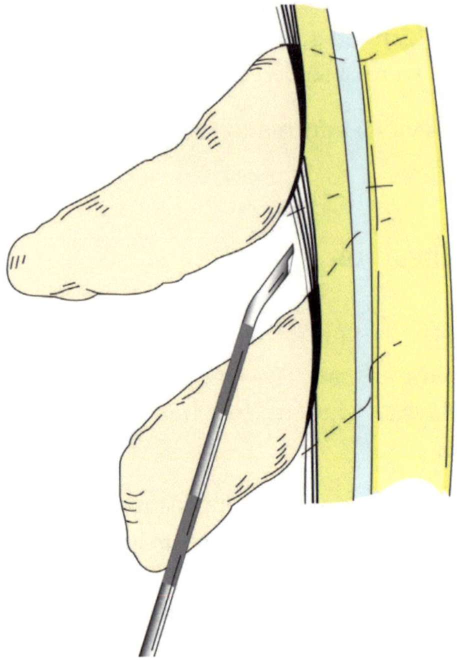

Figure 28. Sequence of stages to place a catheter using the R-X Coude, part 1: The needle is inserted into the epidural space with the tip directed as shown.

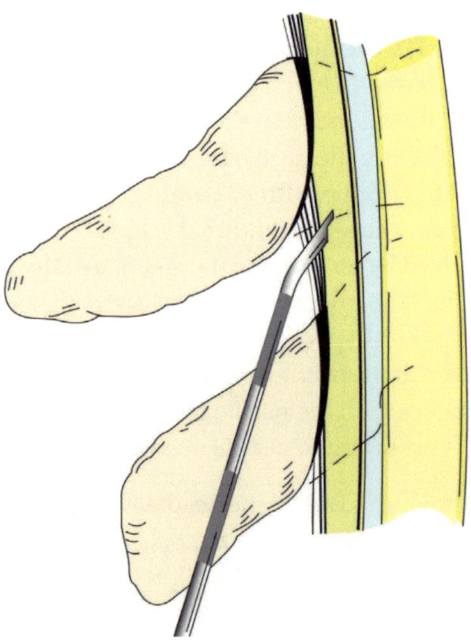

Figure 29. Sequence of stages to place a catheter using the R-X Coude, part 2: The needle is inserted into the epidural space with the tip directed as shown.

http://dx.doi.org/10.5772/58753

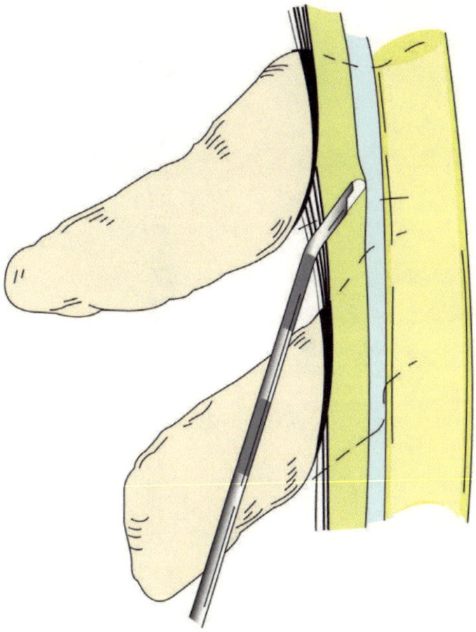

Figure 30. Sequence of stages to place a catheter using the R-X Coude, part 3: The protruding stylet is inserted.

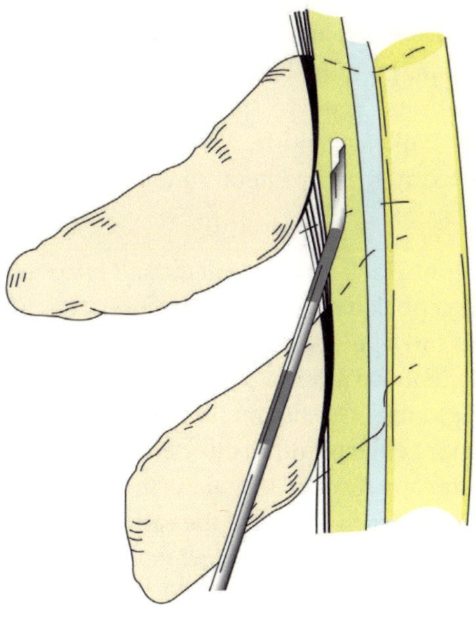

Figure 31. Sequence of stages to place a catheter using the R-X Coude, part 4: Then the needle is rotated so the tip is parallel to the dura.

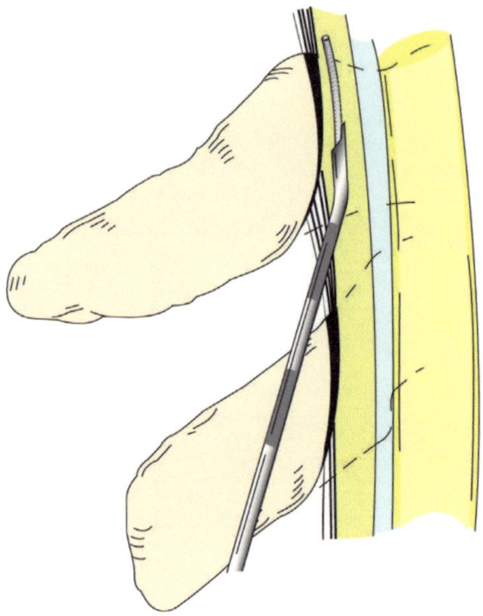

Figure 32. Sequence of stages to place a catheter using the R-X Coude, part 5: The catheter is inserted.

Inject an additional small volume as needed to complete the epidurogram. If there is no free flow of injected contrast, pressure may build up in the lateral epidural space. Characteristic fluid spread by the path of least resistance can be recognized as *perivenous counter spread* (PVCS). Presence of PVCS means pressure builds up in the lateral epidural space that is unable to spread laterally to decompress. The dye spread picks the path of least resistance to the opposite side. Pressure may build up and lead to ischemic spinal cord injury. Flexion and rotation of the head and neck can open up lateral runoff and release the pressure through the enlarged neural foramina (Figure 33) [38].

As with the caudal epidurogram, look for filling defects. It is extremely important to visualize spread of the contrast in the cephalad and caudal directions. Loculation of contrast in a small area must be avoided as this can significantly increase the pressure in the epidural space and can compromise the already tenuous arterial blood supply to the spinal cord. Place a bend on the catheter as previously described for the caudal approach and insert it through the needle (Figure 32). The opening of the needle should be directed toward the target side. Slowly advance the catheter to the lateral gutter and direct it cephalad. Redirect the catheter as needed and once the target level has been reached, turn the tip of the catheter toward the foramen (Figure 34). Inject 0.5 to 1 mL of contrast to visualize the target nerve root. Make sure there is runoff of contrast out of the foramen (Figure 35). Slowly instill 150 U of Hylenex dissolved in 5 mL of preservative-free normal saline. Follow this with 1 to 2 mL of additional contrast and observe for "opening up" of the "scarred in" nerve root. Give a 2 mL test dose of a 6 mL solution of LA/S. Our combination is 5 mL of 0.2% ropivicaine and 4 mg of dexamethasone. If after 5 minutes there is no evidence of intrathecal or intravascular spread, inject the remaining 4 mL. Remove

http://dx.doi.org/10.5772/58753

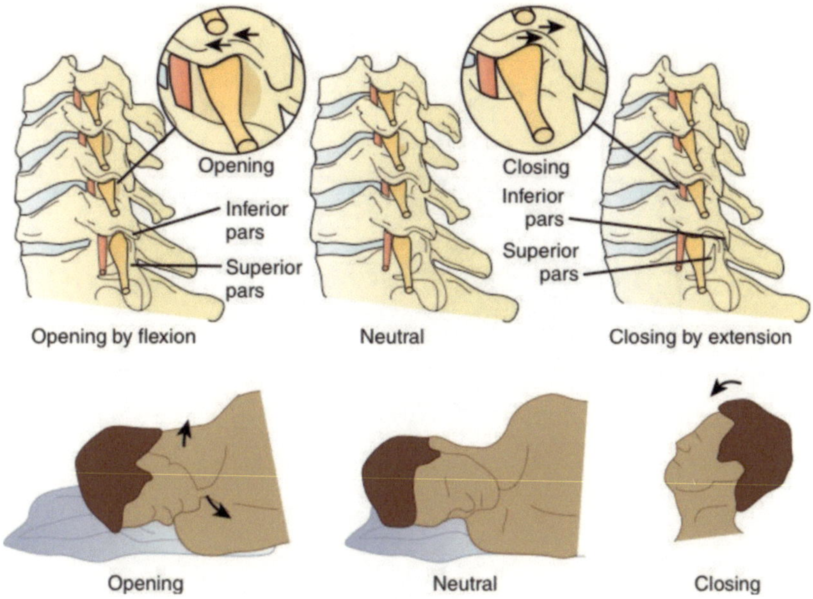

Figure 33. Flexion rotation, left to right regardless patient position. The neural foramen enlarges on flexion rotation and gets smaller with extension. The inferior pars slides forward over the superior pars to enlarge the foramen. This allows lateral run off and pressure release with PVCS.

the needle, and secure and dress the catheter as previously described. Once 20 minutes have passed since the last dose of LA/S solution and there is no evidence of a subarachnoid or subdural block, start an infusion of 5 mL of hypertonic saline over 30 minutes. At the end of the infusion, flush the catheter with 1 to 2 mL of preservative-free normal saline and cap the catheter.

A 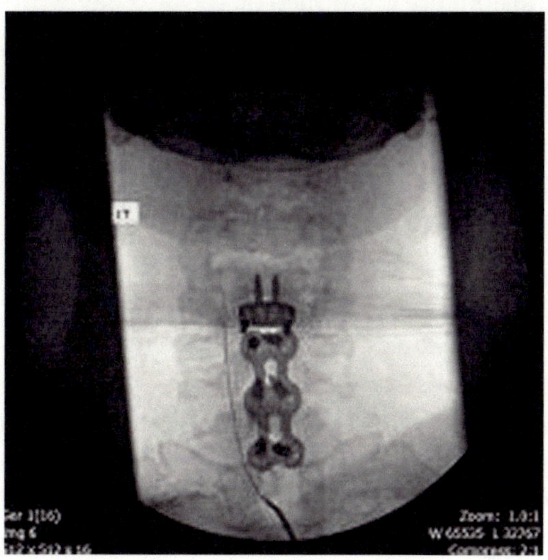

Figure 34. Cervical left ventral lateral catheter to the upper level of fusion C5-7.

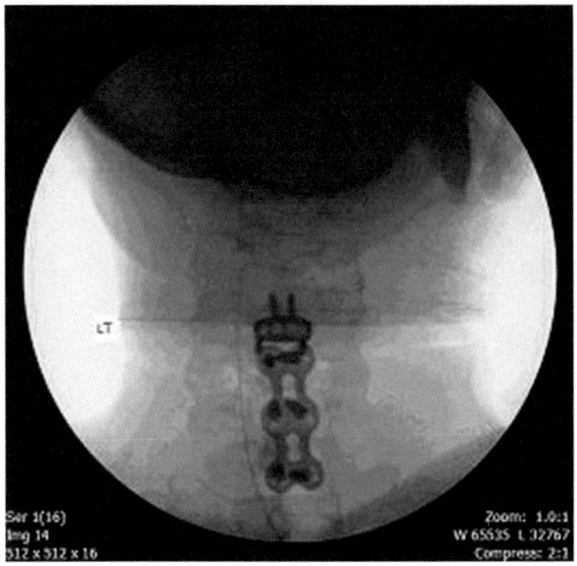

B

Figure 35. Cervical-left ventral lateral catheter threaded to above level of fusion of C4. The dye injection spreads cephalad and lateral.

The second and third infusions are performed on the next day with 6 mL of 0.2% ropivacaine without spread and 5 mL of hypertonic saline using the same technique and precautions described for the first infusion. The catheter is removed and prophylactic antibiotics are prescribed. Clinic follow-up is 30 days.

13. Thoracic lysis of adhesions

The technique for entry into the thoracic epidural space for adhesiolysis is identical to that for the cervical region. Always remember the 3-D technique. Make sure to get a true lateral when checking the depth of the needle. This can be obtained by superimposing the rib shadows on one another. The target is still the ventrolateral epidural space with the tip of the catheter in the foramen of the desired level. The major difference for thoracic lysis compared to the caudal and cervical techniques is the volumes of the various injectates. Volumes of 8 mL are used for the contrast, Hylenex, LA/S, and hypertonic saline. Table 1 lists typical infusion volumes for epidural adhesiolysis.

http://dx.doi.org/10.5772/58753

	Contrast	Hyaluronidase and Normal Saline	Local Anesthetic and Steriod	10% Hypertonic Saline Infusion
Caudal	10 mL	10 mL	10 mL	10 mL
Caudal and transforaminal	5 mL in each catheter	5 mL in each catheter	5 mL in each catheter	8 mL in caudal catheter and 4 mL in transforaminal catheter
Thoracic	8 mL	8 mL	8 mL	8 mL
Cervical	5 mL	6 mL	6 mL	5 mL

Table 1. Typical Infusion Volumes for Epidural Adhesiolysis

14. Neural flossing

The protocol for epidural adhesiolysis has been aided by neural flossing exercises that were designed to mobilize nerve roots by "sliding" them in and out of the foramen (Figure 36). This breaks up weakened scar tissue from the procedure and prevents further scar tissue deposition. If these exercises are done effectively three to four times per day for a few months after the procedure, the formation of scar tissue will be severely restricted.

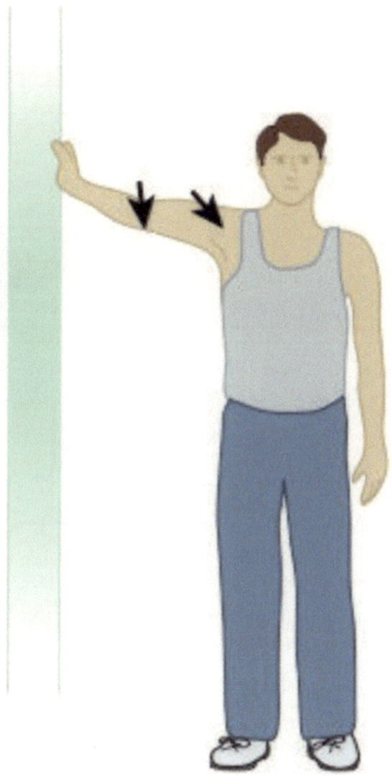

Figure 36. Neural flossing exercises, part 1: Standing erect, firmly grasp a stable surface (e.g., a door frame) with outstretched arm. Press elbow and shoulder forward.

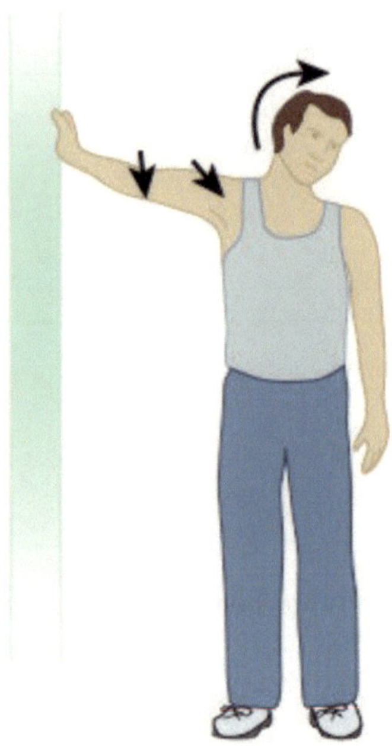

Figure 37. Neural flossing exercises, part 2: Next, slowly tilt head in opposite direction from outstretched arm to achieve gentle tension.

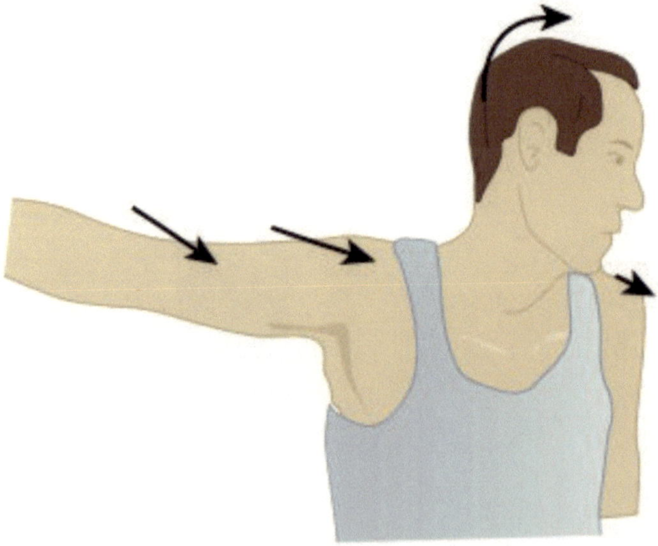

Figure 38. Neural flossing exercises, part 3: Finally, rotate chin toward opposite shoulder as is comfortable. Hold this final position for approximately 20 to 30 seconds.

http://dx.doi.org/10.5772/58753

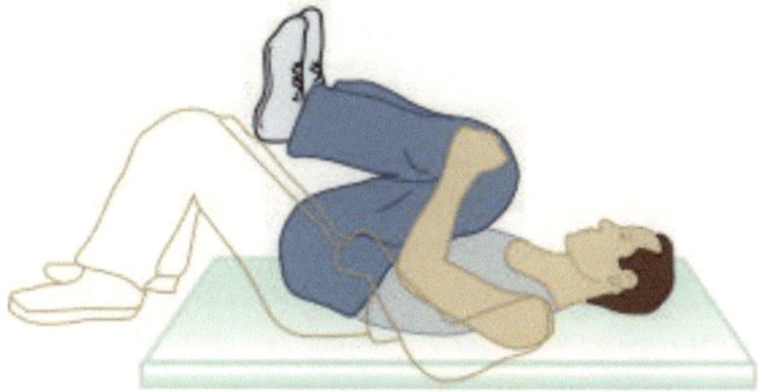

Figure 39. Neural flossing exercises, part 4: Lay down supine on an exercise mat without a pillow. Slowly bring both knees close to the chest with bent legs and hold this position for 20 seconds. Release and assume a neutral position.

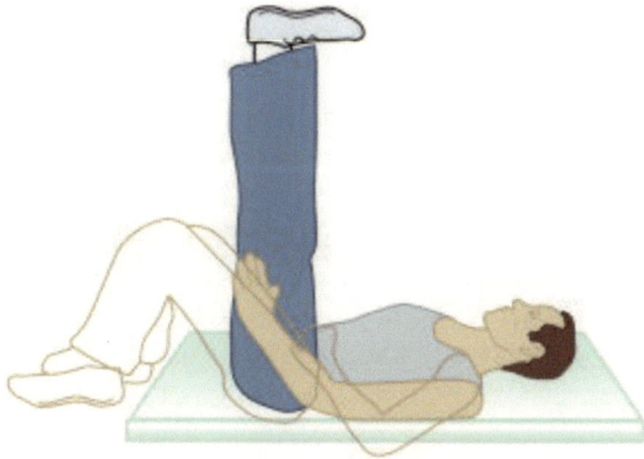

Figure 40. Neural flossing exercises, part 5: Again in supine position, raise both legs to 90 degrees, with knees straight while laying flat on a firm surface. Hold for 20 seconds. Assume a neutral position and rest briefly.

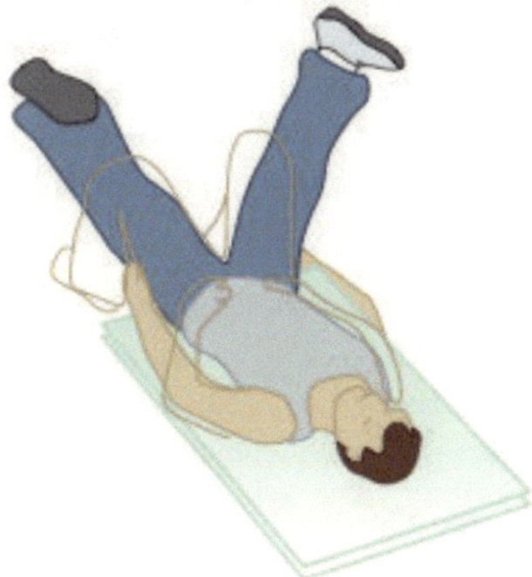

Figure 41. Neural flossing exercises, part 6: Bring both legs to a 90-degree angle while lying supine. Slowly spread legs in a V shape, as much as is comfortable, and hold for 20 seconds.

15. Epidural mapping

In patients with multilevel radiculopathy and complex pain, it can be difficult to determine from where the majority of the pain is emanating. We have been using a technique that we have termed *mapping* to locate the most painful nerve root with stimulation and then carry out the adhesiolysis at that level. There are several references in the literature regarding the use of stimulation to confirm epidural placement of a catheter and for nerve root localization [39]. The TunL Kath and the TunL-XL catheter can be used as stimulating catheters to identify the nerve root(s).

After entering the epidural space, advance the catheter into the ventrolateral epidural space past the suspected target level. Make sure the tip of the catheter is pointing laterally toward the foramina, just below the pedicle. Pull the catheter stylet back approximately 1 cm. Using alligator clips, attach the cathode to the stylet and ground the anode on the needle or ground pad or a 22-gauge needle inserted into the skin. Apply electrical stimulation with a stimulator box with a rate of 50 pulses per second and a pulse width of 450 milliseconds, dialing up the amplitude until a paresthesia is perceived in small increments, usually less than 2 or 3 volts. Inquire of the patient as to whether or not the paresthesia is felt in the area of the patient's recognized greatest pain. This process is repeated at each successive level until the most painful nerve root is identified. Once identified, the adhesiolysis is carried out at that level. The mapping procedure is also useful to identify the optimal site of surgery either before the first surgery or when surgery has failed one or more times.

16. Complications

As with any invasive procedure, complications are possible. These include bleeding, infection, headache, damage to nerves or blood vessels, catheter shearing, bowel/bladder dysfunction, paralysis, spinal cord compression from loculation of the injected fluids or hematoma, subdural or subarachnoid injection of local anesthetic or hypertonic saline, and reactions to the medications used. We also include on the consent form that the patient may experience an increase in pain or no pain relief at all.

Although the potential list of complications is long, the frequency of complications is very rare. However, there is clearly a learning curve, and recent studies reflect this by the significantly improved long-term outcome and the very rare publications of complications and medicolegal consequences when one considers the ever-increasing clinical experience.

Subdural spread is a complication that should always be watched for when injecting local anesthetic. During the caudal adhesiolysis, particularly if the catheter is advanced along the midline, subdural catheter placement is a risk (Figure 42 and 43). Identification of the subdural motor block should occur within 16 to 18 minutes. Catheters used for adhesiolysis should never be directed midline in the epidural space.

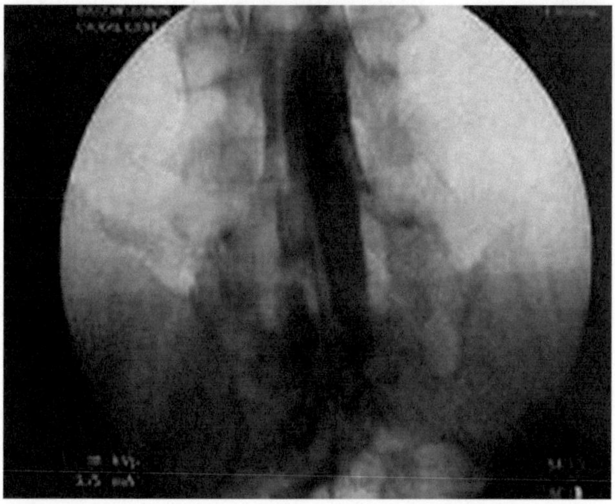

Figure 42. Midline catheter placement enters subdural space. There is also some epidural dye spread. But the patient starts to complain of bilateral leg pain.

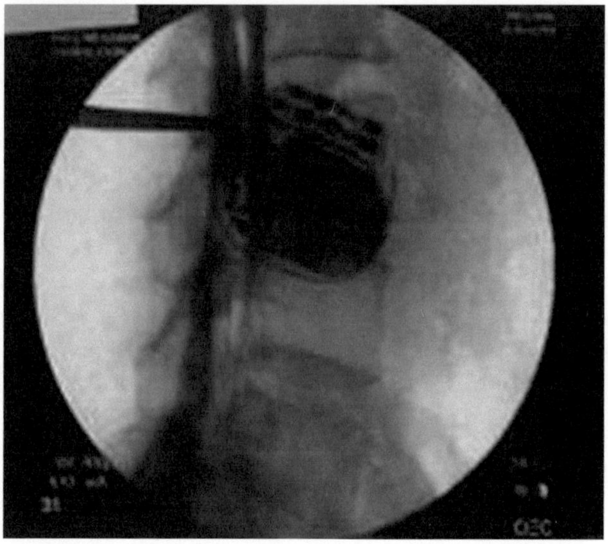

Figure 43. A 22-gauge spinal needle and extension set with syringe placed in the subdural space and 12 mL fluid aspirated. The patient reported immediate reversal of bilateral leg pain. Note the dye in the extension tubing and syringe at the 7-o'clock position.

Most hematomas and other major complications are associated with the use of sharp needles. The use of blunt needles or catheters should be considered to reduce the risk of major complications with the lysis procedure or transforaminal procedures [40].

Venous run off is most common on the first epidural procedure due to high-pressure veins being engorged and large. Following lysis of adhesions and fluid foraminotomy, these high-pressure veins are converted to low-pressure veins and venous run off is less likely. In fact, no cases of hematoma have been reported after lysis of adhesions and fluid foraminotmy in the ventrolateral epidural space [41].

A case of a hematoma has been reported after the MILD procedure before lysis was performed. Lysis should be considered prior to the MILD procedure to achieve fluid foraminotomies and allow fluid to pass out of the spinal canal and avoid venous run off and hematomas [42].

17. Outcomes

Initially in the early 1980s the protocol was designed to direct site-specific medication onto the dorsal root ganglion; however, after performing a number of the procedures, it was found that the dorsal root ganglion was exceptionally hard to reach secondary to developing scar tissue or adhesions. In the early days, our understanding was coming from the use of local anesthetics for surgery giving a 2-to 4-hour block for the surgeon to operate. It was gratifying to see chronic pain patients get months and years of pain relief following the placement of the new steerable x-ray visible catheter. The early report in 1985 by Racz et al [43] described the use of phenol at the dorsal root ganglion followed by an observational listing of outcomes that were clearly not as good as the latest studies on failed back surgery and spinal stenosis showing 75% to 80% improvement at 12 months' follow-up by Manchikanti [38]. Initially we were pleased to see some patients getting 3 to 4 months of relief and report seeing recovery of footdrops. This philosophy still proves to be true even in studies in 2008 by Sakai et al [44] in which they found that adhesiolysis with catheter-directed steroid and local anesthetic injection during epiduroscopy alleviated pain and reduced sensory nerve dysfunction in patients with chronic sciatica. The evolution of these findings has changed the process into what it is today [45]. Racz and Holubec first reported on epidural adhesiolysis in 1989 [46]. There were slight variations in the protocol compared to today's protocol, namely the dose of local anesthetic and the fact that hyaluronidase was not used. Catheter placement was lesion-specific (i.e., the tip of the catheter was placed in the foramen corresponding to the vertebral level and side of the suspected adhesions). The retrospective analysis conducted 6 to 12 months after the procedure reported initial pain relief in 72.2% of patients (*N*=72) at time of discharge. Relief was sustained in 37.5% and 30.5% of patients at 1 and 3 months, respectively. Forty-three percent decreased their frequency and dosage of medication use and 16.7% discontinued their medications altogether. In total, 30.6% of patients returned to work or returned to daily functions. In April 1990, at a presentation of the 7th IASP World Congress on Pain in Adelaide, Austraila, Arthur et al [47] reported on epidural adhesiolysis in 100 patients, 50 of whom received hyaluronidase as part of the procedure. In the hyaluronidase group, 81.6% of the participants had initial pain relief, with 12.3% having persistent relief; 68% of the no hyaluronidase group had relief of pain, with 14% having persistent relief at the end of the 3-year follow-up period from which the study sample was randomly selected.

An informal survey of ophthalmologic anesthesiologists found no cases of anaphylaxis to hyaluronidase used for retrobulbar blocks. In this survey, skin testing for allergy to hyaluronidase was not reported. This implies that severe allergic reactions are rare; however, it is recommended that these procedures be performed in an environment with resuscitative equipment [48].

In 1994 Stolker et al [49] added hyaluronidase to the procedure, but omitted the hypertonic saline. In a study of 28 patients, they reported greater than 50% pain reduction in 64% of patients at 1 year. They stressed the importance of the patient selection and believed that the effectiveness of adhesiolysis was based on the effect of the hyaluronidase on the adhesions and the action of the local anesthetic and steroids on the sinuvertebral nerve.

Devulder et al published a study of 34 patients with failed back surgery syndrome in whom epidural fibrosis was suspected or proved with MRI [50] and an epidural catheter was inserted via the sacral hiatus to a distance of 10 cm into the caudal canal. Injections of contrast dye, local anesthetic, corticosteroid, and hypertonic saline (10%) were carried out daily for 3 days. No hyaluronidase was used. Filling defects were noted in 30 of 34 patients, but significant pain relief was noted in only 7 patients at 1 month, 2 patients at 3 months, and no patients at 12 months. They concluded that epidurography may confirm epidural filling defects for contrast dye in patients with filling defects, but a better contrast dye spread, assuming scar lysis does not guarantee sustained pain relief. This study was criticized for lack of lesion-specific catheter placement resulting in nonspecific drug delivery [51]. The catheter was never directed to the ventral lateral epidural space where the dorsal root ganglion is located and the lateral recess scarring occurs.

Heavner et al [52] performed a prospective randomized trial of lesion-specific epidural adhesiolysis on 59 patients with chronic intractable low back pain. The patients were assigned to one of four epidural adhesiolysis treatment groups: (1) hypertonic (10%) saline plus hyaluronidase, (2) hypertonic saline, (3) isotonic (0.9%) saline, or (4) isotonic saline plus hyaluronidase. All treatment groups received corticosteroid and local anesthetic. Overall, across all four treatment groups, 83% of patients had significant pain relief at 1 month compared to 49% at 3 months, 43% at 6 months, and 49% at 12 months. The hyaluronidase and the hypertonic saline study group had a much lower incidence of additional need for pain procedures than the placebo groups, showing that site-specific catheter placement is important. Active substances and preservative free normal saline were blinded for the placebo effect.

Manchikanti et al [53] performed a retrospective randomized evaluation of a modified Racz adhesiolysis protocol in 232 patients with low back pain. The study involved lesion specific catheter placement, but the usual 3-day procedure was reduced to a 2-day (group 1) or a 1-day (group 2) procedure. Group 1 had 103 patients and group 2 had 129 patients. Other changes included changing the local anesthetic from bupivacaine to lidocaine, substituting methylprednisolone acetate or betamethasone acetate and phosphate for triamcinolone diacetate, and reduction of the volume of injectate. Of the patients in groups 1 and 2, 62% and 58% had greater than 50% pain relief at 1 month, respectively, with these percentages decreasing to 22% and 11% at 3 months, 8% and 7% at 6 months, and 2% and 3% at 1 year. Of significant interest is that the percentage of patients receiving greater than 50% pain relief after four procedures increased to 79% and 90% at 1 month, 50% and 36% at 3 months, 29% and 19% at 6 months, and 7% and 8% at 1 year for groups 1 and 2, respectively. Short-term relief of pain was demonstrated, but long-term relief was not.

Manchikanti, in 1999, evaluated two groups of randomly pulled, 150 patients for a 2-day reinjection procedure, and a second 150 patients for a one-day procedure out of a pool of 536 patients. It was concluded that repeat use of the one-day procedure is also cost effective when evaluated on a 12-month follow-up. The cost effectiveness indicated the lysis procedure to be superior to surgery or the rehabilitation activity program [53].

In a randomized, prospective study, Manchikanti et al [54] evaluated a 1-day epidural adhesiolysis procedure against a control group of patients who received conservative therapy. Results showed that cumulative relief, defined as relief greater than 50% with one to three injections, in the treatment group was 97% at 3 months, 93% at 6 months, and 47% at 1 year. The study also showed that overall health status improved significantly in the adhesiolysis group. Conservative therapy consisted of physical therapy and medications.

In 2004 Manchikanti et al [55] published their results of a randomized, double-blinded, controlled study on the effectiveness of 1-day lumbar adhesiolysis and hypertonic saline neurolysis in treatment of chronic low back pain. Seventy-five patients whose pain was unresponsive to conservative modalities were randomized into one of three treatment groups. Group 1 (control group) underwent catheterization where the catheter was in the sacral canal without adhesiolysis, followed by injection of local anesthetic, normal saline, and steroid. Group 2 consisted of catheterization with site-specific catheter placement being ventral-lateral for adhesiolysis, followed by injection of local anesthetic, normal saline, and steroid. Group 3 consisted of site-specific catheter placement for adhesiolysis, followed by injection of local anesthetic, hypertonic saline, and steroid. Patients were allowed to have additional injections based on the response, either after unblinding or without unblinding after 3 months. Patients without unblinding were offered either the assigned treatment or another treatment based on their response. If the patients in group 1 or 2 received adhesiolysis and injection and injection of hypertonic saline, they were considered withdrawn, and no subsequent data were collected. Outcomes were assessed at 3, 6, and 12 months using visual analog scale pain scores, Oswestry Disability Index, opioid intake, range-of-motion measurement, and P-3. Significant pain relief was defined as average relief of 50% or greater. Seventy-two percent of patients in group 3, 60% of patients in group 2, and 0% of patients in group 1 showed significant pain relief at 12 months. The average number of treatments for 1 year was 2.76 in group 2 and 2.16 in group 3. Duration of significant relief with the first procedure was 2.8+1.49 months and 3.8+3.37 months in groups 2 and 3, respectively. Significant pain relief (>50%) was also associated with improvement in Oswestry Disability Index, range of motion, and psychologic status.

Manchikanti et al [56, 57] furthered this research using comparisons of percutaneous adhesiolysis versus fluoroscopically guided caudal epidural steroid injections. The first study involved a population of patients with chronic low back pain and known spinal stenosis. The results showed a 76% reduction in pain relief at 1 year with epidural adhesiolysis compared to 4% in the control group. The second study performed in a population of patients with post–lumbar surgery syndrome showed a reduction in pain and improvement in functional status in 73% of the epidural adhesiolysis group compared to 12% in the control group.

In 2006 a study by Veihelmann et al [58] evaluated patients with a history of chronic low back pain and sciatica. Inclusion criteria were radicular pain with a corresponding nerve root compressing substrate found on MRI or CT. All patients were randomized to receive physiotherapy, analgesics, or lysis of adhesions. The lysis group had statistically significantly better outcome than the physical therapy treatment group.

Two other prospective evaluations by Chopra et al and Gerdesmeyer et al [59, 60] evaluated patients with monosegmental radiculopathy of the lumbar spine. All the patients suffered from chronic disk herniations or failed back syndrome. All these randomized trials showed positive short-term and long-term relief. Two prospective evaluations also showed positive short-and long-term relief [60, 61].

Gerdesmeyer has published a prospective double blind placebo controlled multicenter trial, which has been the most significant evaluation of the technique. The target site remained ventral lateral at the most likely level of the pain generator. The study continued for over 12 months and the significant finding was that the study arm of the procedure showed better outcome at all points of measurements. The placebo arm was a subcutaneously placed catheter so that the patient could not tell the difference during the three daily reinjections or subsequently. The study has succeeded in differentiating the placebo group from the treatment group in each location. The results have led to the conclusion that percutaneous lysis of adhesions for patients with chronic lumbosacral radicular pain should be offered this procedure as first choice of treatment [62].

A systematic review of percutaneous adhesiolysis for chronic low back pain in post lumbar surgery syndrome and spinal stenosis by S Helm II, et al, found effectiveness of the procedure in both spinal stenosis and in post-lumbar surgery syndrome [59]. Additionally it was noted that there have not been any hematomas reported. The results of the review support the use of the procedure for the conditions listed.

The randomized double blind active control trial by Koh, et al, in patients with lateral spinal canal stenosis demonstrated that the hypertonic saline showed significant short-term pain relief [63]. Post procedure pain after the use of steroids has been a significant problem at the first recognition of the effectiveness of percutaneous lysis of adhesions. Patients reported significant post procedural pain prior to the introduction of hyaluronidase and hypertonic saline to the sequence of injections. The parallel observation from the use of increased volume of injection was that the hypertonic saline addition has not only reduced the radiculopathy pain but also reduced the patient's back pain. The volume increase was from the 2 mL per injection range to the 5 mL range of each fluid component. The sequence of injections is first contrast, followed by hyaluronidase, local anesthetic and steroid, and 20-30 minutes later, if there was no motor block, the injection of hypertonic saline.

Manchikanti's, et al, two-year follow-up of randomized controlled trial compared one-day lysis of adhesions procedure to caudal epidural injection where the reinjection was triggered by the patient's pain relief dropping to below 50%. During the two-year study, the study group received 6.4 ± 2.35 procedures and 82% of the patients received at least 50% pain relief, whereas the caudal epidural injection had 5% similar rating. This strongly supports the effectiveness of the percutaneous epidural lysis of adhesions [64].

Park's, et al, evaluation of severity of spinal stenosis with transforaminal adhesiolysis and lumbar neuroforaminal stenosis showed effectiveness regardless of the intensity of lumbar stenosis [65].

Park, et al, evaluated epidural neuroplasty for cervical disc herniation and demonstrated effectiveness when conservative measures had failed. Park, et al, evaluated epidural neuroplasty for cervical disc herniation and found safety and efficacy. There was no control arm to the study, but the clinical results indicate reduction in cervical radiculopathy. The overall clinical experience has showed us that there is a need for evaluation for cervicogenic facet pain and appropriate treatment. Additionally, the anterior compartment between the anterior and middle scalene muscles may be additional pain generators in patients that have pain secondary to facet joint arthropathy [66].

Choi, et al, compared two patient groups with herniation of intervertebral discs and post lumbar surgery syndrome. These results indicate better outcome in non-operated patients. While not absolute prognostic predictor, the recommendation is that percutaneous adhesiolysis is a reasonable non-operative treatment option of herniation of intervertebral discs, spinal stenosis, and post lumbar surgery syndrome [67].

The cost effectiveness of the Racz procedure compared favorably to other treatments for the same conditions. The cost utility for 1 year of quality-adjusted life year (QALY) of USD is $2,652 for post-lumbar surgery syndrome and USD $2,649 for lumbar central spinal stenosis [68].

Epidural adhesiolysis has evolved over the years as an important treatment option for patients with intractable cervical, thoracic, and low back and leg pain. Studies show that patients are able to experience significant pain relief and restoration of function. Manchikanti's studies show that the amount and duration of relief can be achieved by repeat procedures. Recent prospective randomized double-blind studies on failed back surgery and spinal stenosis show 75% and 80% improvement in visual analog scale scores and functional improvements at 12 months' follow-up. There have been no negative studies to date where the lysis target was the ventral-lateral epidural space. The one negative study used a 10 cm sacral mid-canal catheter placement which was non-target specific [51]. This negative study was subsequently used as the placebo group in a study performed by Manchikanti. Manchikanti's study consisted of 3 treatment groups: placebo (sacral mid-canal catheter placement), target specific ventral-lateral epidural without hypertonic saline and target specific ventral-lateral epidural with hypertonic saline. The later two treatment groups had positive outcomes with the hypertonic saline group superior, whereas, the placebo group did not [55]. The evolution in the recognition of the site-specific importance of the catheter and medication delivery together with the fact that physicians need to acquire the skills to be able to carry out the procedure led to the improved outcomes seen in recent prospective randomized studies.

The management of failed back surgery syndrome and post laminectomy syndrome will likely continue to be controversial among the multitude of practitioners who treat these patients. However, in experienced hands, it is established as a reasonable option for many patients.

Percutaneous neuroplasty via a transforaminal approach evolved from the caudal approach. Lysis of adhesions via the caudal approach involves introducing a catheter through the sacral

http://dx.doi.org/10.5772/58753

hiatus and advancing it to the affected nerve root in the ventral-lateral epidural space. On the other hand, transforaminal percutaneous neuroplasty achieves a midline catheter placement in the epidural space that is able to target the two most heavily innervated structures in the spine—the posterior annulus fibrosus and the posterior longitudinal ligament [5]. Apart from a surgical approach, the ventral epidural structures have been otherwise inaccessible.

Endoscopy offers direct visualization of the affected nerve roots in addition to mechanical adhesiolysis, and may become more mainstream as the technique is refined.

Facet pain is commonly associated with the postlysis period or after provocative testing a month or so later if two-facet diagnostic blocks show efficacy. In addition to epidural lysis of adhesions, the combined use of radiofrequency facet denervation gives us the best long-term outcome.

Epidural adhesiolysis has been accepted as a treatment for post laminectomy syndrome, failed back syndrome, and cervical and thoracic radicular syndromes. Additional studies are underway to further refine the technique and indications. The combined use of long term patient education for neural flossing exercises and the inclusion of the facet delayed treatment in the algorithm further improves patient outcome. The identification of back pain provocation by saline injection and the successful use of percutaneous neuroplasty in the treatment represents hopeful promise for a cost effective treatment of back pain.

The increasing overall evidence is positive in the recommendation for use of percutaneous lysis of adhesions based on high quality and observational clinical studies. The procedure recommendation is for patients that failed conservative therapies. There are no negative studies reported regarding the use of percutaneous adhesiolysis from the sacral to the cervical areas.

The diagnosis and treatment of unusual rare complications must be within the scope of the physician's practice and the postoperative observational periods. Delayed secondary motor block in patients where only caudal catheter is used to treat spinal stenosis needs to be recognized as a consequence of fluid expansion from osmotic effect. Our preferred clinical practice is heading in the direction of caudal and transforaminal catheter use at the level of stenosis based on the utilization of the above-mentioned transforaminal catheter reports [4].

Clearly, additional studies will further prove safety and efficacy. Rare problems will come to light, such as allergies, unusual loculations, or syrinx or congenital malformations. Thus, the field shall become similar to any other advanced medical intervention. The quality of outcome improves with improved training and experience. The most significant hazard is physicians that are not trained, claiming to carry out percutaneous lysis procedure without appropriate catheter placement. Therefore, recommendation is to describe the procedure and/or save procedure fluoroscopic images that will prove appropriate catheter placement on anterior-posterior and lateral views. Midline catheter placement for lysis of adhesions should be avoided.

The treatment algorhythm for patients with leg and back pain, based on accumulating evidence, should focus on radiculopathy and back pain. Next, a month later, the patient must be examined for diagnosis and treatment of other causes of back pain, such as facet joint related, and pain from muscle spasms like gluteus medius, para spinal, quadratus lumborum, psoas, and piriformis muscle related radiculopathy in the lumbosacral area. Significant undiagnosed problems include trochanteric bursa related pain, cluneal nerve entrapments and hip joint arthropathies. Similarly, the order of evaluation and treatment in the upper extremity addressed should begin with radiculopathy, followed by facet joints and interscalene entrapments. Involvement through neural flossing exercises and appropriate instructions as outlined in the above text has been remarkably well accepted by the patients.

Acknowledgements

Racz GB, Day MR, Heavner JE, Scott J. *Lysis of Epidural Adhesions.* In: Waldman S, ed. *Pain Management, 2nd Edition*. Elsevier; 2011: 1258-1272.

Racz GB, Day MR, Heavner JE, Smith JP. The Racz Procedure: Lysis of Epidural Adhesions (Percutaneous Neuroplasty). In: Deer T, ed. The AAPM Text of Pain Medicine. Springer; 2011.

The authors would also like to thank Marzieh N. Brown and Paula Brashear, Katie Clower and Floramay Holidayfor their assistance in the editing of this chapter.

Author details

Gabor B. Racz[1], James E. Heavner[1], Jeffrey P. Smith[1], Carl E. Noe[2], Adnan Al-Kaisy[3], Tomikichi Matsumoto[4], Sang Chul Lee[5] and Laszlo Nagy[6]

*Address all correspondence to: gbracz@yahoo.com

1 Texas Tech University Health Sciences Center, Lubbock, Texas, USA

2 University of Texas Southwestern Medical Center, Dallas, Texas, USA

3 London Bridge Hospital, London, UK

4 Shiga University of Medical Science, Shiga, Japan

5 Department of Anesthesiology and Pain Medicine, Seoul National University Hospital, Seoul, Korea

6 Texas Tech University Health Sciences Center and Covenant Medical Center, Department of Pediatric Neurosurgery, USA

References

[1] Lawrence R., Helmick C., Arnett F., et al: Estimates of the prevalence of arthritis and selected musculoskeletal disorders in the United States. *Arthritis Rheum* 1998; 41(5): 778-799.

[2] Straus B.: Chronic pain of spinal origin: the costs of intervention. *Spine* 2002; 27(22): 2614-2619.

[3] National Center for Health Statistics : *National hospital discharge survey*, Washington, DC, US Department of Health and Human Services, Centers for Disease Control and Prevention, 1990. Report no. PB92-500818

[4] Van Zundert J.: *Personal communication*. 2005.

[5] Kuslich S., Ulstrom C., Michael C.: The tissue origin of low back pain and sciatica. *Orthop Clin North Am* 1991; 22:181-187.

[6] Racz G., Noe C., Heavner J.: Selective spinal injections for lower back pain. *Curr Rev Pain* 1999; 3:333-341.

[7] Anderson S.: A rationale for the treatment algorithm of failed back surgery syndrome. *Curr Rev Pain* 2000; 4:396-406.

[8] Pawl R.: Arachnoiditis and epidural fibrosis: the relationship to chronic pain. *Curr Rev Pain* 1998; 2:93-99.

[9] Cervellini P., Curri D., Volpin L., et al: Computed tomography of epidural fibrosis after discectomy: a comparison between symptomatic and asymptomatic patients. *Neurosurgery* 1988; 23(6):710-713.

[10] Manchikanti L., Staats P., Singh V.: Evidence-based practice guidelines for interventional techniques in the management of chronic spinal pain. *Pain Phys* 2003; 6:3-81.

[11] LaRocca H., Macnab I.: The laminectomy membrane: studies in its evolution, characteristics, effects and prophylaxis in dogs. *J Bone Joint Surg* 1974; 5613:545-550.

[12] Cooper R., Freemont A., Hoyland J., et al: Herniated intervertebral disc–associated periradicular fibrosis and vascular abnormalities occur without inflammatory cell infiltration. *Spine* 1995; 20:591-598.

[13] McCarron R., Wimpee M., Hudkins P., et al: The inflammatory effects of nucleus pulposus; a possible element in the pathogenesis of low back pain. *Spine* 1987; 12:760-764.

[14] Parke W., Watanabe R.: Adhesions of the ventral lumbar dura: an adjunct source of discogenic pain?. *Spine* 1990; 15:300-303.

[15] Viesca C., Racz G., Day M.: Special techniques in pain management: lysis of adhesions. *Anesthesiol Clin North Am* 2003; 21:745-766.

[16] Songer M., Ghosh L., Spencer D.: Effects of sodium hyaluronate on peridural fibrosis after lumber laminectomy and discectomy. *Spine* 1990; 15:550-554.

[17] Key J., Ford L.: Experimental intervertebral disc lesions. *J Bone Joint Surg Am* 1948; 30:621-630.

[18] Olmarker K., Rydevik B.: Pathophysiology of sciatica. *Orthop Clin North Am* 1991; 22:223-233.

[19] Ross J., Robertson J., Frederickson R., et al: Association between peridural scar and recurrent radicular pain after lumbar discectomy; magnetic resonance evaluation. *Neurosurgery* 1996; 38:855-863.

[20] Gilbert K., Brismee J., Collins D., et al: Lumbosacral nerve roots displacements and strain: part 1. A novel measurement technique during straight leg raise in unembalmed calavers. *Spine* 2007; 32(14):1513-1520.Phila Pa 1976

[21] Heavner JE, Chokhavatia S, Kizelshteyn G: Percutaneous evaluation of the epidural and subarachnoid space with a flexible fiberscope, *Reg Anesth* 1991;15:85.

[22] Bosscher HA, Heavner JE: Incidence and severity of epidural fibrosis after back surgery: an endoscopic study, *Pain Pract* 2010; 10: 18-24.

[23] Hatten Jr H.: Lumbar epidurography with metrizamide. *Radiology* 1980; 137:129-136.

[24] Stewart H., Quinnell R., Dann N.: Epidurography in the management of sciatica. *Br J Rheumatol* 1987; 26(6):424-429.

[25] Devulder J., Bogaert L., Castille F., et al: Relevance of epidurography and epidural adhesiolysis in chronic failed back surgery patients. *Clin J Pain* 1995; 11:147-150.

[26] Manchikanti L., Bakhit C., Pampati V.: Role of epidurography in caudal neuroplasty. *Pain Digest* 1998; 8:277-281.

[27] Day M., Racz G.: Technique of caudal neuroplasty. *Pain Digest* 1999; 9(4):255-257.

[28] Horlocker T., Wedel D., Benzon H., et al: Regional anesthesia in the anticoagulated patient: defining the risks (the second ASRA Consensus Conference on Neuraxial Anesthesia and Anticoagulation). *Reg Anesth Pain Med* 2003; 28:172-197.

[29] *Omnipaque product insert*, Princeton, NJ, Nycomed, Inc.

[30] *Isovue product insert*, Princeton, NJ, Bracco Diagnostics, Inc.

[31] *Hypaque product insert*, Princeton, NJ, Amersham Health, Inc.

[32] *Conray product insert*, Phillipsburg, NJ, Mallinckrodt, Inc.

[33] Racz G., Day M., Heavner J., et al: Hyaluronidase: a review of approved formulations, indications and off-label use in chronic pain management. *Expert Opin Biol Ther* 2010; 10(1):127-131.

[34] Teske W., Zirke S., Nottenkamper J., Lichtinger T., Theodoridis T., Kramer J., Schmidt K.: Anatomical and surgical study of volume determination of the anterolateral epidural space nerve root L5/S1 under the aspect of epidural perineural injection in minimal invasive treatment of lumbar nerve root compression. European Spine Journal 2011; 20(4):537-41.

[35] Lauretti G.R., Mattos A.L., Trevellin W., Righeti C.C.F., Resende C.S.: 911 Sacral Neuroplasty for Postlaminectomy Chronic Low Back Pain. *European Journal of Pain* 2009; 13(S1):S258a-S258.

[36] Matsumoto. Treatment of lower back and leg pain using the Racz Catheter-Matsumoto way via S1 foramen. WIP World Congress, Maastricht; 2014.

[37] Paincast.com. Paincast | Paincast [Internet] 2014.

[38] Racz G.B., Heavner J.E.: Cervical spinal canal loculation and secondary ischemic cord injury—PVCS—perivenous counter spread—danger sign!!. *Pain Pract* 2008; 8:399-403.

[39] Larkin T., Carragee E., Cohen S.: A novel technique for delivery of epidural steroids and diagnosing the level of nerve root pathology. *J Spinal Disord Tech* 2003; 16(2): 186-192.

[40] Scanlon G.C., Moeller-Bertram T., Romanowsky S.M., Wallace M.S.: Cervical Transforaminal Epidural Steriod Injections More Dangerous Than We Think?. *Spine;* 32(11):1249-1256.

[41] Jamison A.E., Hsu E., Cohen S.P.: Epidural adhesiolysis: an evidence based review. *J Neurosurg Sci* 2014; 58:65-76.

[42] Racz G.B., Heavner J.E., Bosscher H., Helm II S.: The MILD Procedure. *Pain Practice* 2013; 13(7):594-596.

[43] Racz G.B., Sabonghy M., Gintautas J., et al: Intractable pain therapy using a new type of epidural catheter. *JAMA* 1985; 248:579-580.

[44] Sakai T., Aoki H., Hojo M., et al: Adhesiolysis and targeted steroid/local anesthetic injection during epiduroscopy alleviates pain and reduces sensory nerve dysfunction in patients with chronic sciatica. *J Anesth* 2008; 22(3):242-247.

[45] Anderson S., Racz G., Heavener J.: Evolution of epidural lysis of adhesions. *Pain Physician* 2000; 3(3):262-270.

[46] Racz G., Holubec J.: *Lysis of adhesions in the epidural space*. In: Raj P., ed. *Techniques of neurolysis*, Boston: Kluwer Academic; 1989:57-72.

[47] Arthur J., Racz G., Heinrich R., et al: *Epidural space: identification of filling defects and lysis of adhesions in the treatment of chronic painful conditions. Abstracts of the 7th World Congress on Pain*, Paris: IASP Publications; 1993.

[48] Racz G.B., Day M.R., Heavener J.E., Smith J.P.: "The Racz Procedure: Lysis of Epidural Adhesions (Percutaneous Neuroplasty)." Comprehensive Treatment of Chronic Pain by Medical, Interventional, and Integrative Approaches, Ed. Tim Deer. Springer, 2013.

[49] Stolker R., Vervest A., Gerbrand J.: The management of chronic spinal pain by blockades: a revew. *Pain* 1994; 58:1-19.

[50] Devulder J., Bogaert L., Castille F., et al: Relevance of epidurography and epidural adhesiolysis in chonic failed back surgery patients. *Clin J Pain* 1995; 11:147-150.

[51] Racz G., Heavner J.: In response to article by Drs. Devulder et al. *Clin J Pain* 1995; 11:151-154.

[52] Heavner J., Racz G., Raj P.: Percutaneous epidural neuroplasty: prospective evaluation of 0.9% saline versus 10% saline with or without hyaluronidase. *Reg Anesth Pain Med* 1999; 24:202-207.

[53] Manchikanti L., Pakanati R., Bakhit C., et al: Role of adhesiolysis and hypertonic saline neurolysis in management of low back pain: evaluation of modification of the Racz protocol. *Pain Digest* 1999; 9:91-96.

[54] Manchikanti L., Pampati V., Fellow B., et al: Role of one day epidural adhesiolysis in management of chronic low back pain: a randomized clinical trial. *Pain Phys* 2001; 4:153-166.

[55] Manchikanti L., Rivera J., Pampati V., et al: One day lumbar adhesiolysis and hypertonic saline neurolysis in treatment of chronic low back pain: a randomized, double-blinded trial. *Pain Phys* 2004; 7:177-186.

[56] Manchikanti L., Cash K., McManus C., et al: The preliminary results of a comparative effectiveness of adhesiolysis and caudal epidural injections in managing chronic low back pain secondary to spinal stenosis. *Pain Phys* 2009; 12(6):E341-E354.

[57] Manchikanti L., Singh V., Cash K., et al: A comparative effectiveness evaluation of percutaneous adhesiolysis and epidural steroid injections in managing lumbar post surgery syndrome. *Pain Phys* 2009; 12(6):E355-E368.

[58] Veihelmann A., Devens C., Trouiller H., et al: Epidural neuroplasty versus physiotherapy to relieve pain in patients with sciatica: a prospective randomized blinded clinical trial. *J Orthop Sci* 2006; 11(4):365-369.

[59] Helm II S., Benyamin R., Chopra P., Deer T., Justiz R.: Percutaneous Adhesiolysis in the Management of Chronic Low Back Pain in Post Lumbar Surgery Syndrome and Spinal Stenosis: A Systematic Review. *Pain Physician* 2012; 15:E435-E62.

[60] Gerdesmeyer L., Lampe R., Veihelmann A., et al: Chronic radiculopathy: use of minimally invasive percutaneous epidural neurolysis according to Racz. *Der Schmerz* 2005; 19:285-295.

[61] Gerdesmeyer L., Rechl H., Wagenpfeil S., et al: Minimally invasive epidural neurolysis in chronic radiculopathy: a prospective controlled study to prove effectiveness. *Der Orhopade* 2003; 32:869-876.

[62] Gerdesmeyer L., Wagenpfeil S., Birkenmaier C., Veihelmann A., Hauschild M., Wagner K., Al Muderis M., Gollwitzer H., Diehl P., Toepfer A.: Percutaneous Epidural Lysis of Adhesions in Chronic Lumbar Radicular Pain: A Randomized, Double-Blind, Placebo-Controlled Trial. *Pain Physician* 2013; 16:185-196.

[63] Koh W.U., Choi S.S., Park S.Y., Joo E.Y., Kim S.H., Lee J.D., Shin J.Y., Leem J.G., Shin J.W.: Transforaminal Hypertonic Saline for the Treatment of Lumbar Lateral Canal Stenosis: A Double-Blinded, Randomized, Active-Control Trial. *Pain Physician* 2013; 16: 197-211.

[64] Manchikanti L., Singh V., Cash K., Pampati V.: Assesment of effectiveness of percutaneous adhesiolysis and caudal epidural injection in managing post lumbar surgery syndrome: 2-year follow-up of a randomized, controlled trial. *Journal of Pain Research* 2012; 5: 597-608.

[65] Park C.H., Lee S.H.: Effectiveness of Percutaneous Transforaminal Adhesiolysis in Patients with Lumbar Neuroforaminal Spinal Stenosis. *Pain Physician* 2013; 16: E37-E43.

[66] Park E.J., Park S.Y., Lee S.J., Kim N.S., Koh D.Y.: Clinical Outcomes of Epidural Neuroplasty for Cervical Disc Herniation. *Journal of Korean Medical Science* 2013; 28: 461-465.

[67] Choi E., Nahm F., Lee P.B.: Evaluation of Prognostic Predictors of Percutaneous Adhesiolysis Using a Racz Catheter for Post Lumbar Surgery Syndrome or Spinal Stenosis. *Pain Physician* 2013; 16:E531-E536.

[68] Manchikanti L., Helm II S., Pampati V., Racz G.B.: Cost Utility Analysis of Percutaneous Adhesiolysis in Managing Pain of Post-Lumbar Surgery Syndrome and Lumbar Central Spinal Stenosis. Pain Practice 2014; doi:10.1111/papr.12195.